AF371659

Heart Failure Management: The Neural Pathways

Edoardo Gronda • Emilio Vanoli
Alexandru Costea

Editors

Heart Failure Management: The Neural Pathways

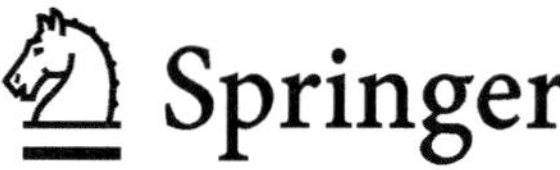 Springer

Editors
Edoardo Gronda
IRCCS MultiMedica
Sesto San Giovanni
Milan
Italy

Emilio Vanoli
IRCCS MultiMedica
Sesto San Giovanni
Milan
Italy

Department of Molecular Cardiology
University of Pavia

Alexandru Costea
University of Cincinnati
Cincinnati
Ohio
USA

ISBN 978-3-319-24991-9   ISBN 978-3-319-24993-3   (eBook)
DOI 10.1007/978-3-319-24993-3

Library of Congress Control Number: 2015960204

Springer Cham Heidelberg New York Dordrecht London

Printed on acid-free paper

Springer International Publishing AG Switzerland is part of Springer Science+Business Media (www.springer.com)

Foreword

The idea of the brain being in command and the heart housing the soul, distracts from the actual primary director of our life: the autonomic nervous system (ANS). It drives breathing, heartbeat, and any other aspect of being alive. Heart transplantations had shown that the removed heart was able to function properly without innervation.

In early 1960, however, a major shift occurred in the understanding of the autonomic control of the heart by the discovery of its specialized and detailed control of all aspects of the cardiovascular system. Specific areas were described in the central nervous system with "highly specialized and sharply localized capacities for regional control of myocardial function" (Randall WC 1977). The evidence that parasympathetic fibers were distributed in the ventricles overcame the dogma that the cardiac vagal control was limited to the supraventricular structures. In 1977, Randall edited a first comprehensive book *Neural Regulation of the Heart* that still stands as a masterpiece in this field. In that period, Italy was one of the most fertile cradles in the field of neural control of cardiac function and of its clinical applications. Extensive research on integrated pathophysiological models described in detail the neural hierarchy of cardiac control and the critical role of the parasympathetic modulation of sympathetic activity. However, the hope for new effective therapies to challenge cardiac diseases such as sudden cardiac death and heart failure were confined to the modulation of single ion channels. It was wrongly thought that the failing heart was only needing inotropic support. The ultimate consequences were a systematic interruption of clinical trials in this field, because of an excessive mortality in the treated group, causing a dramatic delay in the use of adequate integrated approaches to the autonomic control of the heart. The saga of the beta-blockers is the most outstanding example: for 20 years this therapy was denied to heart failure subjects due to the belief that, after a large myocardial infarction, boosting of the residual function of the surviving tissue was the right way to recover hemodynamic stability and autonomic function. The sequence of trials in which mortality in the treated group exceeded the placebo paved the hard way to the truth. Today we appreciate the enormous benefit to the failing heart by modulating the sympathetic hyperactivity by beta-blockers. But we can't stop short here now! It is time to confront the real core of the problem, to the central control of the cardiovascular system. Our current approaches are, indeed, surrendering the progression of the disease. Current device therapy is limited.

The ANS is very much "autonomous" being provided with intrinsic complex systems and circuits which allow a very fast and detailed self-tuning and regulation in order to rapidly adjust the cardiovascular system to the dynamicity of daily challenges and adaptations. The ANS activates a large number of adjustments in a fraction of a second as, for example, to adjust cerebral perfusion when rising to one's feet from laying down. The complexity of the ANS had generated the belief that its external modulation was not possible. This misconception was supported by the failure of trials on central pharmacologic modulation of sympathetic activity.

The concept of direct neural stimulation to treat resistant angina in the pre-revascularization era was conceived and proposed by Braunwald in the 1960s, but it was rapidly abandoned mostly because of the lack of adequate technology. Today the effective use of selective sympathetic denervation to treat arrhythmogenic diseases has opened the path to direct interventions on the autonomic circuits. Accordingly, renal denervation has been proposed as a new approach to the treatment of resistant malignant arterial hypertension. The initial promises of this approached to major frustration when the apparent failure of this treatment was documented by the first controlled trial. These trials, however, suffered from severe flaws regarding conceptualization and design.

This book was conceived uring the international symposium "Heart Failure & Co" held in Milano in 2014 by the chief editor Edoardo Gronda and other participants. The title of the meeting was "Hurting the heart: the partners in crime". The systematic analysis of the leading protagonists in the crime pointed to the deranged ANS as the true director of the plot.

The beauty of ANS complexity is described in this book by contributions of some of the most competent specialists. Their elaborations provide the most updated compendium of the state of the art in the understanding of the functional aspects of the ANS and describe options of its directed modulation to overcome the current growing limitations affecting diagnosis and therapy in the management of heart failure.

Prof. L. Rossi Bernardi, MD, Ph.D.
Past President of the National Research Council of Italy

Contents

Part I

Current Heart Failure Therapies

Introduction

A Second Look at the Autonomic Nervous System: Repurposing Our Lessons Learned

Esther Vorovich and Mariell L. Jessup

The key function of the autonomic nervous system (ANS) in normal cardiac physiology has been known for more than 50 years. Early studies in the 1960s and 1970s by Braunwald and colleagues demonstrated the ANS' role in the maintenance of cardiac output at rest and in response to exercise through modulation of heart rate, contractility, preload, and afterload [1, 2]. Abnormal hyperactivity of the sympathetic nervous system (SNS) and simultaneous dysfunction of the parasympathetic nervous system in heart disease were also recognized during this time period [1–4]. Additional population studies in heart failure (HF) patients showed an association of SNS activation with exercise capacity, hemodynamics, degree of left ventricular dysfunction, as well as mortality, establishing the critical impact of the ANS in cardiovascular dysregulation in the heart failure syndrome [5–9]. However it remained unclear if ANS activation played a truly causative role in myocardial deterioration rather than serving as a marker of the body's attempt to maintain homeostasis in the face of a failing heart.

Since that time, our understanding of HF, the ANS, and their intersection has grown immensely. HF is a progressive disorder characterized by an initial myocardial insult that is followed by activation of multiple regulatory systems including the ANS, renin-angiotensin-aldosterone system (RAAS), and inflammatory pathways that serve to reestablish adequate cardiac output; these compensatory systems, in time, become maladaptive through their effects on hemodynamics as well as biochemical, cellular, and structural changes in the myocardium (Fig. 1.1) [10].

E. Vorovich, MD
Northwestern Memorial Hospital, Division of Cardiology,
Arkes Family Pavilion Suite 600, 676 N Saint Clair, Chicago, IL 60611, USA

M.L. Jessup, MD (✉)
Hospital of the University of Pennsylvania and the Presbyterian
Medical Center of Philadelphia, Philadelphia, PA 19104, USA
e-mail: jessupm@uphs.upenn.edu

© Springer International Publishing Switzerland 2016
E. Gronda et al. (eds.), *Heart Failure Management: The Neural Pathways*,
DOI 10.1007/978-3-319-24993-3_1

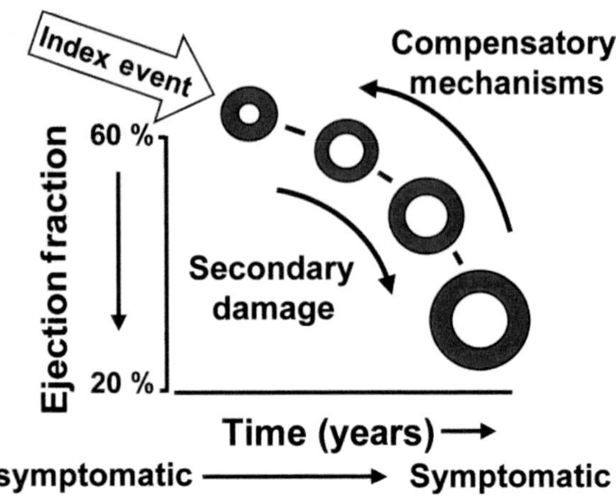

Fig. 1.1 Pathogenesis of heart failure (Mann and Bristow [10])

However, it is important to recognize that this knowledge and understanding evolved over the past two to three decades. Early forays into HF therapy targeted the hemodynamic derangement characteristically seen in severe HF patients [11]. Numerous observational studies were performed evaluating the acute hemodynamic effects of diuretics, hydralazine, nitrates, and other vasodilators. The era of randomized clinical trials in HF was ushered in with the publication of VHEFT-1 in 1986 [12], demonstrating a benefit of combination therapy with isosorbide dinitrate and hydralazine on outcomes in chronic HF. Subsequent clinical trials transitioned our focus from vasodilation to neurohormonal blockade and in particular to agents that inhibited the RAAS. Simultaneously, cautious case series and then larger trials demonstrated the profound benefits of beta-blockers on both mortality and meaningful salutary effects on ventricular remodeling [13–18].

The focus of newer HF trials remained primarily on RAAS antagonists [19–21] until further blockade of the RAAS proved less fruitful and, in certain cases, harmful [22]. Subgroup analyses from Val-HEFT and VALIANT showed increased adverse events in patients taking a combination of ACE inhibitor, angiotensin receptor blocker (ARB), and beta-blocker therapy [21, 23]. Moreover, trials of endothelin antagonists, cytokine antagonists, recombinant natriuretic peptide, centrally acting sympatholytics, and direct renin inhibitors on a background of ACE inhibition and beta blockade were also shown to have either neutral or harmful effects of treatment (Fig. 1.2) [22].

After a decade of mostly negative trials, the PARADIGM-HF trial interrupted this trend in 2014. LCZ696, a novel combination compound of valsartan and sacubitril, a neprilysin inhibitor, led to substantial and significant reductions in mortality and multiple metrics of morbidity [24]. Publication of the PARADIGM-HF underscored the investigative shift away from pure RAAS inhibition and toward novel pathways, new drug delivery methodologies, or a focus on treating comorbidities that negatively affect HF progression. In particular, there has been great interest in drugs that influence cardiomyocyte energetics and/or metabolism and interventions such as gene therapy, stem cell therapy, noncoding RNAs, and ventricular assist devices as a potential route to recovery [25–27].

However, novel therapies are costly and sustain a long delay from conception to Phase III trials to regulatory approval. As an example, the initial studies

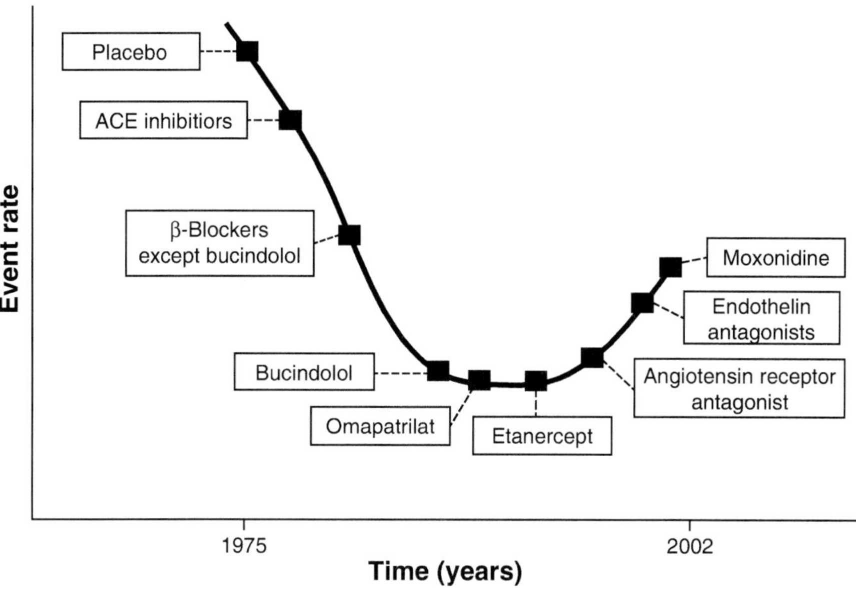

Fig. 1.2 Saturation of benefits with incremental neurohormonal blockade in chronic heart failure (Modified from: Mehra et al. [22])

evaluating neprilysin and RAAS blockage date back to the early 1990s, with publication of the first Phase III trial showing efficacy occurring in 2014 [24, 28]. Accordingly, there exists an increasing motivation to repurpose previously approved therapies for newer indications. Repurposing allows for faster drug delivery to the market and lower costs. In support of this concept, the American National Institutes of Health created an initiative to strengthen the partnership between academic institutions and industry which has already resulted in more than 50 intellectually protected but previously abandoned products becoming available for research [29].

Interestingly, HF as a field has a history of repurposing. In 2005, the AHEFT study reexamined the effect of the combination of hydralazine and isosorbide dinitrate in African-Americans already taking background ACE inhibitor and beta-blocker therapy [30]. AHEFT showed a substantial and sustained benefit on mortality in this subpopulation beyond that is seen in the original VHEFT trials. The drug combination was approved by the FDA in a new formulation in 2005 [31]. In 2007, Costanzo et al. published the UNLOAD study showing that ultrafiltration, shown to have less neurohormonal activation and more total body salt removal than diuretics alone, led to increased weight loss and decreased hospitalization rates as compared to standard therapy [32]. This study ushered in a series of trials examining the outcomes of ultrafiltration in HF patients without renal failure – a repurpose of the technology developed for dialysis. Indeed, ultrafiltration can be thought of as repurposing one of medicine's oldest treatments: bloodletting or venesection. Further repurposing efforts have likewise focused on expanding application of previously approved therapies for severe HF, such as mineralocorticoid antagonists and cardiac resynchronization therapy, to those patients with milder HF symptoms [33–36].

The HF community naturally asked the next question: have we done enough to repurpose previously discovered treatments targeting the ANS? Initial enthusiasm for clonidine, a presynaptic alpha2 agonist that results in central inhibition of the SNS, waned with the publication of the MOXCON study showing harmful effects of its cousin, moxonidine, in HF patients [37, 38]. Animal studies of clenbuterol, a combined beta1 antagonist and beta2 agonist with anabolic characteristics, have been shown to exhibit beneficial effects on cardiac and myocyte remodeling as well as myocyte function [39, 40]. This preceded attempts to repurpose this drug from its initial indication for asthma toward a therapy for HF. In human HF, clenbuterol has largely been investigated in conjunction with ventricular assist devices for myocardial recovery, with promising preliminary results [40, 41]. However, trials have also shown detrimental effects on endurance and exercise duration in HF patients and use of this drug remains limited in HF [40, 42].

Subsequently, focus has shifted to non-pharmacologic, device-based strategies directed at the ANS. To date, investigation of device therapies in HF has targeted four ANS sites: (1) carotid baroreceptor stimulation, (2) vagal nerve stimulation, (3) spinal cord stimulation, and (4) renal sympathetic denervation [37, 43].

Baroreceptor activation therapy (BAT) involves the stimulation of one or both carotid sinuses resulting in inhibition of the sympathetic nervous system, predominantly studied in patients with resistant hypertension. In animal models of HF, BAT has effected improvements in LVEF, LV remodeling, and survival [37, 44]. Human studies are largely in their infancy with pilot data showing improvements in 6 min walk distance and reductions in sympathetic nervous system activation and NT proBNP levels [37]. These findings were recently confirmed in a multicenter, multinational randomized controlled trial [45]. Further trials of BAT in systolic and diastolic HF are planned; development and study of minimally invasive endovascular implantation techniques are scheduled [46].

Like BAT, vagal nerve stimulation (VNS) is performed via surgical implantation and has been used for epilepsy and depression treatment for decades [43]. More recently, this method has been repurposed for HF with animal studies showing improvement in LVEF, hemodynamics, arrhythmias, and survival [37, 43, 46]. Initial studies in human HF have shown improvements in walk distance and quality of life metrics with conflicting results in regard to cardiac remodeling [37, 47]. These promising results have led to the initiation of a large randomized clinical trial of VNS in HF patients [43]. In addition, minimally invasive VNS has shown potential in preclinical and pilot studies in both cardiac and noncardiac conditions [48, 49].

As with vagal nerve stimulation and BAT, spinal cord stimulation is surgically implanted and has been used for peripheral vascular disease, angina, and chronic pain [37]. Animal HF models have shown improved hemodynamics with decreased afterload, lower blood pressure, as well as improvement in LVEF and reduction in arrhythmias and levels of natriuretic peptides [37]. Small pilot studies in HF have suggested improved quality of life, symptoms, peak oxygen consumption, and conflicting results on LV remodeling [43, 50, 51].

The last of the four current treatments is renal sympathetic denervation (RSD), currently the only one addressed by minimally invasive, nonsurgical methods. As with BAT, RSD has been predominantly studied in resistant hypertension. The enthusiasm generated from the immense success of initial RSD trials (SIMPLICTY-1, SIMPLICITY-2) has been greatly curbed with the publication in 2014 of the negative results of the first blinded randomized control trial of RSD, SIMPLICTY-3 [52]. In HF, initial pilot and small randomized trial data have shown procedural safety as well as improvement in symptoms, LVEF, and natriuretic peptide levels with a trend toward a beneficial effect on HF hospitalizations [46]. Both animal and human data exist showing improved natriuresis, hemodynamics, and left ventricular functioning, diastolic dysfunction, as well as reduction in left ventricular hypertrophy, some of which appear to be independent of blood pressure effects [46, 53]. In addition, preliminary data also suggest potential positive effects of RSD on insulin resistance, glucose metabolism, arrhythmias, and obstructive sleep apnea, thereby targeting some of the comorbidities and sequelae of HF [53].

Preclinical and clinical data strongly support a definite pathophysiologic mechanism to validate the benefit of ANS modulation; preliminary data is intriguing. As newer technologies evolve with transition away from surgical implantation to more minimally invasive techniques, the improved safety profile could further tip the scales toward therapeutic benefit. As Dr. Braunwald fittingly quoted Winston Churchill in his call to arms in our war against heart failure, "Now, this is not the end. It is not even the beginning of the end. But it is, perhaps, the end of the beginning" [25]. Certainly, the utility of the current repurposed approach to the neural pathways is an exciting topic for this publication.

References

1. Braunwald E. Regulation of the circulation (second of two parts). N Engl J Med. 1974;290:1420–5.
2. Braunwald E. Regulation of the circulation. I. N Engl J Med. 1974;290:1124–9.
3. Braunwald E, Chidsey CA. The adrenergic nervous system in the control of the normal and failing heart. Proc R Soc Med. 1965;58:1063–6.
4. Eckberg DL, Drabinsky M, Braunwald E. Defective cardiac parasympathetic control in patients with heart disease. N Engl J Med. 1971;285:877–83.
5. Cohn JN, Levine TB, Olivari MT, et al. Plasma norepinephrine as a guide to prognosis in patients with chronic congestive heart failure. N Engl J Med. 1984;311:819–23.
6. Chidsey CA, Harrison DC, Braunwald E. Augmentation of the plasma nor-epinephrine response to exercise in patients with congestive heart failure. N Engl J Med. 1962;267:650–4.
7. Thomas JA, Marks BH. Plasma norepinephrine in congestive heart failure. Am J Cardiol. 1978;41:233–43.
8. Levine TB, Francis GS, Goldsmith SR, Simon AB, Cohn JN. Activity of the sympathetic nervous system and renin-angiotensin system assessed by plasma hormone levels and their relation to hemodynamic abnormalities in congestive heart failure. Am J Cardiol. 1982;49:1659–66.
9. Francis GS, Goldsmith SR, Cohn JN. Relationship of exercise capacity to resting left ventricular performance and basal plasma norepinephrine levels in patients with congestive heart failure. Am Heart J. 1982;104:725–31.

10. Mann DL, Bristow MR. Mechanisms and models in heart failure: the biomechanical model and beyond. Circulation. 2005;111:2837–49.
11. Katz AM. The "modern" view of heart failure: how did we get here? Circ Heart Fail. 2008;1:63–71.
12. Cohn JN, Archibald DG, Ziesche S, et al. Effect of vasodilator therapy on mortality in chronic congestive heart failure. Results of a Veterans Administration Cooperative Study. N Engl J Med. 1986;314:1547–52.
13. Hellawell JL, Margulies KB. Myocardial reverse remodeling. Cardiovasc Ther. 2012;30:172–81.
14. Packer M, Bristow MR, Cohn JN, et al. The effect of carvedilol on morbidity and mortality in patients with chronic heart failure. U.S. Carvedilol Heart Failure Study Group. N Engl J Med. 1996;334:1349–55.
15. The Cardiac Insufficiency Bisoprolol Study II (CIBIS-II): a randomised trial. Lancet. 1999;353:9–13.
16. Effect of metoprolol CR/XL in chronic heart failure: metoprolol CR/XL Randomised Intervention Trial in Congestive Heart Failure (MERIT-HF). Lancet. 1999;353:2001–7.
17. Packer M, Coats AJ, Fowler MB, et al. Effect of carvedilol on survival in severe chronic heart failure. N Engl J Med. 2001;344:1651–8.
18. Swedberg K, Hjalmarson A, Waagstein F, Wallentin I. Beneficial effects of long-term beta-blockade in congestive cardiomyopathy. Br Heart J. 1980;44:117–33.
19. Pitt B, Remme W, Zannad F, et al. Eplerenone, a selective aldosterone blocker, in patients with left ventricular dysfunction after myocardial infarction. N Engl J Med. 2003;348:1309–21.
20. Granger CB, McMurray JJ, Yusuf S, et al. Effects of candesartan in patients with chronic heart failure and reduced left-ventricular systolic function intolerant to angiotensin-converting-enzyme inhibitors: the CHARM-Alternative trial. Lancet. 2003;362:772–6.
21. Pfeffer MA, McMurray JJ, Velazquez EJ, et al. Valsartan, captopril, or both in myocardial infarction complicated by heart failure, left ventricular dysfunction, or both. N Engl J Med. 2003;349:1893–906.
22. Mehra MR, Uber PA, Francis GS. Heart failure therapy at a crossroad: are there limits to the neurohormonal model? J Am Coll Cardiol. 2003;41:1606–10.
23. Cohn JN, Tognoni G, Valsartan Heart Failure Trial I. A randomized trial of the angiotensin-receptor blocker valsartan in chronic heart failure. N Engl J Med. 2001;345:1667–75.
24. McMurray JJ, Packer M, Desai AS, et al. Angiotensin-neprilysin inhibition versus enalapril in heart failure. N Engl J Med. 2014;371:993–1004.
25. Braunwald E. The war against heart failure: the Lancet lecture. Lancet. 2015;385:812–24.
26. Beadle RM, Williams LK, Kuehl M, et al. Improvement in cardiac energetics by perhexiline in heart failure due to dilated cardiomyopathy. JACC Heart Fail. 2015;3:202–11.
27. Jorsal A, Wiggers H, Holmager P, et al. A protocol for a randomised, double-blind, placebo-controlled study of the effect of LIraglutide on left VEntricular function in chronic heart failure patients with and without type 2 diabetes (The LIVE Study). BMJ Open. 2014;4:e004885.
28. Margulies KB, Perrella MA, McKinley LJ, Burnett Jr JC. Angiotensin inhibition potentiates the renal responses to neutral endopeptidase inhibition in dogs with congestive heart failure. J Clin Invest. 1991;88:1636–42.
29. Allarakhia M. Open-source approaches for the repurposing of existing or failed candidate drugs: learning from and applying the lessons across diseases. Drug Des Devel Ther. 2013;7:753–66.
30. Taylor AL, Ziesche S, Yancy C, et al. Combination of isosorbide dinitrate and hydralazine in blacks with heart failure. N Engl J Med. 2004;351:2049–57.
31. Jessup M. Neprilysin inhibition--a novel therapy for heart failure. N Engl J Med. 2014;371:1062–4.
32. Costanzo MR, Saltzberg MT, Jessup M, Teerlink JR, Sobotka PA, Ultrafiltration Versus Intravenous Diuretics for Patients Hospitalized for Acute Decompensated Heart Failure I. Ultrafiltration is associated with fewer rehospitalizations than continuous diuretic infusion in patients with decompensated heart failure: results from UNLOAD. J Cardiac Fail. 2010;16:277–84.
33. Zannad F, McMurray JJ, Krum H, et al. Eplerenone in patients with systolic heart failure and mild symptoms. N Engl J Med. 2011;364:11–21.

34. Tang AS, Wells GA, Talajic M, et al. Cardiac-resynchronization therapy for mild-to-moderate heart failure. N Engl J Med. 2010;363:2385–95.
35. Moss AJ, Hall WJ, Cannom DS, et al. Cardiac-resynchronization therapy for the prevention of heart-failure events. N Engl J Med. 2009;361:1329–38.
36. Linde C, Abraham WT, Gold MR, et al. Randomized trial of cardiac resynchronization in mildly symptomatic heart failure patients and in asymptomatic patients with left ventricular dysfunction and previous heart failure symptoms. J Am Coll Cardiol. 2008;52:1834–43.
37. Patel HC, Rosen SD, Lindsay A, Hayward C, Lyon AR, di Mario C. Targeting the autonomic nervous system: measuring autonomic function and novel devices for heart failure management. Int J Cardiol. 2013;170:107–17.
38. Cohn JN, Pfeffer MA, Rouleau J, et al. Adverse mortality effect of central sympathetic inhibition with sustained-release moxonidine in patients with heart failure (MOXCON). Eur J Heart Fail. 2003;5:659–67.
39. Zhang DY, Anderson AS. The sympathetic nervous system and heart failure. Cardiol Clin. 2014;32:33–45, vii.
40. Triposkiadis F, Karayannis G, Giamouzis G, Skoularigis J, Louridas G, Butler J. The sympathetic nervous system in heart failure physiology, pathophysiology, and clinical implications. J Am Coll Cardiol. 2009;54:1747–62.
41. Birks EJ, George RS, Hedger M, et al. Reversal of severe heart failure with a continuous-flow left ventricular assist device and pharmacological therapy: a prospective study. Circulation. 2011;123:381–90.
42. Kamalakkannan G, Petrilli CM, George I, et al. Clenbuterol increases lean muscle mass but not endurance in patients with chronic heart failure. J Heart Lung Transplant Off Publ Int Soc Heart Transplant. 2008;27:457–61.
43. Gold MR, van Veldhuisen DJ, Mann DL. Vagal nerve stimulation for heart failure: new pieces to the puzzle? Eur J Heart Fail. 2015;17:125–7.
44. Courand PY, Feugier P, Workineh S, Harbaoui B, Bricca G, Lantelme P. Baroreceptor stimulation for resistant hypertension: first implantation in France and literature review. Arch Cardiovasc Dis. 2014;107:690–6.
45. Abraham WT, Zile MR, Weaver FA, Butter C, Ducharme A, Halbach M, Klug DLE, Müller-Ehmsen J, Schafer JE, Senni M, Swarup V, Wachter R, Little WC. Baroreflex activation therapy for the treatment of heart failure with a reduced ejection fraction. JACC Heart Fail. 2015;3(6):487–96.
46. Singh JP, Kandala J, Camm AJ. Non-pharmacological modulation of the autonomic tone to treat heart failure. Eur Heart J. 2014;35:77–85.
47. Zannad F, De Ferrari GM, Tuinenburg AE, et al. Chronic vagal stimulation for the treatment of low ejection fraction heart failure: results of the NEural Cardiac TherApy foR Heart Failure (NECTAR-HF) randomized controlled trial. Eur Heart J. 2015;36:425–33.
48. Ben-Menachem E, Revesz D, Simon BJ, Silberstein S. Surgically implanted and non-invasive vagus nerve stimulation: a review of efficacy, safety and tolerability. Eur J Neurol Off J Eur Fed Neurol Soc. 2015;22(9):1260–8.
49. Wang Z, Yu L, Chen M, Wang S, Jiang H. Transcutaneous electrical stimulation of auricular branch of vagus nerve: a noninvasive therapeutic approach for post-ischemic heart failure. Int J Cardiol. 2014;177:676–7.
50. Tse HF, Turner S, Sanders P, et al. Thoracic spinal cord stimulation for heart failure as a restorative treatment (SCS HEART study): first-in-man experience. Heart Rhythm Off J Heart Rhythm Soc. 2015;12:588–95.
51. Torre-Amione G, Alo K, Estep JD, et al. Spinal cord stimulation is safe and feasible in patients with advanced heart failure: early clinical experience. Eur J Heart Fail. 2014;16:788–95.
52. Bhatt DL, Kandzari DE, O'Neill WW, et al. A controlled trial of renal denervation for resistant hypertension. N Engl J Med. 2014;370:1393–401.
53. Mahfoud F, Luscher TF, Andersson B, et al. Expert consensus document from the European Society of Cardiology on catheter-based renal denervation. Eur Heart J. 2013;34:2149–57.

Therapies in Heart Failure, Tomorrow May Be Too Late

2

Edoardo Gronda and William T. Abraham

2.1 The Heart Failure Pandemic and the "Halfway Technology" Swamp

Heart failure (HF) is a well-recognized, worldwide major and growing health problem. It is known to be the most common and the most socially and economically expensive end product of several clinical conditions that are prevalent in Western societies. Among the many disorders leading to HF are hypertension, chronic kidney disease, diabetes, and, paradoxically, those cardiac diseases that have benefitted most from recent treatments that have lowered mortality in patients with valve diseases, congenital heart diseases, and acute myocardial infarction. Moreover, the incidence of heart failure is intimately related to progressively increasing life expectancy [1] that is the most relevant achievement of the unprecedented quality-of-life improvement enjoyed by Western communities since the end of World War II.

Looking at the big picture, the HF pandemic is largely the result of what we consider the milieu of "progress achievements" of medical science developed to combat what are perceived as threats to our wellness and life.

Contemporary HF management has been established primarily on the basis of two major driving concepts: first, quickly providing the evidence of a statistically significant benefit over an end point that was considered clinically meaningful (survival, hospitalizations, other events, etc.) and second, taking immediate economic advantage of this evidence. Thus, it is not surprising that the approach we have had, thus far, in clinical and experimental research and, in the end, in HF management, has been mainly oriented to a number of mechanisms that were assessed as "running the wheel," instead

E. Gronda, MD (✉)
Cardiology and Heart Failure Research Unit, IRCCS MultiMedica - Sesto San Giovanni, Milan, Italy
e-mail: edoardo.gronda@multimedica.it

W.T. Abraham, MD
Division of Cardiovascular Medicine, The Ohio State University, Columbus, OH, USA

© Springer International Publishing Switzerland 2016

E. Gronda et al. (eds.), *Heart Failure Management: The Neural Pathways*,
DOI 10.1007/978-3-319-24993-3_2

of making the effort to search for the real roots of heart malfunction, to develop a comprehensive approach to the issue, fighting the killer at its source. In this effort, we chose the most immediate use of available tools in the way known as "halfway technology" solutions. Those are technologies able to address disease manifestations and/or symptoms rather the underlying pathological mechanisms that start or perpetuate the disease process [2]. With the exception of pharmacological neurohormonal inhibitors and antagonists, treatment of heart failure has largely focused on the peripheral manifestations of the disease (e.g., fluid retention, peripheral vasoconstriction) or employed pharmacological inotropes at high doses to improve contractility.

The use of inotropes in the treatment of advanced heart failure is an example of the mistaken concepts we applied in managing advanced HF, until recent years. While there is no doubt that decreased contractility is a central component of the pathophysiology of heart failure, attempts to increase contractility with high doses of agents shown to increase myocardial work have not proven to be safe. Perhaps, evidence that the failing heart is an energy-starved pump helps to explain the failure of these prior approaches to directly improve cardiac contractility. The concept was described by analogy to the milk chariot pulled by an exhausted horse [3]. By whipping the horse, we were just killing the animal sooner. Perhaps, newer investigational drugs and devices, which appear to improve contractility without increasing myocardial work or oxygen consumption, will finally get to this root of the HF problem.

Beyond decreased contractility, another central component of heart failure pathophysiology is activation of various neurohormonal vasoconstrictor systems, including the sympathetic and renin-angiotensin-aldosterone systems. On the basis of a more complete understanding of the role of these systems in HF, the therapeutic approach to HF fundamentally changed in the last 25 years. The introduction of angiotensin-converting enzyme inhibitors (ACE I) and, later, of beta-blockers provided stunning evidence of the real potential for medical therapy of HF, at least in its reduced ejection fraction form. The combined action of these pharmacological neural modulators impressively decreased the overall mortality in HF by more than 40 % [4]. These drugs provided most of their benefit by halting the ventricular remodeling and then promoting and consolidating the reversion of this remodeling process both at structural and molecular level, thus reaching the goal of restoring a more efficient heart phenotype, in appropriated cases, by coupling neurohormonal drugs with resynchronization therapy, an almost 60 % decrease of overall HF mortality [4] had been obtained, an achievement that so far has not been matched by any other chronic deadly disease! However, despite this good news, recent large and long-term studies on HF patients who received, on top of optimal pharmacological treatment, the state-of-the-art device therapy reveals a prevailing mortality after a time frame of about 15 years [5]. This observation represents a painful alert that there is more work to be done in improving outcomes in HF patients.

2.2 Current Heart Failure Therapy: The Achievements of Yesterday, the Hurdles of Today

This point is well addressed by challenging the survival gain achieved by the introduction of optimal medical therapy in different HF stages as addressed in multiple HF-controlled trials.

As we have highlighted already, the major achievement in the past was obtained by neurohormonal drugs that primarily counteract the cardiac and end-organ consequences of inappropriate sympathetic nervous system activation. The outstanding benefit in HF outcome has been mostly achieved by adding ACE I to beta-blockers that are able to withdraw or block the inappropriate overstimulation of cardiomyocyte beta-receptors by the excess of cardiac tissue (interstitial) noradrenaline [6, 7]. It is noteworthy that among the adrenergic receptor subpopulations (Beta1, Beta2, Alpha1, Alpha2) that are on the cardiac cell surface, the massive contribution (up to 90 %) to the myocardial dysfunction is generated by the signal alteration provided through the overstimulation of Beta1 receptors [8].

Two considerations then come up. First, in targeting the consequence of sympathetic overactivity, we are on the right track. Second, we have been able to just partially antagonize the deleterious effects of sympathetic activation, without adequately attacking the underlying mechanisms responsible for it. The excess of sympathetic activation in HF, indeed, is ignited by pump failure, but soon, it is maintained and enhanced by multiple scattered neural responses that take place in the cardiorespiratory system under control of the brainstem and involving its specific activity [9]. The matter of fact is that we have not yet been able to implement an effective control of the whole autonomic nervous system that is primarily designed to balance the body's circulation and regulate fluid volume and blood pressure.

This sobering limitation is well addressed by observing the survival gain limitations that we can obtain adding the state-of-the-art therapy in HF subpopulations with progressive disease staging. Despite the fact that the HF populations enrolled in the controlled trials are not entirely comparable on the basis of screening criteria, some hard data cannot be missed. For instance, looking at the mortality in the treated arm of a pivotal beta-blocker study, the MERIT HF (Metoprolol CR/XL Randomised Intervention Trial in Congestive Heart Failure), metoprolol succinate was able to reduce the overall mortality from 11 to 7 % per year [10] and comparable results were achieved in the CIBIS II study (Cardiac Insufficiency Bisoprolol Study II) [11]. Notably in both studies, the prevailing NYHA functional class in the enrolled patients was predominantly stable classes II–III and mean left ventricular ejection fraction (LVEF) in the range of 28 %. Thus, mortality in mild-to-moderate heart failure remains unacceptably high, even in patients on beta-blockers.

Switching to a more advanced HF population with lower left ventricular ejection fraction and/or a recent HF hospital admission in the COPERNICUS (Carvedilol Prospective Randomized Cumulative Survival Study) study population [12], carvedilol administration decreased the annual mortality from 18.5 to 11.4 % per year, a figure that resembles the mortality in the MERIT HF and the CIBIS II studies control arms. This limit of pharmacological therapy is confirmed and someway stressed looking at the Cardiac Resynchronization—Heart Failure (CARE-HF) trial [13]. In the study by adding the wide QRS (in the average 160 msec) to the patient selection criteria (that otherwise closely resemble the selection criteria of MERIT HF and CIBIS II studies but with the addition of an extensive adoption of beta blocker therapy) had a mean LVEF 25 % at enrollment and an annual mortality rate up to 30 % that dropped to 20 % in the resynchronization arm. The figure closely mirrors mortality figure observed in COPERNICUS control arm, i.e., in HFrEF patients not treated with beta-blockers [12] (Fig. 2.1).

Similarly, the implantation of a lifesaving implantable cardiac defibrillator (ICD) following the Multicenter Automatic Defibrillator Implantation Trial (MADIT) criteria does not complete the course of HF therapy as many expected. Adequate prevention of sudden death, indeed, dropped overall mortality of 5.6 %, but, after the effective delivery of the defibrillation therapy, the disease paradoxically progresses [14].

After reputed experts trumpeted outstanding success in HF management, the crude data confirm we are just able to curb disease progression in a portion only of the HF population, but we are unable to fully reverse and definitively cure the disease. More dangerously, we are still led by some misleading concept in daily practice. It is the case of how acute HF management is currently widely performed. After the abrupt development of symptoms driven by lung congestion in the vast majority of cases, indeed, diuretic drugs remain the pivotal therapy [15].

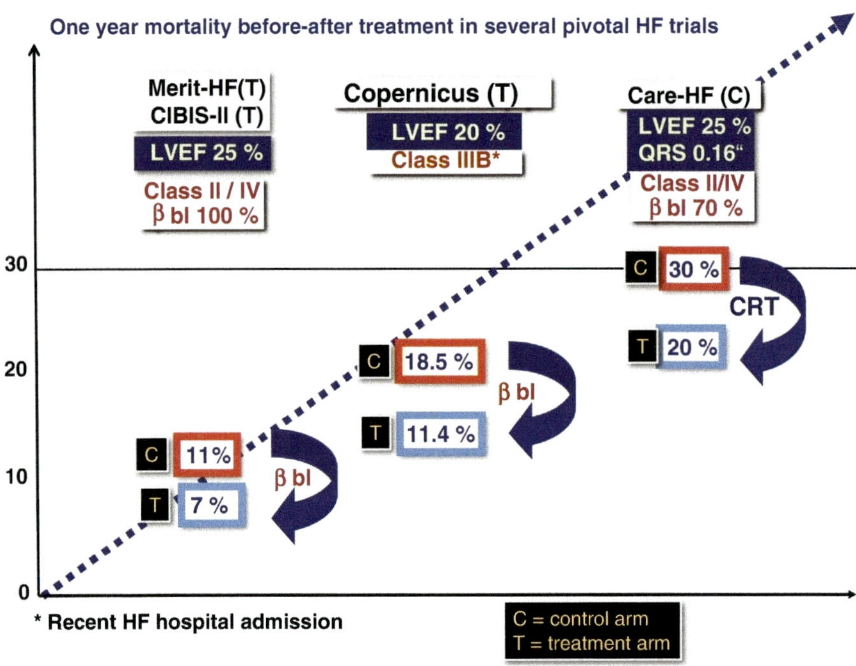

Fig. 2.1 Progressive decrease of overall yearly mortality in successive heart failure (HF) trials, where beta-blockers (beta Bl) [12–14] and, *later*, cardiac resynchronization therapy (CRT) [15] were tested. Notably, over the course of time, the selected HF populations had progressively more severe disease (this was based on patient selection criteria and confirmed by the worse one-year mortality). The key information stands in the fact that, over time, each treatment was able to step back the patient study outcome to the one-year mortality observed in the control arm included in the precedent study

Physicians persist in staggering diuretic drug dosing despite they know congestion is the consequence of a number of failures that overrun compensatory mechanisms of the whole cardiovascular setting. Common knowledge addresses that despite dyspnea is driven by lung congestion, it is a flashing signal of the inadequate pump function that critically pounds kidney perfusion. In the effort to provide rapid relief to the patient's dyspnea, that is poorly treated by rapid diuresis [16], doctors often increase diuretic dose over-sighting that kidney function can deteriorate [17] and that this consequence will decrease drug efficacy [18], worsening patient outcome [19].

On note, the critical balance between the kidney perfusion and the blood pressure becomes a crucial factor in the advanced HF, when even a modest reduction of systolic blood pressure runs disproportionate fall in the renal performance (Fig. 2.2) [20].

These data, collected in an advanced HF population of the CONSENSUS (Cooperative North Scandinavian Enalapril Survival Study) trial, address the relationship between blood pressure and kidney function and may become the critical crossover between therapy benefit and therapy adverse events.

This is because renal dysfunction, per se, plays a direct role in the development and progression of HF and the majority of patients hospitalized for acute decompensated HF have been shown to have already some degree of renal dysfunction [21].

More importantly, renal failure is a more powerful predictor of HF outcome than pump performance indexes like LVEF [22].

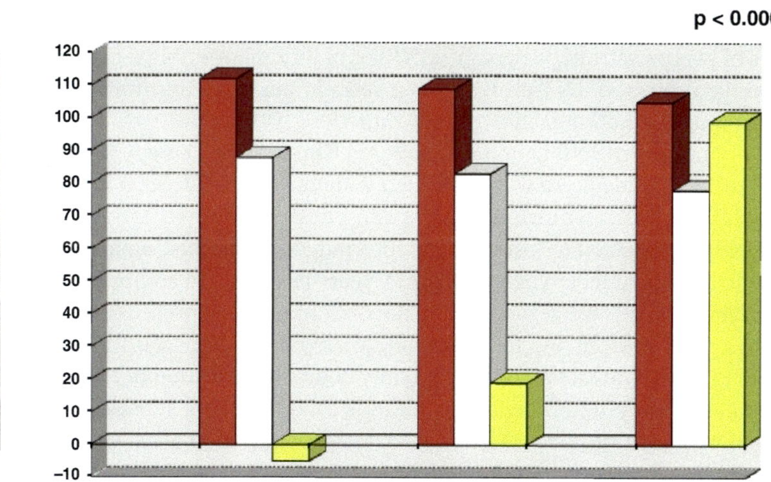

Fig. 2.2 The tight relationship between arterial pressure and renal failure is clearly highlighted by the CONSENSUS study data. When arterial pressure falls below a threshold value, kidney function strikingly worsens. In this figure, the mean arterial pressure fall from 90 to 80 mmHg serum leads to a creatinine increase of 100 % from [20]

Physicians are frequently blurred by patient symptom and they do not mind the underlying pathophysiological key of the disease: the arterial vasculature underfilling. The main consequence of poor cardiac performance, indeed, is the low cardiac output that decreases the kidney perfusion in order to spare the heart and the brain circulation, thereby disproportionately decreasing the renal fraction of cardiac output [23].

One critical consequence of the greater imbalance in renal perfusion is the consequent disproportionate enhancement of renal sympathetic afferent/efferent nerve activity that results in marked increases in renal norepinephrine spillover, with a sympathetically mediated increase in plasma renin activity [9, 23].

In addition to efferent sympathetic activation, activation of renal sensory nerves in HF may cause a reflex increase in sympathetic tone that contributes to the progression of HF by targeting the function of other end-organs, namely, heart and vessels, including venous capacitance in the splanchnic organs [24, 25].

Loop diuretics currently administered in order to clear off fluid volume overload act as a double-edged sword. On one side, they increase water and sodium excretion slowly providing congestion relief [26], but on the other, they promote hypoosmotic diuresis contributing to the water/sodium plasma unbalance [27].

Such an unbalance and fluid loss will eventually have consequences on cardiac output and renal perfusion [17]. This unbalance will indeed create the optimal condition for a vicious circle leading to a further augmentation of the sympathetic/renin-angiotensin system activation with obvious further detrimental consequences on renal perfusion [28] and ultimately in HF outcome. This is the pathophysiology underlying the dramatic negative prognostic consequence of high loop diuretic daily dose [29] and it becomes one more killer in face of the re-uprising of life losses.

More recently, in the effort of improving the patient outcome, several randomized controlled studies have been performed testing plasma concentration of variations of B-type natriuretic peptide (BNP) or of its amino-terminal metabolic product N-terminal-proBNP (NT-proBNP) as a specific guide for up-titration of neurohormonal drugs and optimization of loop diuretics [30].

Only in the ProBNP Outpatient Tailored Chronic HF Therapy (PROTECT trial) NT-proBNP–guided care was associated with a significant reduction in total cardiovascular (CV) events, including worsening heart failure (HF), hospitalization for HF, and CV death. The overall mortality reduction reached almost the statistical significance in patients younger than 75 years but failed to add benefit in the older population [31]. These results should not discourage an appropriate use of biomarkers to optimize lifesaving therapies but do emphasize the need for a better understanding of individual variables that really count in the setting of HF.

In the attempt to turn the tide, today, we can implement sophisticated technologies in treatment of selected cases, such as left ventricular assist devices (LVADs). Those technologies are now a suitable option in experienced HF centers since they displayed impressive implementation involving size, weight, dependability, durability, and implant technique. Skill of surgery team, patient selection criteria, device selection, post-implant patient management, and education are also much improved. Nevertheless bad news are raining again on the end of the story, LVAD chance is most linked to the therapy cost and its burden remains far from a fair cost-effectiveness balance [32].

Moreover, given the need of a major surgical approach and of the complex postoperative management, this sophisticated high-cost "halfway technology" therapy remains, so far, an option only for a tiny minority of patients. The vast majority of those who experience progressive worsening of HF symptoms are old and/or they cluster a number of comorbid conditions (more than three in the average [33] that prevent them to be the ideal LVAD candidates). In the largest advanced HF population, the current prospective remains bleak. The costs due to increased physician visits, hospital admissions, and the extensive need of intensive care units may lead to a figure that is twice as much the need run by other chronic medical conditions [34], adding concerns to its sustainability for even wealthy health-care systems. The apparently never-ending question is: what are we missing, hitherto, in targeting HF outcome?

2.3 Heart Failure Therapy Tomorrow: Looking outside (Beyond) the Current Therapeutic Window

All the therapies that proved to be effective in prolonging HF survival consistently proved to turn down the overexpressed sympathetic-excitatory activity as a primary consequence of pump dysfunction. This is not the only relevant aspect to keep in mind. What we frequently overlook is the pivotal contribution of the autonomic nervous system in maintaining the cardiocirculatory balance by the continuous balancing of its two opposite neuromodulatory systems: the sympathetic or adrenergic system and the parasympathetic or vagal system.

On note, the increased sympathetic activation is coupled to the concomitant, proportional decrease of the counterbalancing vagal nerve activity [35]. This is a critical element for understanding the complex interplay of neurohormonal changes we have learned, since the beta-blocker saga: the autonomic disarray must be stopped and, ideally, reversed.

An intriguing aspect of what we define as autonomic unbalance might reflect the progression of an inherited condition. The findings by Jouven [36] were obtained in a large cohort of persons *without* history of heart disease and highlighted that the individual heart rate profile during exercise and recovery is an important predictor of sudden death even prior to the time when ischemic heart disease becomes evident and symptomatic. Heart rate responses to exercise are under the control of the autonomic nervous system; these data support the concept that the abnormal response of autonomic balance may precede manifestations of cardiovascular disease and may provide relevant information for early identification of persons at high risk for sudden death.

Data from various studies link increased risk of sudden death to increased sympathetic activity and concomitant decreased vagal activity [36–39]. Very importantly, the autonomic imbalance that marked the population at risk in Jouven's study is expressed not only by the decreased vagal activity with a higher heart rate at rest and with a lower heart rate recovery but also by lower sympathetic response under effort with an inadequate heart rate increase. Therefore, it means the occurrence of autonomic impairment involves both sides of the system and this is something we did not expect. As addressed by the authors, the association between altered heart rate responses during exercise and sudden cardiac death without associated non-sudden death from myocardial infarction (MI) suggests this risk factor is linked with a specific cardiac arrhythmia susceptibility and it does not reflect the athero-sclerotic process. It is consistent with the notion that autonomic imbalance is a predisposing factor to life-threatening arrhythmias beyond the critical contribution of the well-known traditional risk factors. Therefore, it is not surprising that the imbalance, highlighted by the decreased heart rate variability and by the impaired baroreflex response, is a well-recognized indicator of a high risk for sudden death after MI [40], but intriguingly, it becomes a marker of the overall risk of death in HF patients [41] and, despite beta-blocker therapy, can predict overall outcome; the lack of baroreflex sensitivity provides comparable prognosis deterioration even in the treated population [42].

This is a relevant framework of HF that reveals how important is the cardiac substrate in determining the double-edged action of autonomic imbalance on sudden death and on HF death. Thus, the current understanding of autonomic reflex control in HF is that in the early stage of the HF syndrome and as long as the hemodynamic balance is maintained, sympathetic afferent information is the critical determinant of the effective vagal contribution to the autonomic cardiac control. However, at the time when the mechanical deterioration progresses toward the end stage of the syndrome, the humoral adrenergic signaling becomes so prevalent to offset the afferent contribution from the dying heart, leading at the end to affect both modes of HF mortality, sudden and progressive pump failure [39].

It is worth noting that all therapies that proved to be effective on prolonging HF survival restore, to some extent, the baroreceptor competence. This beneficial effect was proved to be present after administration of beta-blocker, after resynchronization therapy and after heart transplantation [42–44]. The finding after heart transplantation *is somewhat amazing* as the effect is run only by the hemodynamic balance restoration via replacement of the innervated failing heart with a well-performing denervated heart [44]. The conclusion we can draw is that restoration of normal pump performance is able to reset the autonomic system function while autonomic impairment elicited by pump failure can further derange the cardiac performance and the hemodynamic imbalance. Thus, short of replacing the failing heart with a new one, how can we further improve the autonomic imbalance of HF?

It seems reasonable to look at the sympathetic system as the driver of HF disease progression.

Various approaches to modulating the autonomic nervous system have been investigated in order to tap down the excess of sympathetic activation and/or enhance vagal activity. One approach is via renal denervation, which has been hypothesized to decrease the avid sodium and water retention that takes place along the nephron tubule as soon as the kidney flow is decreased in HF. This notion is being tested in ongoing and future research.

Another approach to neuromodulation in HF is to stimulate the peripheral vagal nerve to override the excessive sympathetic drive. The approach has been tested in several studies, but conflicting results have been generated [45–47], addressing the need for more appropriate study design and size and for a better understanding of the "dose ranging" of vagal nerve stimulation. In this regard, with vagal nerve stimulation, it remains a challenge to find the level of appropriate stimulation to recruit efferent fibers with proactive action and contemporaneous recruitment of the afferent vagal component that has inhibitory effect on sympathetic nerve activity [48].

Another perhaps more physiological approach to neuromodulation in HF may be accomplished by stimulating the baroreceptors that are specifically designed to increase vagal output and inhibit the overall sympathetic drive, acting via afferent neural pathway from the baroreceptors to the central nervous system. This approach may allow a truer rebalancing of the autonomic nervous system. These baroreceptors are located in the atrial wall at the junction with pulmonary veins, in the aortic arch, in the glomerular apparatus, and at the bifurcation of carotid vessels in the carotid sinus. They have a common specific action: to turn down sympathetic activity while turning up vagal activity. The application of this approach via an implanted neurostimulator has been termed baroreflex activation therapy (BAT).

Baroreflex activation therapy has been successfully tested in refractory hypertensive patients on top to optimized medical treatment, providing effective blood pressure lowering in long-term follow-up [49]. Of interest, in the treated subpopulation that underwent echocardiographic assessment, positive structural change of the heart has been documented. Specifically, an impressive 18 % reduction of left ventricular mass was seen in association with a highly significant decrease of systolic and diastolic blood pressure [50].

These findings suggest that BAT can be effective in treatment of HF patients, through its effects on the heart and on peripheral mechanism common to hypertension and HF. The possible positive effects of BAT in HF have been demonstrated by the persistence of decreased sympathetic activation in a prolonged follow-up of a small advanced HF population (9 patients) that received BAT. In this study group, muscle sympathetic nerve activity (MSNA) dropped significantly after 3 and 6 months from starting of the therapy and remained unchanged at an average follow-up of 21 months. The MSNA decrease was coupled with a highly significant decrease in the number of days spent by each patient in the hospital in comparison to the one year before BAT [51].

More recently, a randomized controlled trial was completed in 140 NYHA class III reduced ejection fraction HF patients receiving optimal HF drug and electrophysiological device therapies (OMT) alone ($N=69$) versus OMT plus BAT ($N=71$) [52]. Patients assigned to BAT, compared with control group patients, experienced improvements in the distance walked in 6 min (59.6 ± 14 m vs. 1.5 ± 13.2 m; $p=0.004$), quality-of-life score (-17.4 ± 2.8 points vs. 2.1 ± 3.1 points; $p <0.001$), and NYHA functional class ranking ($p=0.002$ for change in distribution). BAT

Table 2.1 Prominent clinical, biochemical variables changes in baroreflex activation therapy for treatment of heart failure with reduced ejection fraction pivotal study (for details see text) [52]

Variable	Change	P value
Heart failure hospitalizations days per year	From pre to post in BAT patients −6.28 ± 2.7	0.08
BAT vs. OMT NYHA f. class		
Improved %	5 vs. 24	
Stable %	67 vs. 42	0.002
Worsened %	3 vs. 9	
BAT vs. OMT MLWHF QoL score	−17.4 ± 2.8 vs. 2.1 ± 3.1	<0.001
BAT vs. OMT 6-MHD (m)	59.6 ± 14 vs. 1.5 ± 13.2	0.004
NT-proBNP (pg/ml)	From pre to post in BAT patients −342	0.026

BAT baroreflex activation therapy, *OMT* optimal medical therapy, *MLWHF QoL score* Minnesota living with heart failure quality of life score, *6-MHD* 6-minute hall distance, *NT-proBNP* N terminal pro brain natriuretic factor

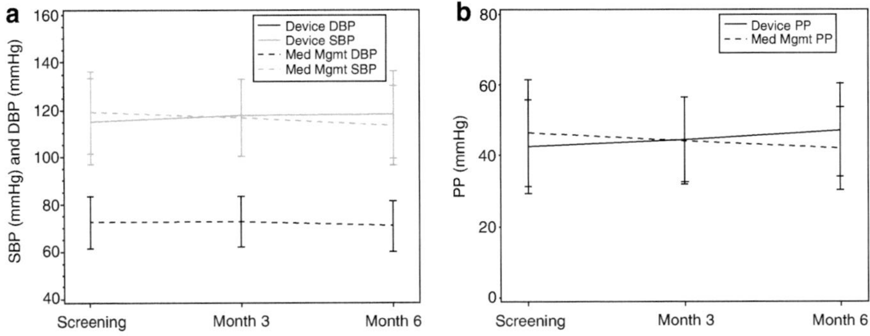

Fig. 2.3 Effect of BAT on blood pressure in heart failure patients with reduced ejection fraction. *DBP* diastolic blood pressure, *Med Mgmt* medical management, *PP* pulse pressure, *SBP* systolic blood pressure. Baroreflex activation therapy (BAT) significantly increased systolic blood pressure (BP) (**a**) and pulse pressure (**b**), with no effect on diastolic BP. In contrast, there were trends toward decreasing systolic BP and pulse pressure in the control group (Reproduced with permission from [52])

significantly reduced N-terminal pro–brain natriuretic peptide ($p = 0.02$) and was associated with a trend toward fewer days hospitalized for HF ($p = 0.08$) (Table 2.1). In addition, BAT significantly increased systolic blood pressure and pulse pressure (Fig. 2.3), correlates of improved survival in HF. Finally, BAT was shown to be safe in this patient population.

These study results support a large multicenter controlled trial focusing on BAT effect in reducing morbidity and mortality in advanced HF patients.

References

1. Stewart S, MacIntyre K, Capewell S, McMurray JJ. Heart failure and the aging population: an increasing burden in the 21st century? Heart. 2003;89:49–53.
2. Brown Physician Exec. Halfway technologies. 1996;22:44–5.
3. Fürstenwerth H. Why whip the starving horse when there is oats for the starving myocardium? Am J Ther. 2014 [Epub ahead of print].
4. Mann DL, Bristow MR. Mechanisms and models in heart failure: the biomechanical Model and Beyond. Circulation. 2005;111:2837–49.
5. Buber J, Klein H, Moss AJ, McNitt S, Eldar M, Padeletti L, Vogt J, Meine M, Brown MW, Barsheshet A, Zareba W, Goldenberg I. Clinical course and outcome of patients enrolled in US and non-US centres in MADIT-CRT. Eur Heart J. 2011;32:2697–704.
6. Cohn JN, Levine TB, Olivari MT, Garberg V, Lura D, Francis GS, Simon AB, Rector T. Plasma norepinephrine as a guide to prognosis in patients with chronic congestive heart failure. N Engl J Med. 1984;311(13):819–23.
7. Lowes BD, Gilbert EM, Abraham WT, Minobe WA, Larrabee P, Ferguson D, Wolfel EE, Lindenfeld J, Tsvetkova T, Robertson AD, Quaife RA, Bristow MR. Myocardial gene expression in dilated cardiomyopathy treated with beta-blocking agents. N Engl J Med. 2002;346:1357–65.
8. Bristow MR, Feldman AM, Adams Jr KF, Goldstein SJ. Selective versus nonselective beta-blockade for heart failure therapy: are there lessons to be learned from the COMET trial? J Card Fail. 2003;9:444–53.
9. Floras JS. Sympathetic nervous system activation in human heart failure: clinical implications of an updated model. J Am Coll Cardiol. 2009;54:375–85.
10. Effect of metoprolol CR/XL in chronic heart failure: Metoprolol CR/XL Randomized Intervention Trial in Congestive Heart Failure (MERIT-HF). Lancet. 1999;353:2001–7.
11. The Cardiac Insufficiency Bisoprolol Study II (CIBIS II): a randomised trial. Lancet. 1999;353(9164):9–13.
12. Packer M, Coats AJ, Fowler MB, Katus HA, Krum H, Mohacsi P, Rouleau JL, Tendera M, Castaigne A, Roecker EB, Schultz MK, DeMets DL, Carvedilol Prospective Randomized Cumulative Survival Study Group. Effect of carvedilol on survival in severe chronic heart failure. N Engl J Med. 2001;344:1651–8.
13. Cleland JG, Daubert JC, Erdmann E, Freemantle N, Gras D, Kappenberger L, Tavazzi L. The effect of cardiac resynchronization on morbidity and mortality in heart failure. N Engl J Med. 2005;352:1539–49.
14. Goldenberg I, Moss AJ, Hall WJ, McNitt S, Zareba W, Andrews ML, Cannom DS. Multicenter Automatic Defibrillator Implantation Trial (MADIT) II Investigators. Causes and consequences of heart failure after prophylactic implantation of a defibrillator in the multicenter automatic defibrillator implantation trial II. Circulation. 2006;113:2810–7.
15. O'Connor CM, Stough WG, Gallup DS, Hasselblad V, Gheorghiade M. Demographics, clinical characteristics, and outcomes of patients hospitalized for decompensated heart failure: observations from the IMPACT-HF registry. J Card Fail. 2005;11:200–5.
16. Costanzo MR, Guglin ME, Saltzberg MT, Jessup ML, Bart BA, Teerlink JR, Jaski BE, Fang JC, Feller ED, Haas GJ, Anderson AS, Schollmeyer MP, Sobotka PA, UNLOAD Trial Investigators. Ultrafiltration versus intravenous diuretics for patients hospitalized for acute decompensated heart failure. J Am Coll Cardiol. 2007;49:675–83.
17. Schrier RW. Blood urea nitrogen and serum creatinine: not married in heart failure. Circ Heart Fail. 2008;1:2–5.
18. Butler J, Forman DE, Abraham WT, Gottlieb SS, Loh E, Massie BM, O'Connor CM, Rich MW, Stevenson LW, Wang Y, Young JB, Krumholz HM. Relationship between heart failure treatment and development of worsening renal function among hospitalized patients. Am Heart J. 2004;147:331–8.
19. Petersson M, Friberg P, Eisenhofer G, Lambert G, Rundqvist B. Long-term outcome in relation to renal sympathetic activity in patients with chronic heart failure. Eur Heart J. 2005;26:906–13.

20. Ljungam S, Kjekshus J, Swedberg K. Renal function in severe congestive heart failure during treatment with enalapril (the Cooperative North Scandinavian Enalapril Survival Study [CONSENSUS] Trial). Am J Cardiol. 1992;70:479.
21. Heywood JT, Fonarow GC, Costanzo MR, Mathur VS, Wigneswaran JR, Wynne J. High prevalence of renal dysfunction and its impact on outcome in 118,465 patients hospitalized with acute decompensated heart failure: a report from the ADHERE database. J Card Fail. 2007;13:422–30.
22. Hillege HL, Girbes AR, de Kam PJ, Boomsma F, de Zeeuw D, Charlesworth A, Hampton JR, van Veldhuisen DJ. Renal function, neurohormonal activation, and survival in patients with chronic heart failure. Circulation. 2000;102:203–10.
23. Shlipak MG, Massie BM. The clinical challenge of cardiorenal syndrome. Circulation. 2004;110:1514–7.
24. Stella A, Zanchetti A. Functional role of renal afferents. Physiol Rev. 1991;71:659–82.
25. Schlaich MP, Socratous F, Hennebry S, Eikelis N, Lambert EA, Straznicky N, Esler MD, Lambert GW. Sympathetic activation in chronic renal failure. J Am Soc Nephrol. 2009;20:933–9.
26. Schrier RW. Use of diuretics in heart failure and cirrhosis. Semin Nephrol. 2011;31:503–12.
27. Gottlieb SS, Brater DC, Thomas I, Havranek E, Bourge R, Goldman S, Dyer F, Gomez M, Bennett D, Ticho B, Beckman E, Abraham WT. BG9719 (CVT-124), an A1 adenosine receptor antagonist, protects against the decline in renal function observed with diuretic therapy. Circulation. 2002;105:1348–53.
28. Bayliss J, Norell M, Canepa-Anson R, Sutton G, Poole-Wilson P. Untreated heart failure: clinical and neuroendocrine effects of introducing diuretics. Br Heart J. 1987;57:17–22.
29. Felker GM, O'Connor CM, Braunwald E. Loop diuretics in acute decompensated heart failure. Necessary? Evil? A necessary evil? Circ Heart Fail. 2009;2:56–62.
30. Januzzi LJ, Troughton R, Are Serial BNP. Measurements useful in heart failure management? Serial natriuretic peptide measurements are useful in heart failure management. Circulation. 2013;127:500–8.
31. Januzzi Jr JL, Rehman SU, Mohammed AA, Bhardwaj A, Barajas L, Barajas J, Kim HN, Baggish AL, Weiner RB, Chen-Tournoux A, Marshall JE, Moore SA, Carlson WD, Lewis GD, Shin J, Sullivan D, Parks K, Wang TJ, Gregory SA, Uthamalingam S, Semigran MJ. Use of amino-terminal pro-B type natriuretic peptide to guide outpatient therapy of patients with chronic left ventricular systolic dysfunction. J Am Coll Cardiol. 2011;58:1881–9.
32. Neyt M, Van den Bruel A, Smit Y, De Jonge N, Vlayen J. The cost-utility of left ventricular assist devices for end-stage heart failure patients ineligible for cardiac transplantation: a systematic review and critical appraisal of economic evaluations. Ann Cardiothorac Surg. 2014;3:439–49.
33. Levy MN, Martin PJ, Stuesse SL. Neural regulation of the heart beat. Annu Rev Physiol. 1981;43:443–53.
34. Ledwidge M, Gallagher J, Conlon C, Tallon E, O'Connell E, Dawkins I, Watson C, O'Hanlon R, Bermingham M, Patle A, Badabhagni MR, Murtagh G, Voon V, Tilson L, Barry M, McDonald L, Maurer B, McDonald K. Natriuretic peptide-based screening and collaborative care for heart failure: the STOP-HF randomized trial. JAMA. 2013;310:66–74.
35. Adler ED, Goldfinger JZ, Kalman J, Park ME, Meier DE. Palliative care in the treatment of advanced heart failure. Circulation. 2009;120:2597–606.
36. Jouven X, Empana JP, Schwartz PJ, Desnos M, Courbon D, Ducimetière P. Heart-rate profile during exercise as a predictor of sudden death. N Engl J Med. 2005;352:1951–8.
37. Lown B, Verrier RL. Neural activity and ventricular fibrillation. N Engl J Med. 1976;294:1165–70.
38. Schwartz PJ, La Rovere MT, Vanoli E. Autonomic nervous system and sudden cardiac death: experimental basis and clinical observations for post-myocardial infarction risk stratification. Circulation. 1992;85(Suppl):I-77–91.
39. Schwartz PJ. The autonomic nervous system and sudden death. Eur Heart J. 1998;19(Suppl F):F72–80.

40. La Rovere MT, Bigger Jr JT, Marcus FI, Mortara A, Schwartz PJ. Baroreflex sensitivity and heart-rate variability in prediction of total cardiac mortality after myocardial infarction. ATRAMI (Autonomic Tone and Reflexes After Myocardial Infarction) Investigators. Lancet. 1998;351(9101):478–84.
41. Mortara A, La Rovere MT, Pinna GD, Prpa A, Maestri R, Febo O, Pozzoli M, Opasich C, Tavazzi L. Arterial baroreflex modulation of heart rate in chronic heart failure: clinical and hemodynamic correlates and prognostic implications. Circulation. 1997;96:3450–8.
42. La Rovere MT, Pinna GD, Maestri R, Robbi E, Caporotondi A, Guazzotti G, Sleight P, Febo O. Prognostic implications of baroreflex sensitivity in heart failure patients in the beta-blocking era. J Am Coll Cardiol. 2009;53:193–9.
43. Gademan MG, van Bommel RJ, Ypenburg C, Haest JC, Schalij MJ, van der Wall EE, Bax JJ, Swenne CA. Biventricular pacing in chronic heart failure acutely facilitates the arterial barore-flex. Am J Physiol Heart Circ Physiol. 2008;295:H755–60.
44. Ellenbogen KA, Mohanty PK, Szentpetery S, Thames MD. Arterial baroreflex abnormalities in heart failure. Reversal after orthotopic cardiac transplantation. Circulation. 1989;79:51–8.
45. De Ferrari GM, Crijns HJ, Borggrefe M, Milasinovic G, Smid J, Zabel M, Gavazzi A, Sanzo A, Dennert R, Kuschyk J, Raspopovic S, Klein H, Swedberg K, Schwartz PJ, CardioFit Multicenter Trial Investigators. Chronic vagus nerve stimulation: a new and promising thera-peutic approach for chronic heart failure. Eur Heart J. 2011;32:847–55.
46. Zannad F, De Ferrari GM, Tuinenburg AE, Wright D, Brugada J, Butter C, Klein H, Stolen C, Meyer S, Stein KM, Ramuzat A, Schubert B, Daum D, Neuzil P, Botman C, Caste MA, D'Onofrio A, Solomon SD, Wold N, Ruble SB. Chronic vagal stimulation for the treatment of low ejection fraction heart failure: results of the neural cardiac therapy for heart failure (NECTAR-HF) randomized controlled trial. Eur Heart J. 2015;36:425–33.
47. Premchand RK, Sharma K, Mittal S, Monteiro R, Dixit S, Libbus I, DiCarlo LA, Ardell JL, Rector TS, Amurthur B, KenKnight BH, Anand IS. Autonomic regulation therapy via left or right cervical vagus nerve stimulation in patients with chronic heart failure: results of the ANTHEM-HF trial. J Card Fail. 2014;20:808–16.
48. Camm AJ, Savelieva I. Vagal nerve stimulation in heart failure. Eur Heart J. 2015;36:404–6.
49. Bisognano JD, Bakris G, Nadim MK, Sanchez L, Kroon AA, Schafer J, de Leeuw PW, Sica DA. Baroreflex activation therapy lowers blood pressure in patients with resistant hyperten-sion: results from the double-blind, randomized, placebo-controlled rheos pivotal trial. J Am Coll Cardiol. 2011;58:765–73.
50. Bisognano JD, Kaufman CL, Bach DS, Lovett EG, de Leeuw P, DEBuT HT, Rheos Feasibility Trial Investigators. Improved cardiac structure and function with chronic treatment using an implantable device in resistant hypertension: results from European and United States trials of the Rheos system. J Am Coll Cardiol. 2011;57:1787–8.
51. Gronda E, Seravalle G, Quarti-Trevano F, Costantino G, Casini A, Alsheraei A, Lovett EG, Vanoli E, Mancia G, Grassi G. Long-term chronic baroreflex activation: Persistent efficacy in patients with heart failure and reduced ejection fraction. J Hyperten. 2015 (accepted).
52. Abraham WT, Zile MR, Weaver FA, Butter C, Ducharme A, Halbach M, Klug D, Lovett EG, Müller-Ehmsen J, Schafer JE, Senni M, Swarup V, Wachter R, Little WC. Baroreflex activation therapy for the treatment of heart failure with a reduced ejection fraction. JACC Heart Fail. 2015;3(6):487–96.

Atrial Fibrillation, Heart Failure, and the Autonomic Nervous System

3

Omeed Zardkoohi, Gino Grifoni, Luigi Padeletti, and Alexandru Costea

In 1628, William Harvey described the importance of the auricle during the motion of the heart: "First the auricle contracts, and this force the abundant blood it contains as the cistern and reservoir of the veins, into the ventricle. This being filled, the heart raises itself, makes its fibers tense, contracts, and beats. By this beat it at once ejects into the arteries the blood received from the auricle." Three centuries later, Gesell described the association between atrial fibrillation and a drop in the arterial pressure, further describing that the blood pressure effects were reversed with restoration of sinus rhythm [1] (Fig. 3.1).

Atrial fibrillation (AF) affects more than 2 million patients in the United Sates, and the prevalence will continue to increase as the population ages [2]. Atrial fibrillation and heart failure have an intimate and bidirectional relationship: atrial fibrillation exacerbates heart failure, and heart failure increases the risk of atrial fibrillation. Many of the risk factors for atrial fibrillation such as diabetes, hypertension, and coronary artery disease are common risk factors for heart failure [2]. In a study by Wang et al., 1470 patients were followed for 5.6 years after atrial fibrillation diagnosis, and 4.2 years after heart failure diagnosis, finding that 42 % of patients with AF developed or had congestive heart failure (CHF), and 41 % of CHF patients developed AF. In addition, the prevalence of AF increases with advancing New York Heart Association (NYHA) functional class, from <10 % in NYHA Class I to 50 % in those with NYHA functional Class IV [3, 4].

O. Zardkoohi, MD (✉)
Department of Medicine Division of Cardiology, Cadence Health Northwestern Medicine Winfield, Winfield, IL, USA
e-mail: Omeed.Zardkoohi@cedencehealth.org

G. Grifoni, MD • L. Padeletti, MD, PhD
Department of Experimental and Clinical Medicine, University of Florence, Florence, Italy

University of Milano, Milan, Italy

A. Costea, MD
Department of Medicine Division of Cardiology, University of Cincinnati, Cincinnati, OH, USA

© Springer International Publishing Switzerland 2016
E. Gronda et al. (eds.), *Heart Failure Management: The Neural Pathways*,
DOI 10.1007/978-3-319-24993-3_3

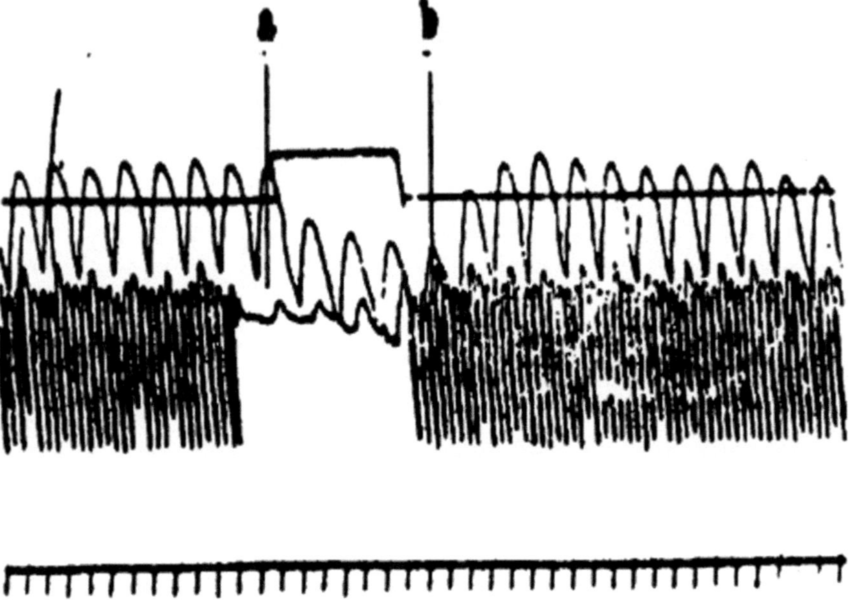

Fig. 3.1 Gesell's description of the association between atrial fibrillation and a drop in the arterial pressure

Numerous clinical trials have demonstrated that AF increases mortality in patients with heart failure. For instance, in the SOLVD trial, patients with AF had higher mortality than patients with sinus rhythm at baseline (34 % vs. 23 %; p <0.001), even after adjusting for clinical parameters such as left ventricular ejection fraction (LVEF), NYHA functional class, and age [5].

Beneath the surface of the epidemiological relationship, translational experiments have elucidated the direct relationship between elevated atrial pressure and the threshold for AF initiation. Increased atrial pressure not only reduces the atrial effective refractory period but also increases the dispersion of atrial refractoriness [6]. These two factors work in concert to promote a substrate for AF inducibility and sustainability.

Atrial fibrillation leads to several physiological consequences: loss of atrial systole, irregular ventricular rhythm, increased ventricular rate, and loss of physiological control of the heart rate. These physiological changes during atrial fibrillation underlie the clinical effects, such as reduced cardiac output, exacerbation of diastolic and systolic heart failure, imbalance between myocardial oxygen supply and demand as a result of impaired coronary perfusion and reduced exercise capacity [2].

Pardeans et al. demonstrated that AF is associated with a 20 % lower peak VO_2 in heart failure patients, highlighting the importance of maintaining cardiac output and exercise performance in patients with impaired ventricular function [7].

Naturally, the relationship between AF and CHF is far more complex than simply pressure overload-induced electrical changes. A schematic representation of the complex and multifaceted relationship between the pathophysiology of AF and CHF was elegantly described by Maisel et al. [2]. Heart failure leads to volume and pressure overload, irregular ventricular filling, neurohormonal activation, atrial enlargement, atrial interstitial fibrosis, calcium dysregulation, and altered atrial electrical properties, all of which promote atrial fibrillation. In terms of fibrosis, it has been noted on histological studies that it is mostly distributed in the posterior wall, has a direct correlation with fractionated potentials found during mapping and ablation while the dominant frequency is lower with a higher organizational index [3]. The location of fibrosis has a major impact in techniques of AF ablation in CHF patients as illustrated later. Atrial fibrillation leads to cellular and extracellular remodeling, loss of AV synchrony, rapid ventricular response, and lower cardiac output, promoting heart failure [2, 8] (Fig. 3.2).

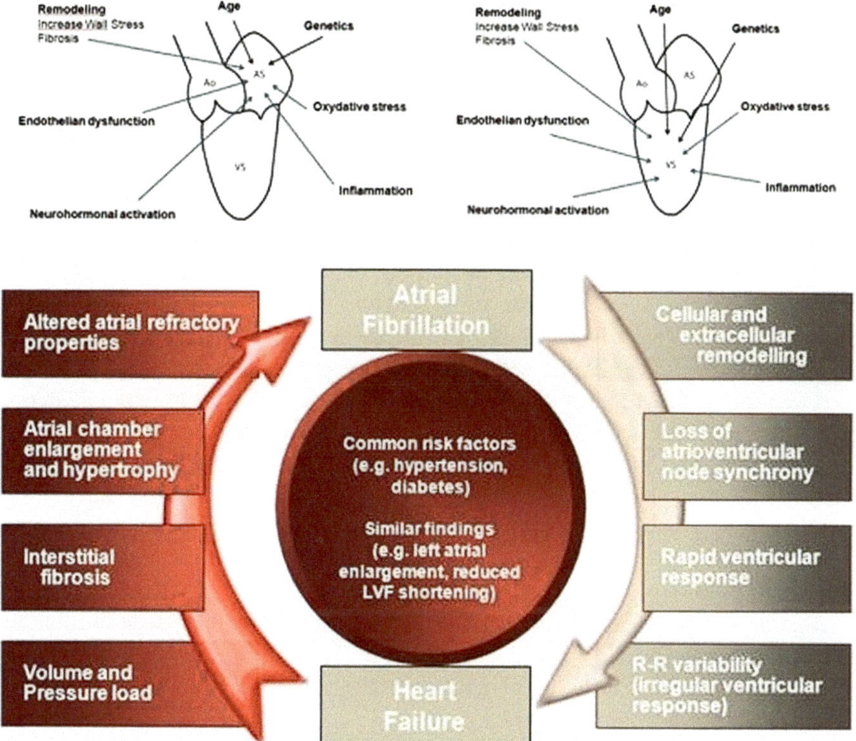

Fig. 3.2 There are multiple facets underlying the common pathophysiology of heart failure and atrial fibrillation. Heart failure leads to volume and pressure overload in the atrium and ventricle. This leads to neurohormonal activation, promoting interstitial fibrosis, atrial chamber enlargement, and endothelial dysfunction, which can alter atrial refractory properties and lead to atrial fibrillation. Atrial fibrillation leads to loss of atrioventricular synchrony, rapid ventricular response, and variable R-R intervals, which thereby promote heart failure. This can lead to a vicious cycle in which heart failure begets atrial fibrillation, and atrial fibrillation begets heart failure (center panel) (Reproduced with permission from [2])

One of the important links between AF and CHF is the upregulation of the neurohormonal system. Neurohormonal activation is a well-established consequence of heart failure and represents the most important target of pharmacotherapy. Angiotensin II, a critical octapeptide hormone of the renin-angiotensin-aldosterone cascade, can cause increased extracellular matrix fibrosis, which can alter atrial conduction properties and refractory periods, predisposing to the development of atrial fibrillation [9].

3.1 Treatment of Atrial Fibrillation in the Heart Failure Population

Having the pathophysiologic changes in mind, it is obvious that optimal medical therapy for heart failure may also help improve atrial fibrillation, including the use of medications targeting the renin-angiotensin-aldosterone pathway. For example, angiotensin-converting enzyme inhibitors (ACE-I), a mainstay of afterload reduction in heart failure, have been shown to reduce atrial fibrillation risk in heart failure. Clinical studies and pathological correlation demonstrate that ACE inhibition may help decrease left atrial fibrosis and the risk of AF recurrence after cardioversion [10]. In addition, angiotensin receptor blockade has also been shown to reduce the incidence of atrial fibrillation in patients with heart failure [11].

Beta-blockers, another mainstay of pharmacotherapy for heart failure, improve atrial fibrillation as well. In a meta-analysis of seven studies including 11,952 patients receiving angiotensin-converting enzyme inhibitors, treatment with beta-blockers was associated with 27 % relative risk reduction in the incidence of AF (RR 0.73, 95 % CI:0.61–0.86, $p = 0.001$) [12].

Given the increased morbidity and mortality associated with growing epidemic of both heart failure and atrial fibrillation, it is of particular scientific and clinical importance to find optimal treatment strategies. For atrial fibrillation treatment, these can be divided into two main categories: rate control or rhythm control.

Rate control entails medical therapy for suppression of rapid ventricular response, or can involve, in some cases, atrioventricular node ablation and pacemaker implantation.

Rhythm control includes antiarrhythmic drugs and ablation of atrial fibrillation. The optimal strategy has been the subject of numerous clinical trials in the atrial fibrillation population at large, as well as in the subgroup of patients with heart failure.

The presence of systolic heart failure renders the treatment pharmacological strategies with rate control or rhythm control more complex. Systolic heart failure, for example, precludes the use of certain antiarrhythmic medication, such as Class Ic drugs (flecainide and propafenone), that may have a negative inotropic effect. In addition, rate control medications may be limited by poor tolerance and hypotension. Several clinical trials in the atrial fibrillation population at large have failed to show benefit of rhythm control over rate control. For instance, the AFFIRM trial compared rate control strategy with a rhythm control strategy. In the trial, 4060 patients were enrolled and randomized to either rate control (digoxin, beta-blocker, diltiazem, verapamil) or rhythm control (most commonly amiodarone and sotalol). At 5-year follow-up, the mortality rate in the rhythm control arm vs. the rate control arm was 23.8 % vs. 21.3 %, respectively, HR 1.15 (95 % CI 0.99–1.34; $P=0.08$) [13].

Therefore, a rhythm control strategy showed no benefit over a rhythm control strategy, and there was a nonsignificant trend toward increased mortality in the rhythm control arm. Of note, the increased mortality in the antiarrhythmic group was due to increased frequency of malignancies, unlikely related to medications, but rather a possible coincidence.

As a result of the AFFIRM trial, it was thought that the clinical benefit of restoring sinus rhythm is typically offset by the negative side effects of antiarrhythmic drugs. It is important to recognize that the AFFIRM trial was performed in the early era of ablation, and therefore, a very small proportion of patients received catheter or surgical ablation for atrial arrhythmia (total of 18 patients). Finally, a minority of the patients in AFFIRM had depressed left ventricular function and/or advanced NYHA Class, making it difficult to extrapolate these findings to patients with systolic heart failure.

Additional studies aimed to answer this question and included the Pharmacological Intervention in Atrial Fibrillation (PIAF), How to Treat Chronic Atrial Fibrillation (HOT CAFE), and Strategies of Treatment of Atrial Fibrillation (STAF). These trials had similar findings that rhythm and rate control strategies were equivalent, although a high proportion of patients in the rhythm control arms did not maintain sinus rhythm long term [8].

Because the rhythm control arm of the AFFIRM trial had a low proportion of patients maintaining sinus rhythm, a subsequent study analyzed the subgroup of patients who maintained sinus rhythm, using an on-treatment analysis. Interestingly, covariates that were associated with improved survival include maintenance of sinus rhythm (HR 0.54, 95 % CI 0.42–0.70, P <0.0001) and warfarin use (HR 0.47, 95 % CI 0.36–0.61, P <0.0001) [14].

However, it is possible that sinus rhythm was simply a confounder for a healthier patient population. Consistent with prior studies, antiarrhythmic drug use was associated with increased mortality [14]. It is also important to recognize that patients with highly symptomatic atrial fibrillation would not likely be randomized to such clinical trials or alternatively would have typically crossover from the rate control to the rhythm control arms. The Atrial Fibrillation and Congestive Heart failure (AF-CHF) trial sought to examine the rhythm vs. rate control question in the heart failure population. In this multicenter, randomized trial of patients with left ventricular ejection fraction of 35 % or less and AF, there was no difference in cardiovascular mortality between the rhythm control group and the rate control group (27 % vs. 25 %, respectively (HR 1.06; 95 % CI 0.86–1.30; $P=0.59$) [15].

In addition, there was no significant difference between the groups with regard to death from any cause, stroke, or worsening heart failure. The vast majority of the patients in the rhythm control arm were taking amiodarone, and maintenance of sinus rhythm was roughly 80 % in the rhythm control arm. The proportion of patients in the rhythm control group requiring hospitalization was higher than the rate control group, which was statistically significant in the first year, likely due to the need for repeat cardioversion or medication adjustments (46 % vs. 39 %, $P=0.001$). However, patients did not undergo catheter ablation of atrial fibrillation as part of the rhythm control strategy. Therefore, the AF-CHF study extends the findings of AFFIRM to the systolic heart failure population, showing no benefit of a rhythm control strategy over a rate control strategy [8, 14].

A relatively newer Class III agent, dofetilide, was approved by the FDA in 1999 and today is one of the cornerstones of antiarrhythmic drug therapy in patients with systolic heart failure. This medication requires inpatient loading of the medication for close QT interval and arrhythmia monitoring. In the DIAMOND congestive failure substudy, dofetilide was more effective than placebo in maintaining sinus rhythm in patients with AF and heart failure (79 % with dofetilide versus 42 % with placebo $P=0.001$) and also reduced the hospitalization rate for heart failure [16].

While prior trials of AAD and heart failure show a signal for increased mortality or heart failure, the DIAMOND substudy showed no effect on all-cause mortality; restoration and maintenance of sinus rhythm was associated with a reduction of mortality (RR 0.44, 95 % CI 0.30–0.64; $P <0.0001$), consistent with the AFFIRM substudy described above. The risk for torsade de pointes (TDP) among patients treated with dofetilide was relatively small, 2.1 %. Independent predictors of the development of Tdp were female gender, NYHA Class III/IV, and higher QTc [17].

Finally, in an observational study assessing the effects of CRT and AV node ablation vs. CRT and rate control in patients with atrial fibrillation, CRT and AV node ablation was associated with a ninefold lower heart failure mortality compared to patients with AF who were received CRT and rate control medications only. This was thought to be due to "complete" heart rate control and hence maximal CRT benefit [18].

Based on our current knowledge, it appears that the benefits of sinus rhythm may be neutralized by the negative effects of antiarrhythmic medication is a recurrent theme of debate in the rate vs. rhythm control. In addition, antiarrhythmic drugs do not have high efficacy in the long term, the options of drugs are limited, and the side effects can be considerable.

Catheter ablation for AF has rapidly been recognized as a highly effective treatment option for AF that is refractory to pharmacological therapy. Many patients undergoing successful ablation may cease their antiarrhythmic medication, avoiding then the potential negative side effects encountered with long-term use. Catheter-based AF ablation is focused not only on pulmonary vein isolation but also associated additional linear ablation or complex fractionated electrogram ablation in patients with CHF, as these patients typically have a different mechanism of atrial fibrillation. While in paroxysmal atrial fibrillation it has been recognized that pulmonary vein foci are the main triggers, in persistent AF usually associated with CHF, there are additional substrates for AF – posterior wall fibrosis, foci outside the pulmonary veins, and extensive scarring in the left atrium. A newer technology, cryoballoon ablation for pulmonary vein isolation, has also recently been approved and is also widely being used clinically; however, its utility in persistent AF and CHF remains to be determined.

In radiofrequency catheter ablation, various lesion sets and techniques have been applied [19] (Fig. 3.3).

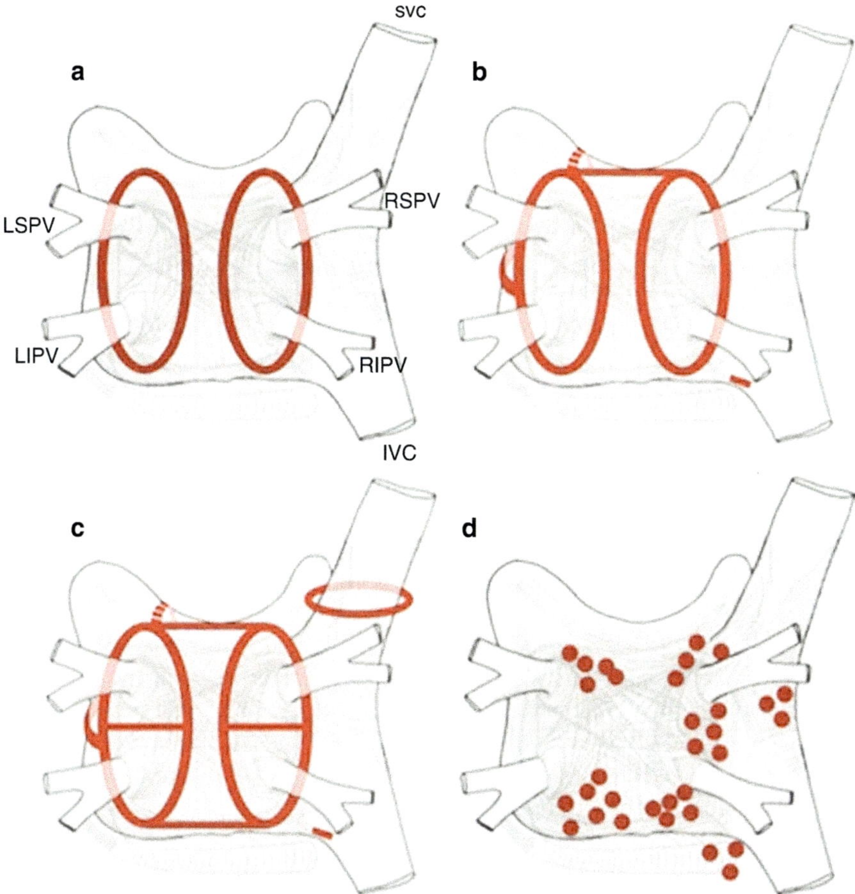

Fig. 3.3 Schematic of common lesion sets employed in AF ablation. A: The circumferential ablation lesions that are created in a circumferential fashion around the right and the left PVs. The primary endpoint of this ablation strategy is the electrical isolation of the PV musculature. B: Some of the most common sites of linear ablation lesions. These include a "roof line" connecting the lesions encircling the left and/or right PVs, a "mitral isthmus" line connecting the mitral valve and the lesion encircling the left PVs at the level of the left inferior PV, and an anterior linear lesion connecting either the "roof line" or the left or right circumferential lesion to the mitral annulus anteriorly. A linear lesion created at the cavotricuspid isthmus is also shown. This lesion is generally placed in patients who have experienced cavotricuspid isthmus-dependent atrial flutter clinically or have it induced during EP testing. C: Similar to 3B but also shows additional linear ablation lesions between the superior and inferior PVs resulting in a figure of 8 lesion set as well as a posterior inferior line allowing for electrical isolation of the posterior left atrial wall. An encircling lesion of the superior vena cava (SVC) directed at electrical isolation of the SVC is also shown. SVC isolation is performed if focal firing from the SVC can be demonstrated. A subset of operators empirically isolates the SVC. D: Some of the most common sites of ablation lesions when complex fractionated electrograms are targeted (these sites are also close to the autonomic GP) (Reproduced with permission from [18])

Several studies have been performed to evaluate the benefits of AF ablation in the systolic heart failure population.

In a small study of patients with atrial fibrillation and systolic heart failure (mean EF 42 %), atrial fibrillation ablation increased LVEF from 42 % +/−9 % to 56+/−8 %, (P <0.001) [20] (Fig. 3.4).

In another study, 58 patients with LVEF <45 % and NYHA Class II or higher underwent catheter-based radiofrequency ablation; maintenance of sinus rhythm was associated with significant improvement in LV function, exercise capacity, and quality of life [21]. The improvement in EF was highest in patients with inadequate rate control before the ablation (24+/−8 %), highlighting the potential role for tachycardia-mediated cardiomyopathy in this population. The majority of patients remained in sinus rhythm at the 12 months follow-up (69 % without antiarrhythmic drugs and 78 % with antiarrhythmic medications). Interestingly, the success rate of ablation at 12 months was no different between patients with systolic heart failure and patients without systolic heart failure (69 % vs. 71 %, respectively, $P=0.84$). Although this study was small and not randomized, compelling evidence exists for the efficacy of catheter ablation in patients with heart failure. It is very important to note that the ablation technique involved additional lines in the left atrium besides pulmonary vein isolation, allowing correction of substrates typically involved in CHF and AF.

Results from a larger nonrandomized trial (94 patients) demonstrated slightly different results [22]. Patients with LVEF <40 % who underwent atrial fibrillation ablation had a higher AF recurrence rate (27 %) than patients with normal LVEF

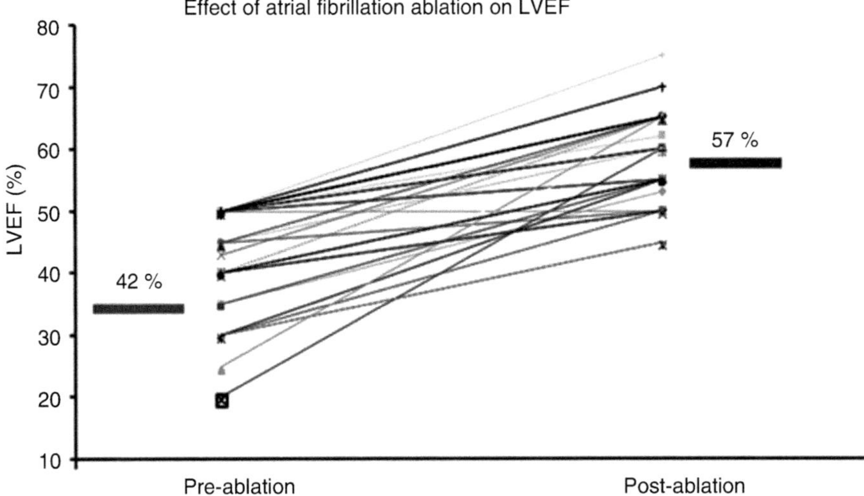

Fig. 3.4 Graph demonstrating effects of AF ablation on left ventricular ejection fraction in patients undergoing atrial fibrillation who have preexisting systolic heart failure. In this population, ablation increased the mean LVEF from 42 % ± 9 % to 56 ± 8 %, P <0.001 (Reproduced with permission from [20])

(13 %). Overall, there was no significant increase in EF in patients with systolic heart failure after successful catheter ablation (36 % before ablation to 41 % after ablation, $P=0.1$) [22]. One possible reason for the lack of EF improvement in this study despite similar AF ablation success rates as in prior studies is that the patients in this study had better rate control pre-ablation than in prior studies; however, the main difference with the previous study consists in the technique of performing the ablation: Natale's group focused only on pulmonary vein isolation without additional lines. Among the patients who did show improvements in EF, the average increase in EF was 7 %.

The need for a randomized clinical study was answered by the CAMTAF trial [23] which enrolled 52 patients with persistent AF predominantly and EF below 35 %.

The hypothesis of this trial was that restoration of sinus rhythm with ablation improves LV function and HF symptoms compared to a rate control strategy in patients with AF and heart failure.

The primary endpoint was EF at 6 months follow-up. Of these 50 patients, 26 patients underwent catheter ablation and 24 patients underwent rate control. In the patients undergoing AF ablation, the freedom from AF was 81 % off of antiarrhythmic drugs. The LVEF at baseline was 32+/−8 % in the ablation arm and 34+/−12 % in the rate control arm [23].

The LVEF at 6 months was 39.9 % (CI 35.2 %–44.7 %) in the catheter ablation group compared with 31.0 % (CI, 25.5–36.6 %) in the medical group ($P=0.015$). Therefore, the mean increase in EF was 8.1 % in the ablation arm compared with a decrease in 3.6 % in the rate control arm. This improvement remained significant at 12 months. In addition, peak VO_2 max and Minnesota living with heart failure score were significantly improved in the catheter ablation as compared with the rate control group [23]. This is the first randomized clinical trial to demonstrate that catheter ablation for AF in patients with heart failure may be a better strategy than rhythm control. However, larger studies should be performed to evaluate important clinical endpoints such as heart failure hospitalization, mortality, and cost-effectiveness.

Finally, a study entitled the Ablation vs. Amiodarone for Treatment of Atrial Fibrillation in Patients with Congestive Heart Failure and Implanted ICD/CRT-D, AATAC-AF in Heart Failure Trial, tested the hypothesis that catheter ablation for persistent AF in patients with HF is superior to amiodarone [24]. This trial enrolled patients with persistent AF, EF <=40 %, and who had either an ICD or CRT-D implant. The presence of the implantable defibrillators allowed for very accurate detection of atrial arrhythmia postablation. Two hundred and three patients were randomized to either catheter ablation or amiodarone. Patients in the catheter ablation group had a 70 % recurrence-free rate, while the amiodarone group had a 34 % recurrence-free rate. Of the 102 patients randomized to AF ablation, the majority (80 patients) underwent combination PVI ablation, posterior wall ablation, and non-pulmonary vein trigger ablation, while 22 patients underwent PVI alone [24]. Of note, the more extensive ablation had a freedom from AF rate of 78.8 %, while patients who had straightforward PVI had a freedom from AF rate of 36.4 % (P <0.001), demonstrating that more extensive ablation beyond PVI had a higher success rate. At 2-year follow-up, the patients who maintained sinus rhythm ($N=105$) compared to the patients who had AF recurrence ($N=98$) had a significantly lower hospitalization rate, higher ejection fraction improvement, longer 6-min walk distance, and lower Minnesota Living with Heart Failure scores. Finally, all-cause mortality was statistically lower in the AF ablation group as compared to the amiodarone group (8 % vs. 18 %), respectively, ($P=0.032$).

While data is accumulating to support that an extensive ablation of AF in CHF patients is better for symptom control and rehospitalizations compared to medication rhythm control or "ablate-and-pace" approach, there is, as of now, no survival benefit. The understanding of the best ablation technique is advancing and the mapping systems able to detect microreentrant and macroreentrant circuits in the left atrium become more accurate and easy to use. As such, there is hope that this complex procedure will become a standard approach for the ever-increasing number of patients with CHF and AF.

3.2　Autonomic Nervous System and AF

Upregulation of the autonomic nervous system is another common theme between heart failure and atrial fibrillation. Heart failure is characterized by countermeasures to support cardiac output, one of which is activation of the sympathetic nervous system [25]. The important role of the autonomic nervous system in the genesis and modulation of atrial fibrillation has been recognized for some time.

Epidemiological data supports the role of the autonomic nervous system in triggering AF. In a study of 1517 patients in the Euro Heart Survey on AF, adrenergic triggers were identified in 15 % of patients, vagal triggers in 6 % of patients, and mixed (adrenergic and vagal) in 12 % of patients [26].

Early experiments in animal models showed that spontaneous atrial fibrillation was preceded by a significant increase in plasma norepinephrine concentration [27].

In addition, studies have suggested that exercise-induced AF may be sympathetically driven [28]. Isoproterenol infusion has been shown to cause triggered activity in the vein of Marshall leading to induction of atrial fibrillation in a canine model [29].

The parasympathetic nervous system may also be responsible for AF – this instance is more frequently seen in young, otherwise healthy patients with no structural heart disease (the so called "vagal" atrial fibrillation) [30].

While the anatomy of the cardiac nervous system was really well known before, the relationship between ANS and arrhythmias has just recently become obvious. The autonomic nervous consists of the duality of the extrinsic and the intrinsic components. The extrinsic refers to the neural fibers that bridge the nervous system and the heart, and the intrinsic refers to the fibers within the heart itself [31]. The two arms of the extrinsic cardiac ANS are the sympathetic and parasympathetic components. The cardiac sympathetic nervous system consists of the regional ganglia spanning from the cervical spinal cord to the thoracic spinal cord. These include the superior cervical ganglia (C1–3), the cervicothoracic or stellate ganglia (C7–8 to T1–2), and the thoracic ganglia (to T7). The axons emanating from these ganglia comprise the superior, middle, and inferior cardiac nerves that terminate on the cardiac surface. The superior and middle branches innervate the atria [31].

Conversely, the vagal arm of the extrinsic cardiac ANS originates in the brainstem at the level of the medulla oblongata (brainstem) and innervates the heart via the vagus nerve, which is divided also into superior, middle, and inferior branches.

The intrinsic cardiac ANS consists of a complex array of clustered ganglionic plexi (GP), which relay signals from the sympathetic and parasympathetic inputs of the extrinsic ANS. In the atria, GP are clustered in specific anatomic locations. An important anatomic region for atrial fibrillation involves the pulmonary vein-left atrial junction, which is also a region harboring a high density of ganglionic plexi. These ganglionic plexi are named the superior left GP (near the left superior pulmonary vein), the inferior left GP (near the left inferior pulmonary vein), anterior right GP (near the right superior pulmonary vein), and the inferior right GP (near the right inferior pulmonary vein) (Fig. 3.5).

Additional sites of atrial GP include the right atrial GP that innervates the sinus node and the inferior atrial GP at the junction of the left atrium and inferior vena cava that innervates the AV node. The ligament of Marshall is also known to contain ganglionic plexi and may play a role in the initiation of atrial fibrillation [29].

Note that the ganglionic plexi are near the LA-PV junctions and may be affected during routine pulmonary vein antral isolation techniques (SVC: superior vena cava. LSPV: left superior pulmonary vein. RSPV: right superior pulmonary vein. LIPV: left inferior pulmonary vein. RIPV: right inferior pulmonary vein).

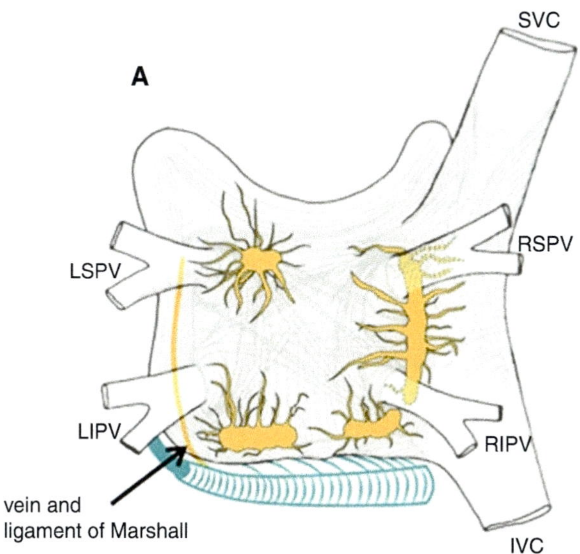

Fig. 3.5 Posterior view of the left atrium shows the major left atrial ganglionic plexi and as well as the nerve bundle of the ligament of Marshall. These ganglionic plexi are named the superior left GP (near the left superior pulmonary vein), the inferior left GP (near the left inferior pulmonary vein), anterior right GP (near the right superior pulmonary vein), and the inferior right GP (near the right inferior pulmonary vein). Note that the ganglionic plexi are near the LA-PV junctions and may be affected during routine pulmonary vein antral isolation techniques. *SVC* superior vena cava, *LSPV* left superior pulmonary vein, *RSPV* right superior pulmonary vein, *LIPV* left inferior pulmonary vein, *RIPV* right inferior pulmonary vein (Reproduced with permission from [19])

However, rather than a single arm of the ANS contributing to AF, it is likely that the duality of the ANS and the parasympathetic and the sympathetic nervous systems have complementary roles in the promotion of atrial fibrillation. For example, cardiac sympathetic stimulation increases the calcium current in the pulmonary sleeves, while vagal simulation shortens the atrial effective refractory period [31]. The confluence of these two electrophysiological effects leads to an ultimate increase in the forward Na/Ca exchanger current, which promotes early afterdepolarizations in the pulmonary veins, important drivers of AF.

A further mechanistic understanding of the role of the ANS in the initiation and maintenance of AF has relied in part on elegant animal studies, which have demonstrated that stimulation of the ganglionic plexi results in rapid firing from the pulmonary veins which can trigger atrial fibrillation. In addition, inhibition of the GP by lidocaine injection can blunt this response [32, 33].

3.3 Ganglionic Plexi: Autonomic Modulation in the Treatment of Atrial Fibrillation

Because of importance of the autonomic nervous system triggering AF, and the predictable anatomic location of the GP, ablation of GP has been proposed as an attractive adjunct to standard ablation for atrial fibrillation.

The method for identification of the particular anatomic target for GP ablation varies from a purely empirical anatomic approach (ablation at sites known to house the GPs), to a more deliberate physiological approach for GP identification by inducing a vagal response during high-frequency stimulation [34].

However, studies incorporating GP ablation for the treatment of AF have demonstrated mixed results. Initial studies were promising, demonstrating high freedom from AF in patients with PVI and GP ablation [35].

However, subsequent studies showed a very low success rate for anatomic ganglionic plexi ablation to treat PAF (34.3 %) as compared to PVI (65.7 %), $P=0.008$ [36].

Additional information about the ANS modulation on AF came from a more recent study where it was shown that autonomic denervation added to PVI increased the success rate of PVI in the paroxysmal AF population [37]. In this particular group of patients, a total of 242 subjects with symptomatic PAF were randomized to PVI alone, anatomic ablation of the left atrial GPs, or PVI followed by anatomic ablation of the left atrial GPs. Freedom from atrial fibrillation or atrial tachycardia was achieved in 56 %, 48 %, and 74 % in the patients with PVI alone, GP alone, and PVI+GP groups, respectively, with no difference in the occurrence of left atrial flutter in follow-up among the groups [37]. The important findings from this study include the fact that GP ablation alone does not appear to be adequate, and GP in addition to PVI appears to be superior to PVI alone. However, there are many questions that remain unanswered. Because catheter-based AF ablation is endocardially performed and the GP is housed epicardially, it is unclear if endocardial ablation is adequate to eliminate GP activity. Furthermore, GP could simply be an innocent bystander clustered near sites of complex fractionations or rotors in the endocardium of the left atrium, whose ablation would increase the success of the procedure without affecting the epicardial GP. The GP remains an active area of research to ultimately establish its future role in the armamentarium for the treatment of AF.

3.4   Renal Denervation

The electrophysiology community has recently become interested in renal denervation as the next frontier in neuromodulation in the treatment of AF along with CHF and ventricular arrhythmias. The renal afferent and efferent nerves play an important role in the sympathetic nervous system (SNS) response. Efferent nerves from the second sympathetic ganglion innervate the adventitia of the renal arteries. Afferents from the kidney feed back to the hypothalamus and regulate central sympathetic activity [38]. Initial enthusiasm of this modality in the treatment of hypertension was deflated after the results of the SIMPLICITY-HTN 3 trial showed no benefit of renal denervation compared to sham procedure in the treatment of patients with resistant hypertension [38]. However, given the renal sympathetic nervous systems importance in the overall sympathetic cascade, other applications in which neuromodulation may play a role are actively being investigated, such as atrial fibrillation.

Animal models have demonstrated that renal denervation can reduce sympathetic innervation to the kidney [39]. The current approach for selective renal denervation is a catheter-based treatment aimed at decreasing renal SNS response. A series of radiofrequency ablations are performed bilateraly disrupting the nerve endings surrounding the renal arteries. While renal denervation has been shown to decrease AF inducibility in a porcine model [39], just recently these findings were explored in humans.

In a meta-analysis by Pokushalov of two prospective randomized studies of patients with moderate or severe resistant hypertension and paroxysmal or persistent atrial fibrillation, in which patients either underwent PVI or PVI with renal denervation, at 12 months, patients in the PVI+renal denervation group had 63 % freedom from AF recurrence, while the PVI-only group had only 41 % freedom from AF recurrence, ($P=0.014$) [40]. The differences were more dramatic in patients with severe hypertension: 61 % AF free in the PVI+ renal denervation group vs. 28 % in the PVI-only group ($P=0.03$). Total procedure time was not significantly different between the two groups. Although this combined meta-analysis only included 80 patients, it provides compelling evidence that in hypertensive patients with AF, adjunctive renal denervation may improve success of PVI by neuromodulation.

3.5   Alternative Therapies for Neuromodulation

Lakkireddy et al. incorporated an age-old practice, yoga, which has long-been touted as a form of exercise that can have pleiotropic health benefits, potentially by way of salutatory effects on autonomic function, to study the effects on atrial fibrillation, mental health, and quality of life [41].

In this study, 52 patients with symptomatic PAF received twice weekly 1 hour structured yoga training over 3 months after an initial 3-month control phase (patients acted as their own control).

Yoga training reduced symptomatic AF episodes (3.8 ± 3 vs. 2.1 ± 2.6, $p < 0.001$), symptomatic non-AF episodes (2.9 ± 3.4 vs. 1.4 ± 2.0; $p < 0.001$), asymptomatic AF episodes (0.12 ± 0.44 vs. 0.04 ± 0.20; $p < 0.001$), and depression and anxiety ($p < 0.001$) and improved the quality-of-life parameters. There was significant decrease in heart rate and systolic and diastolic blood pressure before and after yoga ($p < 0.001$). Also, 22 % of patients with AF during the control phased did not have any AF episodes during the yoga phase. The conclusion was that the effects may have been related to yoga's increase in parasympathetic tone and overall autonomic tone stabilization. However, this study did not specifically study variations in autonomic tone as this would have been relatively difficult to measure.

Further support of the autonomic modulation hypothesis reducing AF burden comes from a study in which patients received acupuncture after cardioversion [42].

In traditional Chinese medicine, stimulation of the Neiguan spot has been thought to reduce palpitations. Patients were divided into four groups after cardioversion: a group who was already taking amiodarone and continued it, an acupuncture group, a sham acupuncture group, and the no-acupuncture and no-antiarrhythmic drug group.

Recurrence rates after cardioversion were 27 % (amiodarone), 35 % (acupuncture), 69 % (sham acupuncture), and 54 % (no treatment), respectively ($P = 0.0075$) [42]. Compared with the amiodarone group, the acupuncture group had similar recurrence rate (HR 1.15, 95 % CI: 0.38–3.49; $P = 0.81$). This is of particular interest as acupuncture is generally well tolerated and not associated with side effects of amiodarone. Although this was a small study, it provide further intriguing insight into the possibility that autonomic stabilization by treatments outside of the heart can actually affect arrhythmogenesis within the heart.

Conclusions

Atrial fibrillation and heart failure have become a "dual epidemic." The treatment of atrial fibrillation in the heart failure population is particularly important and challenging. Clinical trials addressing the optimal treatment for patients with AF and heart failure remains ongoing, but historically, the majority of studies show no significant difference between rhythm control with the use of antiarrhythmic drugs and rate control. However, subgroup analyses have suggested that the presence of sinus rhythm not only provides hemodynamic benefit but may in fact decrease heart failure hospitalizations and mortality. Because many of the benefits of sinus rhythm may be offset by the negative side effects of antiarrhythmic drugs, efforts at rhythm control without the use of or minimizing the use of antiarrhythmic drugs continues to improve. Through this perspective, AF ablation represents a promising modality to achieve that goal. With the recently published data on AF ablation in the setting of CHF, it is likely that as the procedure continues to improve in efficacy and safety, it will emerge as the superior treatment option. Cost-effective analysis should also be considered given the healthcare costs burden of AF, heart failure, and AF ablation procedures as there is already evidence that frequent readmissions and cost of monitoring antiarrhythmic medication might be a more expensive route compared to a successful AF ablation.

More recently, the importance of autonomic nervous system in the pathogenesis and maintenance of AF has gained rekindled interest, and adjunctive treatments to modulate the ANS such as renal denervation, GP ablation, or even yoga and acupuncture are being explored. As our understanding of the pathogenesis of AF improves, the future may provide a more customized approach to the treatment of patients with an array of these various modalities.

References

1. Gesell RA. Auricular systole and its relation to ventricular output. Am J Physiol. 1911;29:32–63.
2. Maisel WH, Stevenson LW. Atrial fibrillation in heart failure: epidemiology, pathophysiology, and rationale for therapy. Am J Cardiol. 2003;91(6A):2D–8.
3. Wang TJ, Larson MG, Levy D, Vasan RS, Leip EP, Wolf PA, D'Agostino RB, Murabito JM, Kannel WB, Benjamin EJ. Temporal relations of atrial fibrillation and congestive heart failure and their joint influence on mortality: the Framingham Heart Study. Circulation. 2003;107(23):2920–5.
4. Ehrlich JR, Nattel S, Hohnloser SH. Atrial fibrillation and congestive heart failure: specific considerations at the intersection of two common and important cardiac disease sets. J Cardiovasc Electrophysiol. 2002;13(4):399–405.
5. Dries DL, Exner DV, Gersh BJ, Domanski MJ, Waclawiw MA, Stevenson LW. Atrial fibrillation is associated with an increased risk for mortality and heart failure progression in patients with asymptomatic and symptomatic left ventricular systolic dysfunction: retrospective analysis of the SOVLD trials. J Am Coll Cardiol. 1998;32:695–703.
6. Calkins H, el-Atassi R, Kalbfleisch S, Langberg J, Morady F. Effects of an acute increase in atrial pressure on atrial refractoriness in humans. Pacing Clin Electrophysiol. 1992;15(11 Pt 1):1674–80.
7. Pardaens K, Van Cleemput J, Vanhaecke J, Fagard RH. Atrial fibrillation is associated with a lower exercise capacity in male chronic heart failure patients. Heart. 1997;78(6):564–8.
8. Anter E, Jessup M, Callans DJ. Atrial fibrillation and heart failure. Treatment considerations for a dual epidemic. Circulation. 2009;119:2516–25.
9. Li D, Shingawa K, Pang L, Leung TK, Cardin S, Wang Z, Nattel S. Effects of angiotensive-converting enzyme inhibition on the development of the atrial substrate in dogs with ventricular tachy-pacing induced heart failure. Circulation. 2001;104:2608–14.
10. Ueng KC, Tsai TP, Yu WC, Tsai CF, Lin MC, Chan KC, Chen CY, Wu DJ, Lin CS, Chen SA. Use of enalapril to facilitate sinus rhythm maintenance after external cardioversion of long-standing persistent atrial fibrillation. Results of a prospective and controlled study. Eur Heart J. 2003;24(23):2090.
11. Maggioni AP, Latini R, Carson PE, Singh SN, Barlera S, Glazer R, Masson S, Cerè E, Tognoni G, Cohn JN, Val-HeFT Investigators. Valsartan reduces the incidence of atrial fibrillation in patients with heart failure: results from the Valsartan Heart Failure Trial (Val-HeFT). Am Heart J. 2005;149:548–57.
12. Nasr IA, Bouzamondo A, Hulot JS, Dubourg O, Le Huezey HY, Lechat P. Prevention of atrial fibrillation onset by beta-blocker treatment in heart failure: a meta-analysis. Eur Heart J. 2007;28(4):457–62.
13. Wyse DG, Waldo AL, DiMarco JP, Domanski MJ, Rosenberg Y, Schron EB, Kellen JC, Greene HL, Mickel MC, Dalquist JE, Corley SD. A comparison of rate control and rhythm control in patients with atrial fibrillation. N Engl J Med. 2002;347(23):1825–33.
14. Corley SD, Epstein AE, DiMarco JP, Domanski MJ, Geller N, Greene HL, Josephson RA, Kellen JC, Klein RC, Krahn AD, Mickel M, Mitchell LB, Nelson JD, Rosenberg Y, Schron E,

Shemanski L, Waldo AL, Wyse DG, AFFIRM Investigators. Relationships between sinus rhythm, treatment, and survival in the Atrial Fibrillation Follow-Up Investigation of Rhythm Management (AFFIRM) Study. Circulation. 2004;109:1509–13.

15. Roy D, Talajic M, Nattel S, Wyse DG, Dorian P, Lee KL, Bourassa MG, Arnold JM, Buxton AE, Camm AJ, Connolly SJ, Dubuc M, Ducharme A, Guerra PG, Hohnloser SH, Lambert J, Le Heuzey JY, O'Hara G, Pedersen OD, Rouleau JL, Singh BN, Stevenson LW, Stevenson WG, Thibault B, Waldo AL, Atrial Fibrillation and Congestive Heart Failure Investigators. Rhythm control versus rate control for atrial fibrillation and heart failure. N Engl J Med. 2008;358:2667–77.

16. Pedersen OD, Bagger H, Keller N, Marchant B, Køber L, Torp-Pedersen C. Efficacy of dofetilide in the treatment of atrial fibrillation-flutter in patients with reduced left ventricular function: a Danish Investigations of Arrhythmia and Mortality on Dofetilide(DIAMOND substudy). Circulation. 2001;104:292–6.

17. Pedersen HS, Elming H, Seibaek M, Burchardt H, Brendorp B, Torp-Pedersen C, Køber L, DIAMOND Study Group. Risk factors and predictors of Torsade de pointes ventricular tachycardia in patients with left ventricular systolic dysfunction receiving Dofetilide. Am J Cardiol. 2007;100(5):876–80.

18. Gasparini M, Auricchio A, Metra M, Regoli F, Fantoni C, Lamp B, Curnis A, Vogt J, Klersy C, Multicentre Longitudinal Observational Study (MILOS) Group. Long-term survival in patients undergoing cardiac resynchronization therapy: the importance of performing atrio-ventricular junction ablation in patients with permanent atrial fibrillation. Eur Heart J. 2008;29(13):1644–52.

19. Calkins H, Kuck KH, Cappato R, Brugada J, Camm AJ, Chen SA, Crijns HJ, Damiano Jr RJ, Davies DW, DiMarco J, Edgerton J, Ellenbogen K, Ezekowitz MD, Haines DE, Haissaguerre M, Hindricks G, Iesaka Y, Jackman W, Jalife J, Jais P, Kalman J, Keane D, Kim YH, Kirchhof P, Klein G, Kottkamp H, Kumagai K, Lindsay BD, Mansour M, Marchlinski FE, McCarthy PM, Mont JL, Morady F, Nademanee K, Nakagawa H, Natale A, Nattel S, Packer DL, Pappone C, Prystowsky E, Raviele A, Reddy V, Ruskin JN, Shemin RJ, Tsao HM, Wilber D. 2012 HRS/EHRA/ECAS Expert Consensus Statement on Catheter and Surgical Ablation of Atrial Fibrillation: recommendations for patient selection, procedural techniques, patient management and follow-up, definitions, endpoints, and research trial design. Europace. 2012;14(4):528–606.

20. Gentlesk PJ, Sauer WH, Gerstenfeld EP, Lin D, Dixit S, Zado E, Callans D, Marchlinski FE. Reversal of left ventricular dysfunction following ablation of atrial fibrillation. J Cardiovasc Electrophysiol. 2007;18(1):9–14.

21. Hsu LF, Jaïs P, Sanders P, Garrigue S, Hocini M, Sacher F, Takahashi Y, Rotter M, Pasquié JL, Scavée C, Bordachar P, Clémenty J, Haïssaguerre M. Catheter ablation for atrial fibrillation in congestive heart failure. N Engl J Med. 2004;351(23):2373–83.

22. Chen MS, Marrouche NF, Khaykin Y, Gillinov AM, Wazni O, Martin DO, Rossillo A, Verma A, Cummings J, Erciyes D, Saad E, Bhargava M, Bash D, Schweikert R, Burkhardt D, Williams-Andrews M, Perez-Lugones A, Abdul-Karim A, Saliba W, Natale A. Pulmonary vein isolation for the treatment of atrial fibrillation in patients with impaired systolic function. J Am Coll Cardiol. 2004;43(6):1004–9.

23. Hunter RJ, Berriman TJ, Diab I, Kamdar R, Richmond L, Baker V, Goromonzi F, Sawhney V, Duncan E, Page SP, Ullah W, Unsworth B, Mayet J, Dhinoja M, Earley MJ, Sporton S, Schilling RJ. A randomized controlled trial of catheter ablation versus medical treatment of atrial fibrillation in heart failure (the CAMTAF trial). Circ Arrhythm Electrophysiol. 2014;7(1):31–8.

24. http://www.clinicaltrialresults.org/Slides/ACC2015/DiBiase_AATAC.pdf

25. Triposkiadis F, Karayannis G, Giamouzis G, Skoulargis J, Lourida G, Butler J. The sympathetic nervous system in heart failure physiology, pathophysiology, and clinical implications. J Am Coll Cardiol. 2009;54(19):1747–62.

26. de Vos CB, Nieuwlaat R, Crijns HJ, Camm AJ, LeHeuzey JY, Kirchhof CJ, Capucci A, Breithardt G, Vardas PE, Pisters R, Tieleman RG. Autonomic trigger patterns and antiarrhythmic treatment of paroxysmal atrial fibrillation: data from the Euro Heart Survey. Eur Heart J. 2008;29(5):632–9.

27. Tisdale JE, Borzak S, Sabbah HN, Shimoyama H, Goldstein S. Hemodynamic and neurohormonal predictors and consequences of the development of atrial fibrillation in dogs with chronic heart failure. J Card Fail. 2006;12(9):747–51.
28. Shen MJ, Choi EK, Tan AY, Lin SK, Fishbein MC, Chen LS, Chen PS. Neural mechanisms of atrial arrhythmias. Nat Rev Cardiol. 2012;9(1):30.
29. Doshi RN, Wu TJ, Yashima M, Kim YH, Ong JJ, Cao JM, Hwang C, Yashar P, Fishbein MC, Karagueuzian HS, Chen PS. Relation between ligament of Marshall and adrenergic atrial tachyarrhythmia. Circulation. 1999;100(8):876–83.
30. Chen PS, Tan AY. Autonomic nerve activity and atrial fibrillation. Heart Rhythm. 2007;4(3 Suppl):S61–4.
31. Shen MJ, Zipes DP. Role of the autonomic nervous system in modulating cardiac arrhythmias. Circ Res. 2014;114:1004–21.
32. Lu Z, Scherlag BJ, Lin J, et al. Autonomic mechanism for initiation of rapid firing from atria and pulmonary veins: evidence by ablation of ganglionated plexi. Cardiovasc Res. 2009;84:245–52.
33. Scherlag BJ, Yamanashi W, Patel U, Lazzara R, Jackman WM. Autonomically induced conversion of pulmonary vein focal firing into atrial fibrillation. J Am Coll Cardiol. 2005;45:1878–86.
34. Chugh A. Ganglionated plexus ablation in patients undergoing pulmonary vein isolation for paroxysmal atrial fibrillation: here we go again. J Am Coll Cardiol. 2013;62(24):2326–8.
35. Pappone C, Santinelli V, Manguso F, Vicedomini G, Gugliotta F, Augello G, Mazzone P, Tortoriello V, Landoni G, Zangrillo A, Lang C, Tomita T, Mesas C, Mastella E, Alfieri O. Pulmonary vein denervation enhances long-term benefit after circumferential ablation for paroxysmal atrial fibrillation. Circulation. 2004;109(3):327–34.
36. Mikhaylov E, Kanidieva A, Sviridova N, Abramov M, Gureev S, Szili-Torok T, Lebedev D. Outcome of anatomic ganglionated plexi ablation to treat paroxysmal atrial fibrillation: a 3-year follow-up study. Europace. 2011;13(3):362–70.
37. Katritsis D, Pokushalov E, Romanov A, et al. Autonomic denervation added to pulmonary vein isolation for paroxysmal atrial fibrillation: a randomized clinical trial. J Am Coll Cardiol. 2013;62:2318–25.
38. McArdle MJ, deGoma EM, Cohen DL, Townsend RR, Wilensky RL, Giri J. Beyond blood pressure: percutaneous renal denervation for the management of sympathetic hyperactivity and associated disease states. J Am Heart Assoc. 2015;4(3):e001415.
39. Linz D, Mahfoud F, Schotten U, Ukena C, Neuberger HR, Wirth K, Böhm M. Effects of electrical stimulation of carotid baroreflex and renal denervation on atrial electrophysiology. J Cardiovasc Electrophysiol. 2013;24(9):1028–33.
40. Pokushalov E, Romanov A, Katritsis DG, Artyomenko S, Bayramova S, Losik D, Baranova V, Karaskov A, Steinberg JS. Renal denervation for improving outcomes of catheter ablation in patients with atrial fibrillation and hypertension: early experience. Heart Rhythm. 2014;11(7):1131–8.
41. Lakkireddy D, Atkins D, Pillarisetti J, Ryschon K, Bommana S, Drisko J, Vanga S, Dawn B. Effect of yoga on arrhythmia burden, anxiety, depression, and quality of life in paroxysmal atrial fibrillation the YOGA My Heart Study. J Am Coll Cardiol. 2013;61(11):1177–82.
42. Lomuscio A, Belletti S, Battezzati PM, Lombardi F. Efficacy of acupuncture in preventing atrial fibrillation recurrences after electrical cardioversion. J Cardiovasc Electrophysiol. 2011;22:241–7.

Current Therapies for Ventricular Tachycardia: Are there Autonomic Implications of the Arrhythmogenic Substrate?

4

Alexandru Costea and Omeed Zardkoohi

In the last two decades, significant advances have been made in diagnosis, understanding, and treatment of various ventricular arrhythmias (VA). Years ago, in its infancy, the field of cardiac electrophysiology was limited to the study of the effects of antiarrhythmic drugs on ventricular programmed stimulation in the setting of various disease states. However, modern scientific and technological advances not only have improved the characterization of the arrhythmia substrate but also have provided an opportunity to potentially cure many ventricular arrhythmias. Contemporary mapping systems, ablation catheters, and advanced intracardiac ultrasound technology have also significantly improved the efficacy and safety of ablation procedures. An increasing number of centers are embarking on a very exciting journey of ventricular tachycardia ablation programs, focusing on high-risk patients with low ejection fractions, as well as complex ablations involving epicardium, aortic cusps, and epicardial vessels. Patients who in the past would have otherwise had little chance of survival, now, with improvements in complex ablations, procedures can benefit from improved longevity and quality of life. Another recent significant advance has been the use of ventricular assist devices during the ablation of ventricular arrhythmias for high-risk patients with cardiogenic shock.

In such exciting times, have we reached the pinnacle of ventricular arrhythmia management? Do we completely understand all the mechanisms of VA, their substrates, and their most effective and safest treatment? Are all the VA the same? Although the answer to these questions may not be a resounding yes, the

A. Costea, MD (✉)
Division of Cardiology, Department of Medicine, University of Cincinnati Medical Center, 231 Albert Sabin Way, Cincinnati, OH 45219, USA
e-mail: ionutcostea1972@gmail.com

O. Zardkoohi, MD
Northwestern Medicine West Region, Faculty, Northwestern Feinberg School of Medicine, 25 North Winfield Road, Winfield, IL 60190, USA
e-mail: Omeed.Zardkoohi@cadencehealth.org

© Springer International Publishing Switzerland 2016
E. Gronda et al. (eds.), *Heart Failure Management: The Neural Pathways*,
DOI 10.1007/978-3-319-24993-3_4

momentum of the field's prior discoveries will continue to drive further pathophysiological understanding and improved procedural success.

While VAs share certain common features, there are many differentiating factors that play a crucial role in their management.

When one evaluates a patient with ventricular arrhythmia, the most important predictor of outcomes is the associated cardiac comorbidities. The absence of organic heart disease (i.e., coronary artery disease, congestive heart failure, or congenital abnormalities) portends a more positive prognosis. The well-known entities of outflow tract VA (right and left ventricular outflow tract) as well as the fascicular or papillary muscle VA are benign arrhythmias that rarely pose a life-threatening risk and can be easily corrected with either beta-blockers, calcium channel blockers, or ablation.

Conversely, VAs in the settings of ischemic heart disease, congestive heart failure, and low ejection fraction are potentially life-threatening conditions. Such patients may be candidates for implantable cardioverter–defibrillators (ICDs). Occasionally, these patients may present with ventricular tachycardia storm (multiple shocks delivered by the ICD for incessant, repetitive ventricular tachycardia of ventricular fibrillation). In these cases, additional antiarrhythmic agents and even ventricular tachycardia ablation may be necessary in order to stabilize the patient.

Congenital abnormalities are also responsible for VA, and although many of them have been described more than 20 years ago, standard risk stratification methodology and treatment approach are still under debate. Management of patients with hypertrophic cardiomyopathy, long QT syndrome, short QT syndrome, Brugada syndrome, and arrhythmogenic right ventricular dysplasia continues to evolve and usually involves highly specialized management and follow-up.

When VAs are limited to premature ventricular contractions (PVCs), the management may range from no treatment and observation to catheter-based ablation. The first step in the management of PVCs is to evaluate for structural heart disease. The next step would be to determine the patient's symptoms and the overall burden of PVCs. While symptom management with either medication or ablation is recommended, it is now well established that a high premature ventricular contraction burden (10–20 % of total beats) can lead to a form of "tachycardia-induced cardiomyopathy." In this category of patients in which PVCs are thought to be responsible for the systolic heart failure, aggressive treatment with medication or ablation should be strongly considered to potentially reverse this condition.

Is it possible that all these conditions listed above are solely due to abnormalities intrinsic to the heart, or is it possible that external forces, such as the nervous system, could be playing an important role?

As early as seventeenth century, William Harvey suspected a link between the brain and the heart when he wrote, "For every affection of the mind that is attended with either pain or pleasure, hope or fear, is the cause of an agitation whose influence extends to the heart." [1] After more than five decades of research, it is now known that the brain, through autonomic activation, alters heart rate, conduction, contractility, and interestingly also electrical and mechanical properties of individual myocytes [2–6]. Moreover, studies more than a century ago [7–9] have demonstrated the critical role of the autonomic nervous system in cardiac arrhythmogenesis.

This topic has gained much recent interest because of mounting evidence showing that neural modulation, either by ablation or stimulation, can effectively control a wide spectrum of cardiac arrhythmias [10–13].

While extensive anatomical studies of the autonomic system of the heart have been performed, the knowledge pertinent to arrhythmias has been summarized by Shen et al. [14]. According to this review article, the cardiac autonomic nervous system (ANS) can be divided into extrinsic and intrinsic components. The extrinsic cardiac ANS comprises fibers that mediate connections between the heart and the nervous system, whereas the intrinsic cardiac system consists of primarily autonomic nerve fibers once they enter the pericardial sac.

The extrinsic cardiac autonomic nervous system may be subdivided into sympathetic and parasympathetic components. The sympathetic fibers are largely derived from major autonomic ganglia along the cervical and thoracic spinal cord. The parasympathetic preganglionic fibers are carried almost entirely within the vagal nerve and are divided into superior, middle, and inferior branches. Most of the vagal nerve fibers converge at a distinct fat pad between the superior vena cava and the aorta (known as the third fat pad) en route to the sinus and atrioventricular nodes.

In addition to the extrinsic cardiac autonomic nervous system, the heart is also innervated by a complex intrinsic system. Armour et al. [6] provided a detailed map of the distribution of autonomic nerves in human hearts. Throughout the heart, numerous cardiac ganglia, each of which contains 200–1000 neurons, form synapses with the sympathetic and parasympathetic fibers that enter the pericardial space. The vast majority of these ganglia are organized into ganglionated plexi (GP) on the surface of the atria and ventricles (Fig. 4.1).

Atrial ganglionated plexuses were identified on (1) the superior surface of the right atrium, (2) the superior surface of the left atrium, (3) the posterior surface of the right atrium, (4) the posterior medial surface of the left atrium (the latter two fuse medially where they extend anteriorly into the interatrial septum), and (5) the inferior and lateral aspect of the posterior left atrium. Ventricular ganglionated plexuses were located in fat (1) surrounding the aortic root, (2) at the origins of the right and left coronary arteries (the latter extending to the origins of the left anterior descending and circumflex coronary arteries), (3) at the origin of the posterior descending coronary artery, (4) adjacent to the origin of the right acute marginal coronary artery, and (5) at the origin of the left obtuse marginal coronary artery [6].

Sympathetic influences on cardiac electrophysiology are complex and can be modulated by myocardial function. In the normal heart, sympathetic stimulation shortens action potential duration [4] and reduces transmural dispersion of repolarization [15]. In contrast, in pathological states such as heart failure (HF) [16] and long QT syndrome (LQTS) [17], sympathetic stimulation is a potent stimulus for the generation of arrhythmias, perhaps by enhancing the dispersion of repolarization or by generation of afterdepolarizations. In the ventricles, vagal stimulation prolongs action potential duration and effective refractory period [4, 18], whereas in the atria, vagal activation reduces the atrial effective refractory period [19, 20], augments spatial electrophysiological heterogeneity [21], and promotes early

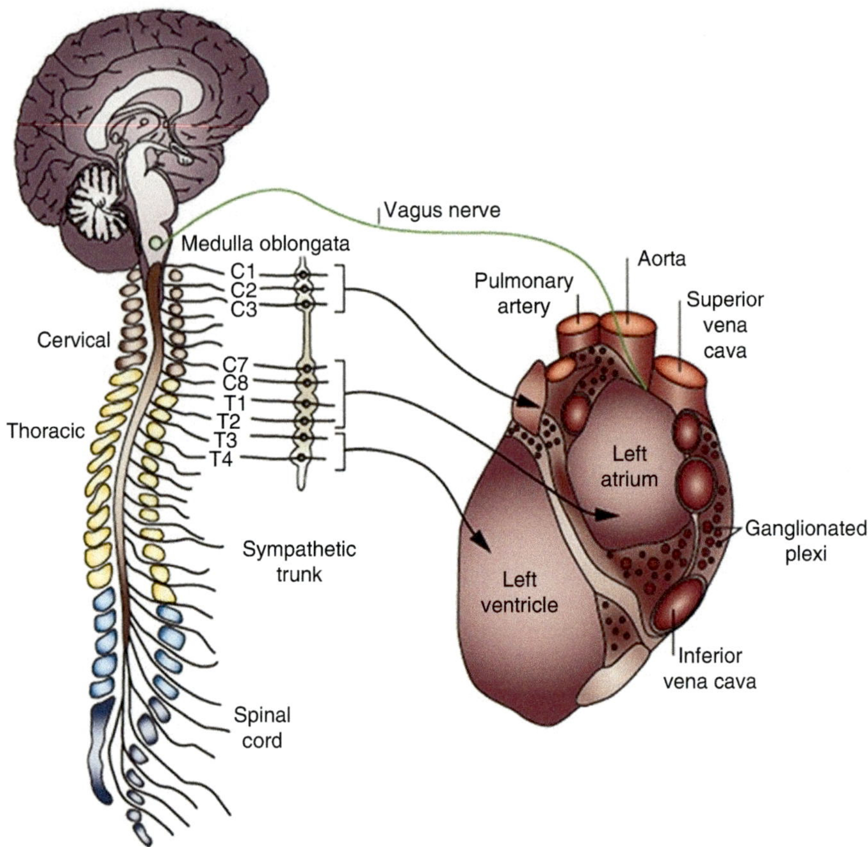

Fig. 4.1 Scheme of autonomic innervation of the heart. The cardiac sympathetic ganglia consist of cervical ganglia, stellate ganglia, and thoracic ganglia. Parasympathetic innervation comes from the vagal nerve (Reproduced with permission from Shen et al. [12])

afterdepolarization (EAD) toward the end of phase 3 in the action potential [22]. This differential effect may explain why parasympathetic stimulation is proarrhythmic in the atria but antiarrhythmic in the ventricles, whereas sympathetic stimulation seems to be proarrhythmic for both chambers [23].

What happens when we apply the knowledge about the autonomic nervous system to ventricular arrhythmias?

Ischemic Cardiomyopathy Experimentally, sympathetic stimulation induces changes in ECG repolarization and reduction of fibrillation threshold, facilitating the initiation of VF [24]. These effects are magnified in the presence of cardiac ischemia [25]. The ischemic and infarcted myocardium becomes a substrate exquisitely sensitive to arrhythmia triggers because of not only regional cellular and tissue remodeling [26] but also heterogeneity of sympathetic nervous system innervation [27].

Contributing to the heterogeneity is the phenomenon of nerve sprouting [28, 29]. By examining explanted hearts, Cao et al. [30] found that patients who had a history of ventricular arrhythmias had augmented sympathetic nerve sprouting as compared with patients with similar structural heart disease but no arrhythmias.

They also showed that there is inhomogeneous distribution of sympathetic nerve fibers in the ventricles with myocardial injury, which is characterized by regional hyperinnervation in the perivascular regions or in the periphery of injured myocardium and regional denervation in the regions with necrosis or dense fibrosis. These results suggest that there are increased sympathetic nerves after MI and that the density of these sympathetic nerves directly correlates with the occurrence of life-threatening ventricular arrhythmia.

Both infusion of nerve growth factor into the left stellate ganglia (LSG) [28] and subthreshold electric stimulation of the LSG [31] in dogs with myocardial infarction resulted in sympathetic nerve sprouting with increased ventricular fibrillation (VF) and sudden cardiac death (SCD), suggesting a causal relationship. Follow-up studies demonstrated that myocardial infarction causes the upregulation of proteins that contributed to nerve growth (nerve growth factor, growth-associated protein 43, and synaptophysin) in both the infarcted site [32] and the more upstream bilateral stellate ganglia [33]. Interestingly, sympathetic nerve sprouting itself can lead to an increased incidence of VF without concomitant cardiac ischemia.

A very original study by Liu et al. [34] found that the nerve sprouting encountered in ischemia could be induced by other stimuli, for example, a high cholesterol diet. Density of growth-associated protein 43 and tyrosine hydroxylase–positive nerves in the heart was significantly higher in high cholesterol than in control rabbits. Compared with controls, the high cholesterol rabbits had longer QTc intervals, more QTc dispersion, a longer action potential duration, and increased heterogeneity of repolarization. It was also found that rabbits given a high-cholesterol diet developed myocardial hypertrophy and cardiac sympathetic hyperinnervation without coronary artery disease along with an increased vulnerability to VF [34].

The possible explanation for this finding is based on the fact that in both human and animal studies, a high cholesterol level was associated with increased oxidative stress. Oxidative stress can cause neurodegeneration, neurite retraction, and mitochondrial dysfunction of the neurons in the central nervous system. It is therefore possible that oxidative stress causes cardiac nerve injury, which triggers the re-expression of nerve growth factor or other neurotrophic factor genes in the nonneural cells around the site of injury, leading to nerve regeneration through nerve sprouting [34].

While data from anesthetized animals suggests that sympathetic nerve activity is responsible for the development of ventricular arrhythmias, a direct temporal relationship in patients has not been established. Clinically, increased sympathetic activity, as suggested by heart rate variability analysis, was found to be in the 30 min before the onset of ventricular tachyarrhythmias [35]. With direct nerve activity recordings in a canine model of SCD, Zhou et al. [36] observed that VF and SCD were immediately preceded by spontaneous sympathetic nerve discharge from the LSG. Moreover, as the stellate ganglion nerve activity can directly be recorded with thoracotomy, the same group developed a valid technique to predict susceptibility of VT and VF in the same canine model by recording subcutaneous nerve activity. The latency from the onset of stellate ganglia activity and the subcutaneous recordings of discharges to the development of ventricular tachycardia or fibrillation was about 17 s, slightly longer than the latency of 10 s to the development of atrial arrhythmias [36]. Although increased stellate ganglion nerve activity contributes to VF and SCD in myocardial infarction, acute myocardial infarction itself can cause an increase in nerve activity and nerve density of the LSG—electroanatomic remodeling [33]. This generates a vicious cycle that can lead to more ischemia, VF, and SCD.

As the vast majority of ventricular arrhythmias in the settings of ischemia are provoked by increased sympathetic activity, early treatment with beta-blockers has been proven to reduce recurrences. Furthermore, various invasive approaches have been taken to decrease the occurrence of VT or VF.

While VT ablation has been long established treatment for organized arrhythmia in chronic ischemic cardiomyopathy, the invasive ablative approach for arrhythmias in acute ischemic events—VF or polymorphic VT—has just been recently entertained. Emerging evidence in patients with ventricular fibrillation (VF) in a variety of clinical scenarios implicates an important role for triggers originating from the distal Purkinje arborization in the initiation of this malignant arrhythmia, triggers not surprisingly sensitive to high sympathetic tone. Haissaguerre's group was able to show on 5 patients with VF post MI that ablation of the local Purkinje network allows suppression of polymorphic VT and VF [37].

Renal denervation (RDN) is a new approach to reduce sympathetic activity. RDN reduces not only renal norepinephrine spillover by 48 % but also muscle sympathetic nerve activity by 37 %. This certainly suggests a reduction in local and central sympathetic activity after RDN by a process of modulation of efferent and afferent renal signaling. On that basis, Linz et al. elegantly showed that RDN reduced the occurrence of ventricular arrhythmias and attenuated the rise in left ventricular diastolic pressure during left ventricular ischemia created by left anterior descending artery ligation in anesthetized pigs. Therefore, RDN may protect from ventricular arrhythmias during ischemic events [38]. The same group reported their results on two cases of advanced nonischemic cardiomyopathy and incessant ventricular arrhythmias resistant to ablation and/or antiarrhythmic medication. While the patients did not have acute ischemic events, the mechanism of arrhythmia shared common features, specifically increased sympathetic tone. Renal denervation was performed successfully in these very unstable patients and led to a significant reduction in their ventricular arrhythmia load [39].

Along the same lines of neuromodulation as an alternative therapy, cardiac sympathetic denervation (CSD) has been shown to be effective in animal models and case series of patients with and without cardiomyopathy. Vaseghi et al. [40] elegantly demonstrate that left and bilateral sympathectomies, involving removal of the lower third to lower half of the stellate ganglion and T2–T4 sympathetic ganglia, have a clear benefit in the setting of VT storm and VT refractory to medical therapy in a small number of patients with cardiomyopathy. In patients with VT storm, bilateral CSD is more beneficial than left CSD. The beneficial effects of bilateral CSD extend beyond the acute postsympathectomy period, with continued freedom from ICD shocks in 48 % of patients, and a significant reduction in ICD shocks in 90 % of patients.

Conversely, studies with anesthetized dogs have shown that vagal nerve stimulation (VNS) reduces the occurrence of ventricular tachyarrhythmias after acute coronary artery occlusion. In dogs that survived an acute myocardial infarction, Vanoli et al. [41] demonstrated that VNS during the process of coronary artery occlusion reduced the occurrence of VF from 100 to 10 %.

Nonischemic Cardiomyopathy Even though the pathophysiology of nonischemic cardiomyopathy is very different from ischemic cardiomyopathy, the provoking factors for lethal arrhythmias as well as their treatment are very similar. Because the ANS activity regulates cardiac ion channel function, it is possible that specific ANS activity might be responsible for triggering cardiac arrhythmias in congestive heart failure. Ogawa et al. [42] developed a pacing-induced CHF model in dogs and simultaneously recorded the left stellate ganglion nerve activity (SGNA), vagal nerve activity (VNA), and electrocardiography before and after pacing-induced CHF. The reduction of sympathovagal balance at night in ambulatory dogs was due to reduced sympathetic discharge rather than a net increase of vagal discharge. The tachy–brady syndrome in CHF may be triggered by intermittent short burst of SGNA that resulted in tachycardia and sinus node suppression. Simultaneous sympathovagal discharge is a cause of long paroxysmal atrial tachycardia episodes. Moreover, it was again confirmed that VA is always preceded by SGNA discharges. Importantly, when SGNA occur on the background of continuous, heightened vagal tone observed in nonischemic cardiomyopathy, the risk of VAs is increased.

While the novel neuromodulation methods used to treat arrhythmias in ischemic cardiomyopathy focused on reducing sympathetic discharges in the myocardium, the overall CHF treatment shifted attention to vagal nerve stimulation (VNS).

VNS also results in modulation of the renin–angiotensin system, reduced heart rate, modulation of inflammatory cytokines, less likelihood of spontaneous or induced ventricular arrhythmias, and reduced mortality. A single-center pilot study of eight patients with severe heart failure [seven in New York Heart Association (NYHA) class III] showed that right-sided VNS with the CardioFit system (BioControl Medical, Yehud, Israel), synchronized at 70 ms after the R wave with a duty cycle of no more than 25 %, was safe and tolerable. Sinus bradycardia was noted but was not a limiting factor since it was patient discomfort that generally prevented further increase of the stimulus intensity. There were significant and clinically important improvements in NYHA class, quality of life, and echocardiogram-derived end-systolic volume when compared with baseline values [43].

Due to encouraging positive results of the above study, three other randomized trials are ongoing (NECTAR-HF, ANTHEM-HF, and INOVATE-HF) and are assessing different outcomes in different patients. The details of the stimulation protocols are not completely clear, nor is it certain whether the protocols' specified electrode spacing, polarity, and positioning are more likely to recruit afferent or efferent vagal fibers, whether sympathetic activity will also be suppressed, or what effect there may be on ventricular contractility. However, there is hope that this will be an important step in management of congestive heart failure and associated arrhythmias through neuromodulation mechanisms.

Inherited Arrhythmia Syndromes In the past decade, the discovery of ventricular arrhythmias and SCD in young individuals, and the fact that they could be caused by genetic abnormalities, has defined a new subset of cardiac conditions: inherited arrhythmia syndromes. Patients with inherited arrhythmia syndromes may have a "structurally normal" heart but typically have an abnormal ECG suggesting electric abnormalities with the potential for life-threatening arrhythmias.

As in previously described conditions, the sympathetic stimulation can create a substrate for micro reentry and VF or polymorphic VT.

Long QT syndromes (LQTS) In normal individuals, high adrenergic tone or sympathetic stimulation shortens the ventricular action potential duration and hence the QT interval. In contrast, in congenital LQTS types 1 and 2, increased adrenergic tone can prolong the QT interval. However, there is some variability in terms of the degree of response to sympathetic activation depending on the type of LQTS and, thus, the type of channel and current affected. Noda et al. [44] observed that sympathetic stimulation by infusion of epinephrine caused more prominent and prolonged effects on QT prolongation in patients with congenital LQTS type 1 (characterized by an abnormality in KCNQ1 and the I_{Ks} current) than in type 2 (characterized by an abnormality in KCNH2 and the I_{Kr} current). In contrast, type 3 of LQTS is characterized by an abnormality on SCN5A and Na current; therefore, it responds much less to sympathetic stimulation [44–46]. As expected, LQTS 3 manifests itself by ventricular arrhythmias triggered by increased vagal tone, similar to Brugada syndrome.

The hypothesis proposed to explain the development of LQTS-related torsades de pointes (TdP) maintains that the various mutations that underlie the syndrome amplify the transmural dispersion of repolarization (TDR) by producing a net reduction in repolarizing current. Conditions leading to a reduction in I_{Kr} (e.g., LQT2) or augmentation of late I_{Na} (e.g., LQT3) amplify transmural electrical heterogeneities by producing a preferential prolongation of the M cell action potential. Thus, QT interval prolongation is accompanied by a dramatic increase in TDR, which creates a vulnerable window for the development of reentry across the ventricular wall. The reduction in net repolarizing current also predisposes to the development of early afterdepolarization (EAD)-induced triggered activity in M and Purkinje cells, which provide the extrasystole that triggers TdP when it arrives during the vulnerable period [47].

CPVT Catecholaminergic polymorphic ventricular tachycardia (CPVT) is a rare syndrome characterized by bidirectional or polymorphic ventricular arrhythmias under conditions of increased sympathetic activity in patients with structurally normal hearts. Most of the patients have mutations in the genes encoding proteins involved in calcium handling from the sarcoplasmic reticulum (ryanodine receptor or calsequestrin2 mutations) with inappropriate calcium leak that generates delayed afterdepolarizations (DAD), triggered activity, and ventricular arrhythmias [48].

Recently, research groups have identified the therapeutic effects of flecainide in CPVT. Flecainide directly inhibits the ryanodine channel and suppresses DADs and triggered activity in mutant cardiomyocytes in which Ryr2 or Casq2 loci are modified. In a recent study, Watanabe et al. found that flecainide suppressed ventricular arrhythmias during exercise testing in patients with genotype-negative CPVT, similar to that in patients with genotype-positive CPVT. Flecainide was highly effective in preventing arrhythmia events during a long-term follow-up [49].

Since both LQTS and CPVT are sympathetically mediated, in order to prevent cardiac events, β-blocker pharmacotherapy is the cornerstone of medical therapy while high-risk patients will benefit from ICDs. Additionally, the left cardiac sympathetic denervation (LCSD) procedure, in which the first 3–4 thoracic ganglia are removed, has emerged as a treatment modality for patients with LQTS, and more recently patients with CPVT, who continue to have cardiac events despite maximally tolerated β-blocker therapy, and has been proved to be a safe and effective treatment option [50]. Potential adverse effects of this procedure could include Horner's syndrome and altered sweating patterns in the face and upper extremities.

Brugada Syndrome The Brugada syndrome is an inherited arrhythmia disorder characterized by its typical ECG changes (right bundle branch block and persistent ST segment elevation) and an increased risk of VF and SCD in young patients.

Most episodes of VF in patients with Brugada syndrome are observed during periods of high vagal tone, such as at rest, during sleep, or from 12 am to 6 am. Similarly to LQTS 3, sudden increase of vagal activity just before the episodes of VF has been noted. This suggests that an increased vagal tone or decreased sympathetic tone may be important mechanisms in the arrhythmogenesis of this lethal disease [51]. Additionally, as the epicardium of right ventricular outflow tract serves as a substrate that mediates and sustains ventricular arrhythmias triggered by altered autonomic tones, the arrhythmia may be ablated successfully while also eliminating the repolarization abnormalities [52].

Arrhythmogenic right ventricular cardiomyopathy (ARVC) is a frequent underlying disease in young patients with ventricular tachycardia (VT) and sudden death. These arrhythmias often occur during physical exercise or mental stress and may be provoked by intravenous catecholamine infusion during electrophysiological study (catecholamine sensitivity). In contrast, VAs are frequently suppressed by an antiarrhythmic drug regimen with antiadrenergic properties [53].

Wichter et al. [53] have investigated the neuronal reuptake of norepinephrine and beta-adrenergic receptor density in eight patients with ARVC using quantitative [11] PET C-HED and [11] C-CGP-12177 as compared to twenty-nine matched controls.

The results provide clear evidence of abnormal sympathetic myocardial innervation in patients with ARVC and demonstrate a severe and highly significant reduction of postsynaptic beta-adrenergic receptor density. Additionally, this confirms regional reduction of transporter-mediated neuronal catecholamine reuptake in ARVC. Moreover, increased synaptic concentrations of norepinephrine not only may increase the risk of ventricular arrhythmias but also may contribute to progression of myocardial atrophy mediated by apoptotic cell death.

While ablation of reentrant arrhythmias is performed in highly experienced centers by accessing the epicardial surface of the scarred right ventricle [54], implantable defibrillators and treatment with beta-blockers and class III antiarrhythmic agents remain the mainstay of management at this time.

Idiopathic VF with repolarization abnormalities, the so-called J-point elevation syndromes, is characterized by ST segment elevation in the inferior and/or lateral leads. While this ECG finding is fairly frequently seen in young athletic adults, identifying the high-risk population is, of course, extremely important as those are at risk for sudden cardiac death due to VF. While most of the congenital abnormalities bear high risk of arrhythmias in the settings of high adrenergic tone, this rare syndrome seems to be triggered by increased vagal tone while exercise and increased sympathetic tone or isoproterenol infusion decrease the chance of arrhythmias.

For example, Mizumaki et al. [55] recently observed that in patients with idiopathic VF as compared with control subjects, J-wave augmentation was associated with an increase in vagal activity. This data suggests a critical role of cardiac ANS in the occurrence of VF in patients with J-wave syndromes. The differential responses of characteristic ECG changes to autonomic input may provide a useful tool in the identification of high-risk patients within the broad population of healthy individuals with this specific ECG pattern. While at this time autonomic modulation approaches for this condition are not available, treatment options are on the horizon.

Premature ventricular contractions can, as mentioned above, also pose diagnosis and management problems, as their impact on patients varies from asymptomatic PVCs to mild palpitations to acquired "PVC-induced cardiomyopathy" with heart failure and even VF and sudden cardiac death.

In the setting of ischemic and nonischemic cardiomyopathy, the PVCs seem to originate from areas around the scar and surviving Purkinje fibers. Their triggering factors and treatment options, including neuromodulation techniques, are similar to the management of VF and VT.

When conservative medical therapy fails, ablation of these PVCs provides additional and significant benefit. Marchlinski et al. recently published a retrospective study focused on the location of the PVCs which induce VF both structurally normal and abnormal hearts.

Ventricular fibrillation and polymorphic ventricular tachycardia (PMVT) triggered by monomorphic PVCs were the presenting arrhythmias in 30 of 1132 patients (2.7 %) undergoing ablation for VT/PVCs. Analysis of the study cohort revealed that in 21 patients, VF/PMVT occurred in the setting of ischemic ($n=14$) or nonischemic CMP ($n=7$). In 9 patients, there were no cardiac structural abnormalities, and VF/PMVT was idiopathic. The PVC triggers were found to originate from the Purkinje network ($n=9$), left and right ventricle papillary muscles ($n=8$), left ventricular outflow tract (LVOT) ($n=9$), and other low-voltage areas (without evidence of Purkinje system involvement [scar triggers]; $n=4$). Each distinct anatomic area of origin was associated with VF/PMVT trigger in patients with and without heart disease. Acute PVC elimination was accomplished in 26 patients (87 %) with a significant decrease in PVCs in another 3 patients (97 %). In structurally normal heart patients, the PVCs originated predominantly from left ventricular outflow tract as well as Purkinje fibers. Conversely, in patients with cardiomyopathies, the VF inducing PVCs originated from scar borders and Purkinje fibers as expected. While no cases of VF triggered by PVCs from the papillary muscles (PM) have been previously described, this group found six patients with cardiomyopathy and two patients with structurally normal heart and reproducible arrhythmias originate in the PM (Figs. 4.2 and 4.3) [56].

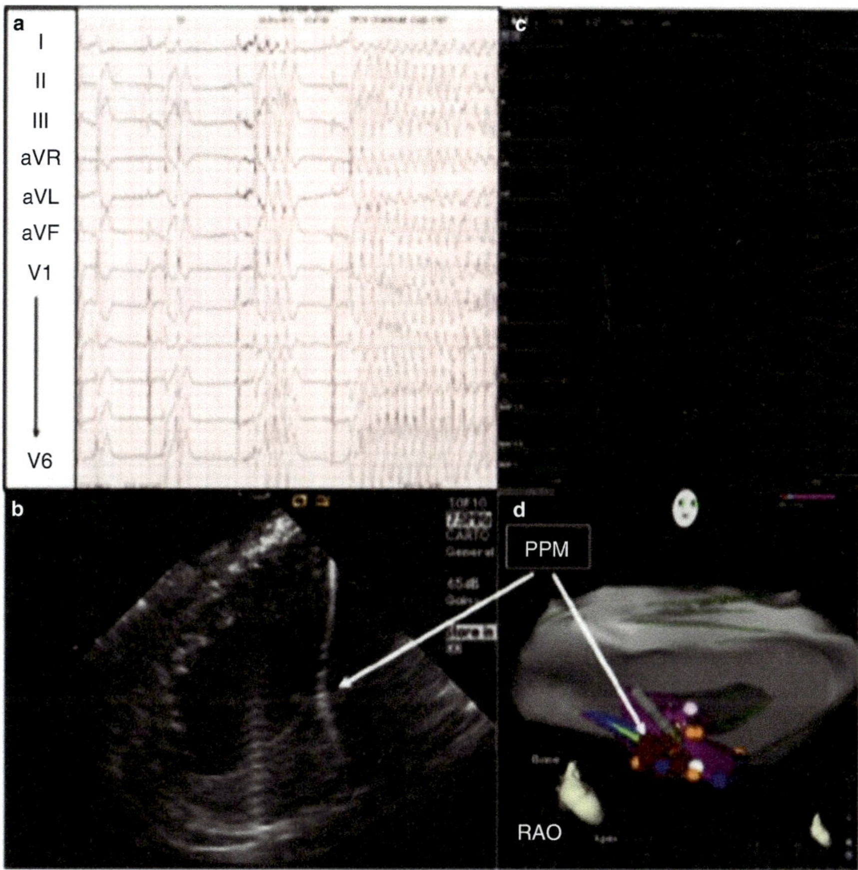

Fig. 4.2 Example of recurrent ventricular fibrillation in patient with triggering ventricular premature depolarization (VPD) arising from the left ventricular posteromedial papillary muscle after inferior wall myocardial infarction. Twelve-lead ECG obtained during episodes of nonsustained and sustained ventricular fibrillation (**a**) and with the same VPD in the electrophysiology laboratory (**b**). Intracardiac echocardiography (**c**) and electroanatomic map (**d**) with the catheter on the posteromedial papillary muscle (*PPM, arrows*). *RAO* right anterior oblique (Reproduced with permission from Van Herendael et al. [56])

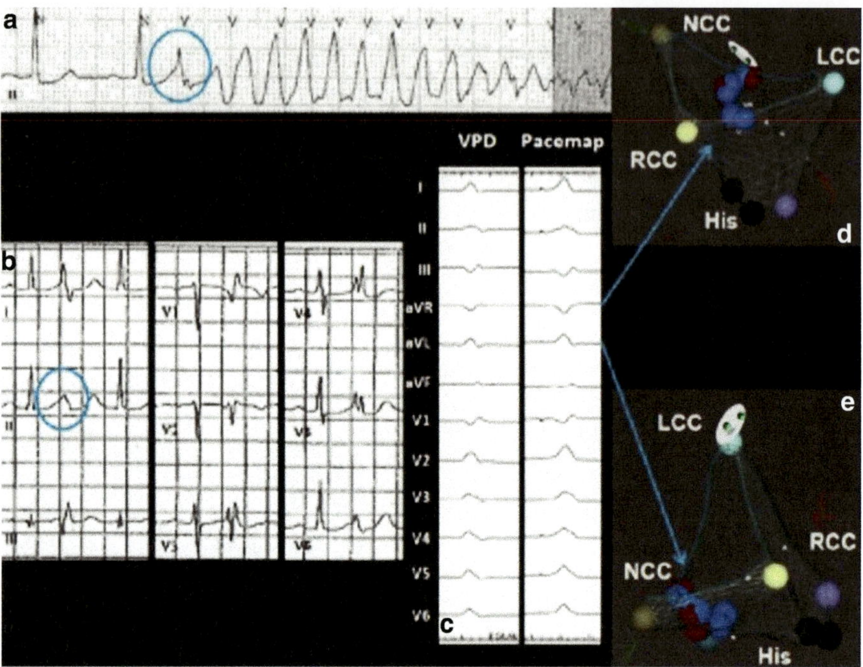

Fig. 4.3 Example of ventricular fibrillation initiated by a ventricular premature depolarization (*VPD*) originating just below the aortic cusp. (**a**) Initiation of ventricular fibrillation (*VF*) documented on telemetry. (**b**) Similar VPD on 12-lead ECG without initiating VF. (**c**) Good pace-map from the blue dots displayed in electroanatomic maps in the left anterior oblique (**d**) and right anterior oblique € views. *LCC* left coronary cusp, *NCC* noncoronary cusp, *RCC* right coronary cusp (Reproduced with permission from Van Herendael et al. [56])

Interestingly enough, Natale's research group almost simultaneously published their results on 6 patients. In these series, PVCs originating from papillary muscles induced VF episodes (Fig. 4.4).

The main findings of the study suggested that VF can be triggered by PVCs arising from PMs of both the right and left ventricles and VF can be successfully corrected long term with ablation of PVCs arising from PM. No complication was present in this series [57]. While the right ventricular outflow tract (RVOT) is the most common origin of monomorphic VT in structurally normal hearts, it is occasionally also the origin for triggers of polymorphic VT, which rapidly degenerates into VF. This type of ablation is essentially no different than the ablation of idiopathic RVOT PVCs or VT. The ablation targets the site of earliest activation, and pace-mapping may be of additional benefit to localize the exit site. Success in eliminating VF is not only by the elimination of the triggering PVCs but also potentially by the creation of conduction block between the pulmonary artery and RVOT [58].

Benign PVCs While the frequency of VF induced by PVCs is relatively rare, those originating from the RVOT and LVOT are frequently encountered in clinical practice and usually do not pose significant problems. As a matter of fact, there is recent

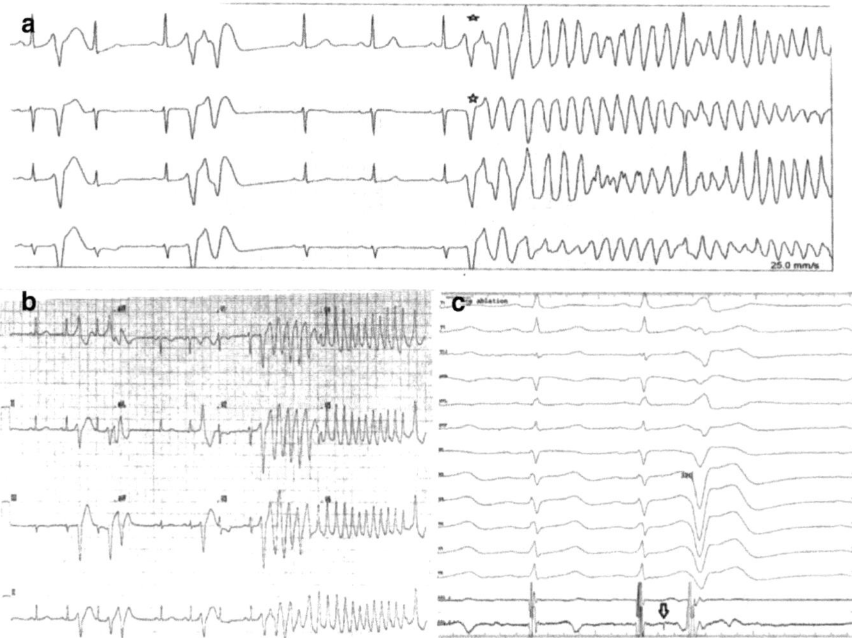

Fig. 4.4 Images are from the same patient, with a normal structural heart, having frequent PVCs from RV posterolateral papillary muscle (*PM*). (**a**) ECG strips recorded during hospitalization showing a monomorphic premature ventricular contraction (*PVC*, *), initiating polymorphic ventricular tachycardia. (**b**) 12-lead ECG showing sinus rhythm interrupted by the same PVC initiating an episode of polymorphic ventricular tachycardia. (**c**) Surface ECG and intracardiac recordings from the ablation catheter (ABL p, ABL d). Surface ECG showing sinus rhythm and a PVC, and intracardiac recording showing a PVC preceded by a Purkinje-like potential (*arrow*) (Reproduced with permission from Santoro et al. [57])

evidence suggesting that these PVCs originating from the outflow tracts are intricately connected with the autonomic function of the heart. It is by now very well known that when performing atrial fibrillation ablation using a wide area of circumferential ablation and when targeting fractionated potentials and ganglia around the left atrial structures, there is a significant cardiac autonomic modulation [59–62]. In this setting, Patel et al. set out to evaluate the incidence of increased outflow tract PVCs after atrial fibrillation ablation. They prospectively examined 53 consecutive patients undergoing wide-area circumferential antral pulmonary vein isolation (PVI); no patients had evidence of PVCs originating from the outflow tract on 24 h of pre-procedural telemetry monitoring. The results showed that in an unselected population of patients with paroxysmal or persistent atrial fibrillation referred for PVI, 11 % of patients had new onset of outflow trace ventricular premature depolarizations (OT VPDs) after AF ablation. Interestingly, the patients with OT VPDs had a significant increase in mean heart rate post-procedure compared to the patients without PVCs. Long-term follow-up showed that both increased heart rate and PVC load persisted for up to 1 year [63].

These findings may be explained by a more extensive collateral ablation of autonomic ganglionated plexi in the patients with increased PVCs originating from the outflow tract and highlight the impact of the autonomic tone on cardiac function. As mentioned previously, when the amount of PVCs exceed 10 or 20 % of the normal beats, there is a significant concern for tachycardia/PVC cardiomyopathy. While medications can be used, ablation of the outflow tract PVCs has been successful not only in correcting the arrhythmia and symptoms but also in reversing the cardiomyopathy [64–66]. Mountantonakis et al. [67] were able to prove on 69 patients with outflow tract PVC and secondary cardiomyopathy that even a reduction of the PVC load to less than 5000 per day or less than 80 % of the initial frequency is effective in allowing the ejection fraction to recover. In their series, most of the PVCs originated from the LVOT area or even epicardial origin within the coronary sinus.

Ablating PVCs from the areas situated in close proximity of the cardiac autonomic plexi and considering that there is an increase in PVCs after extensive atrial fibrillation ablation, a question begs answering: is the reason for success partially due to injuring the cardiac innervation responsible for these arrhythmias? Could this be a similar mechanism with paroxysmal atrial fibrillation where the origin of arrhythmia is a combination of "extension digits" within the pulmonary veins as well as exacerbation of vagal or sympathetic tone?

With current data available, one can hope that in the near future, we might be able to complement our medical and ablation therapy with autonomic manipulation for the various conditions described in this section. It is also possible that some of the approaches already available to us, such as renal denervation, carotid stimulation, or stellate ganglia resection, could lead to a "remote control" of the arrhythmias without having to actually place a catheter within the heart. These are exciting prospects for both patients and cardiac electrophysiologists alike, and we must continue our research efforts to improve our understanding of the "brain–heart connection" and its role in cardiac arrhythmias.

References

1. Harvey W. Exercitatio Anatomica de Motu Cordis et Sanguinis in Animalibus. Springfield: Charles C Thomas; 1929.
2. Levy MN, Manuel NG, Martin P, Zieske H. Sympathetic and para- sympathetic interactions upon the left ventricle of the dog. Circ Res. 1966;19:5–10.
3. Levy MN. Sympathetic-parasympathetic interactions in the heart. Circ Res. 1971;29:437–45.
4. Martins JB, Zipes DP. Effects of sympathetic and vagal nerves on recovery properties of the endocardium and epicardium of the canine left ventricle. Circ Res. 1980;46:100–10.
5. Yuan BX, Ardell JL, Hopkins DA, Losier AM, Armour JA. Gross and microscopic anatomy of the canine intrinsic cardiac nervous system. Anat Rec. 1994;239:75–87.
6. Armour JA, Murphy DA, Yuan BX, Macdonald S, Hopkins DA. Gross and microscopic anatomy of the human intrinsic cardiac nervous system. Anat Rec. 1997;247:289–98.
7. Leriche R, Herman L, Fontaine R. Ligature de la coronaire gauche et fonction du coeur après énervation sympathique. C R Soc Biol. 1931;107:547.
8. McEachern CG, Manning GW, Hall G. Sudden occlusion of coronary arteries following removal of cardiosensory pathways: experimental study. Arch Intern Med. 1940;65:661–70.

9. Harris AS, Estandia A, Tillotson RF. Ventricular ectopic rhythms and ventricular fibrillation following cardiac sympathectomy and coronary occlusion. Am J Physiol. 1951;165:505–12.

10. Kapa S, Venkatachalam KL, Asirvatham SJ. The autonomic nervous system in cardiac electrophysiology: an elegant interaction and emerging concepts. Cardiol Rev. 2010;18:275–84.

11. Taggart P, Critchley H, Lambiase PD. Heart-brain interactions in cardiac arrhythmia. Heart. 2011;97:698–708.

12. Shen MJ, Choi EK, Tan AY, Lin SF, Fishbein MC, Chen LS, Chen PS. Neural mechanisms of atrial arrhythmias. Nat Rev Cardiol. 2012;9:30–9.

13. Schwartz PJ. Cutting nerves and saving lives. Heart Rhythm. 2009;6:760–3.

14. Shen M, Zipes D. Role of the autonomic nervous system in modulating cardiac arrhythmias. Circ Res. 2014;114:1004–21.

15. Dukes ID, Vaughan Williams EM. Effects of selective alpha 1-, alpha 2-, beta 1-and beta 2-adrenoceptor stimulation on potentials and contractions in the rabbit heart. J Physiol. 1984;355:523–46.

16. Lukas A, Antzelevitch C. Differences in the electrophysiological response of canine ventricular epicardium and endocardium to ischemia. Role of the transient outward current. Circulation. 1993;88:2903–15.

17. Shimizu W, Antzelevitch C. Cellular basis for the ECG features of the LQT1 form of the long-QT syndrome: effects of beta-adrenergic agonists and antagonists and sodium channel blockers on transmural dispersion of repolarization and torsade de pointes. Circulation. 1998;98:2314–22.

18. Ng GA, Brack KE, Coote JH. Effects of direct sympathetic and vagus nerve stimulation on the physiology of the whole heart–a novel model of isolated Langendorff perfused rabbit heart with intact dual autonomic innervation. Exp Physiol. 2001;86:319–29.

19. Zipes DP, Mihalick MJ, Robbins GT. Effects of selective vagal and stellate ganglion stimulation of atrial refractoriness. Cardiovasc Res. 1974;8:647–55.

20. Wijffels MC, Kirchhof CJ, Dorland R, Allessie MA. Atrial fibrillation begets atrial fibrillation. A study in awake chronically instrumented goats. Circulation. 1995;92:1954–68.

21. Fareh S, Villemaire C, Nattel S. Importance of refractoriness heterogeneity in the enhanced vulnerability to atrial fibrillation induction caused by tachycardia-induced atrial electrical remodeling. Circulation. 1998;98:2202–9.

22. Burashnikov A, Antzelevitch C. Reinduction of atrial fibrillation immediately after termination of the arrhythmia is mediated by late phase 3 early after depolarization-induced triggered activity. Circulation. 2003;107:2355–60.

23. Zipes DP, Rubart M. Neural modulation of cardiac arrhythmias and sudden cardiac death. Heart Rhythm. 2006;3:108–13.

24. Yanowitz F, Preston JB, Abildskov JA. Functional distribution of right and left stellate innervation to the ventricles. Production of neurogenic electrocardiographic changes by unilateral alteration of sympathetic tone. Circ Res. 1966;18:416–28.

25. Opthof T, Misier AR, Coronel R, Vermeulen JT, Verberne HJ, Frank RG, Moulijn AC, van Capelle FJ, Janse MJ. Dispersion of refractoriness in canine ventricular myocardium. Effects of sympathetic stimulation. Circ Res. 1991;68:1204–15.

26. Tomaselli GF, Zipes DP. What causes sudden death in heart failure? Circ Res. 2004;95:754–63.

27. Barber MJ, Mueller TM, Henry DP, Felten SY, Zipes DP. Transmural myocardial infarction in the dog produces sympathectomy in noninfarcted myocardium. Circulation. 1983;67:787–96.

28. Karagueuzian HS, Wolf PL, Fishbein MC, Chen PS. Nerve sprouting and sudden cardiac death. Circ Res. 2000;86:816–21.

29. Chen PS, Chen LS, Cao JM, Sharifi B, Karagueuzian HS, Fishbein MC. Sympathetic nerve sprouting, electrical remodeling and the mechanisms of sudden cardiac death. Cardiovasc Res. 2001;50:409–16.

30. Cao JM, Fishbein MC, Han JB, Lai WW, Lai AC, Wu TJ, Czer L, Wolf PL, Denton TA, Shintaku IP, Chen PS, Chen LS. Relationship between regional cardiac hyperinnervation and ventricular arrhythmia. Circulation. 2000;101:1960–9.

31. Swissa M, Zhou S, Gonzalez-Gomez I, Chang CM, Lai AC, Cates AW, Fishbein MC, Karagueuzian HS, Chen PS, Chen LS. Long-term subthreshold electrical stimulation of the left stellate ganglion and a canine model of sudden cardiac death. J Am Coll Cardiol. 2004;43:858–64.

32. Zhou S, Chen LS, Miyauchi Y, Miyauchi M, Kar S, Kangavari S, Fishbein MC, Sharifi B, Chen PS. Mechanisms of cardiac nerve sprouting after myocardial infarction in dogs. Circ Res. 2004;95:76–83.

33. Han S, Kobayashi K, Joung B, Piccirillo G, Maruyama M, Vinters HV, March K, Lin SF, Shen C, Fishbein MC, Chen PS, Chen LS. Electroanatomic remodeling of the left stellate ganglion after myocardial infarction. J Am Coll Cardiol. 2012;59:954–61.

34. Liu YB, Wu CC, Lu LS, Su MJ, Lin CW, Lin SF, Chen LS, Fishbein MC, Chen PS, Lee YT. Sympathetic nerve sprouting, electrical remodeling, and increased vulnerability to ventricular fibrillation in hypercholesterolemic rabbits. Circ Res. 2003;92:1145–52.

35. Shusterman V, Aysin B, Gottipaty V, Weiss R, Brode S, Schwartzman D, Anderson KP. Autonomic nervous system activity and the spontaneous initiation of ventricular tachycardia. ESVEM Investigators. Electrophysiologic Study Versus Electrocardiographic Monitoring Trial. J Am Coll Cardiol. 1998;32:1891–9.

36. Doytchinova A, Patel J, Zhou S, Chen LS, Lin H, Shen C, Everett TH 4th, Lin SF, Chen PS. Subcutaneous nerve activity and spontaneous ventricular arrhythmias in ambulatory dogs. Heart Rhythm. 2015;12(3):612–20.

37. Szumowski L, Sanders P, Walczak F, Hocini M, Jais P, Kepski R, Szufladowicz E, Urbanek P, Derejko P, Bodalski R, Haissaguerre M. Mapping and ablation of polymorphic ventricular tachycardia after myocardial infarction. J Am Coll Cardiol. 2004;44:1700–6.

38. Linz D, Wirth K, Ukena C, Mahfouf F, Poss J, Linz B, Bohm M, Neuberger HR. Renal denervation suppresses ventricular arrhythmias during acute ventricular ischemia in pigs. Heart Rhythm. 2013;10:1525–30.

39. Ukena C, Bauer A, Mahfoud F, Schreieck J, Neuberger HR, Eick C, Sobotka P, Gawaz M, Bohm M. Renal sympathetic denervation for the treatment of electrical storm: first in man experience. Clin Res Cardiol. 2012;101:63–7.

40. Vaseghi M, Gima J, Kanaan C, Ajijola O, Marmureanu A, Mahajan A, Shivkumar K. Cardiac sympathetic denervation in patients with refractory ventricular arrhythmias or electrical storm: intermediate and long term follow up. Heart Rhythm. 2014;11:360–6.

41. Vanoli E, De Ferrari GM, Stramba-Badiale M, Hull Jr SS, Foreman RD, Schwartz PJ. Vagal stimulation and prevention of sudden death in conscious dogs with a healed myocardial infarction. Circ Res. 1991;68:1471–81.

42. Ogawa M, Zhou S, Tan A, Song J, Gholmieh G, Fishbein M, Luo H, Siegel R, Karagueuzian H, Chen L, Lin S, Chen P. Left stellate ganglion and vagal nerve activity and cardiac arrhythmias in ambulatory dogs with pacing induced congestive heart failure. J Am Coll Cardiol. 2007;50:335–43.

43. Schwartz PJ, De Ferrari GM, Sanzo A, Landolina M, Rordorf R, Raineri C, Campana C, Revera M, Ajmone-Marsan N, Tavazzi L, Odero A. Long- term vagal stimulation in patients with advanced heart failure: first experience in man. Eur J Heart Fail. 2008;10:884–91.

44. Noda T, Takaki H, Kurita T, et al. Gene-specific response of dynamic ventricular repolarization to sympathetic stimulation in LQT1, LQT2 and LQT3 forms of congenital long QT syndrome. Eur Heart J. 2002;23:975–83.

45. Antzelevitch C, Sun ZQ, Zhang ZQ, Yan GX. Cellular and ionic mechanisms underlying erythromycin-induced long QT intervals and torsade de pointes. J Am Coll Cardiol. 1996;28:1836–48.

46. Huffaker R, Lamp ST, Weiss JN, Kogan B. Intracellular calcium cycling, early after depolarizations, and reentry in simulated long QT syndrome. Heart Rhythm. 2004;1:441–8.

47. Antzelevitch C. Sympathetic modulation of the long QT syndrome. Eur Heart J. 2002;23:1246–52.

48. Cerrone M, Noujaim SF, Tolkacheva EG, Talkachou A, O'Connell R, Berenfeld O, Anumonwo J, Pandit SV, Vikstrom K, Napolitano C, Priori SG, Jalife J. Arrhythmogenic mechanisms in a

mouse model of catecholaminergic polymorphic ventricular tachycardia. Circ Res. 2007;101:1039–48.

49. Watanabe H, Werf C, Roses-Noguer F, Adler A, Sumitomo N, Veltman C, Rosso R, Till J, Wilde A. Effects of flecainide on exercise- induced ventricular arrhythmias and recurrences in genotype-negative patients with catecholaminergic polymorphic ventricular tachycardia. Heart Rhythm. 2013;10:542–7.

50. Collura CA, Johnson JN, Moir C, Ackerman MJ. Left cardiac sympathetic denervation for the treatment of long QT syndrome and catecholaminergic polymorphic ventricular tachycardia using video-assisted thoracic surgery. Heart Rhythm. 2009;6:752–9.

51. Brugada P, Brugada J. Right bundle branch block, persistent st segment elevation and sudden cardiac death: a distinct clinical and electrocardiographic syndrome. J Am Coll Cardiol. 1992;20:1391–6.

52. Nademanee K, Veerakul G, Chandanamattha P, Chaothawee L, Ariyachaipanich A. Prevention of ventricular fibrillation episodes in Brugada syndrome by catheter ablation over the anterior right ventricular outflow tract epicardium. Circulation. 2011;123(12):1270–9.

53. Wichter T, Schäfers M, Rhodes CG, Borggrefe M, Lerch H, Lammertsma AA, Hermansen F, Schober O, Breithardt G, Camici PG. Abnormalities of cardiac sympathetic innervation in arrhythmogenic right ventricular cardiomyopathy: quantitative assessment of presynaptic norepinephrine reuptake and postsynaptic beta-adrenergic receptor density with positron emission tomography. Circulation. 2000;101:1552–8.

54. Philips B, Madhavan S, James C, Tichnell C, Murray B, Dalal D, Bhonsale A, Nazarian S, Judge DP, Russell SD, Abraham T, Calkins H, Tandri H. Outcomes of catheter ablation of ventricular tachycardia in arrhythmogenic right ventricular dysplasia/cardiomyopathy. Circ Arrhythm Electrophysiol. 2012;5(3):499–505.

55. Mizumaki K, Nishida K, Iwamoto J, Nakatani Y, Yamaguchi Y, Sakamoto T, Tsuneda T, Kataoka N, Inoue H. Vagal activity modulates spontaneous augmentation of J-wave elevation in patients with idiopathic ventricular fibrillation. Heart Rhythm. 2012;9:249–55.

56. Van Herendael H, Zado E, Haqqani H, Tschabrunn C, Callans D, Frankel D, Lin D, Garcia D, Hutchinson M, Riley M, Bala R, Dixit S, Yadava M, Marchlinki F. Catheter ablation of ventricular fibrillation: importance of left ventricular outflow tract and papillary muscle triggers. Heart Rhythm. 2014;11:566–73.

57. Santoro F, Di Biase L, Hranitzky P, Sanchez J, Santangeli P, Paoletti Perini A, Burkhardt J, Natale A. Ventricular fibrillation triggered by PVCS from papillary muscles: clinical features and ablation. J Cardiovasc Electrophysiol. 2014;25:1158–64.

58. Nogami A. Mapping and ablating ventricular premature contractions that trigger ventricular fibrillation: trigger elimination and substrate modification. J Cardiovasc Electrophysiol. 2015;26:110–5.

59. Doll N, Pritzwald-Stegmann P, Czesla M, Kempfert J, Stenzel MA, Borger MA, et al. Ablation of ganglionic plexi during combined surgery for atrial fibrillation. Ann Thorac Surg. 2008;86(5):1659–63. Evaluation studies.

60. McClelland JH, Duke D, Reddy R. Preliminary results of a limited thoracotomy: new approach to treat atrial fibrillation. J Cardiovasc Electrophysiol. 2007;18(12):1289–95. Clinical trial.

61. Mehall JR, Kohut Jr RM, Schneeberger EW, Taketani T, Merrill WH, Wolf RK. Intraoperative epicardial electrophysiologic mapping and isolation of autonomic ganglionic plexi. Annals of Thorac Surgery. 2007;83(2):538–41.

62. Po SS, Nakagawa H, Jackman WM. Localization of left atrial ganglionated plexi in patients with atrial fibrillation. J Cardiovasc Electrophysiol. 2009;20(10):1186–9. Review.

63. Patel P, Ahlemeyer L, Freas M, Cooper J, Marchlinski F, Callans D, Hutchinson M. Outflow tract premature ventricular depolarizations after atrial fibrillation ablation may reflect autonomic influences. J Interv Card Electrophysiol. 2014;41:187–92.

64. Yarlagadda RK, Iwai S, Stein KM, et al. Reversal of cardiomyopathy in patients with repetitive monomorphic ventricular ectopy originating from the right ventricular outflow tract. Circulation. 2005;112:1092–7.

65. Sekiguchi Y, Aonuma K, Yamauchi Y, et al. Chronic hemodynamic effects after radiofrequency catheter ablation of frequent monomorphic ventricular premature beats. J Cardiovasc Electrophysiol. 2005;16:1057–63.
66. Bogun F, Crawford T, Reich S, et al. Radiofrequency ablation of frequent, idiopathic premature ventricular complexes: comparison with a control group without intervention. Heart Rhythm. 2007;4:863–7.
67. Mountantonankis S, Frankel D, Gerstenfeld E, Dixit S, Lin D, Hutchingson M, Riley M, Bala R, Cooper J, Callans D, Garcia F, Zado E, Marchlinski F. Reversal of outflow tract ventricular premature depolarization-induced cardiomyopathy with ablation: effect of residual arrhythmia burden and preexisting cardiomyopathy on outcome. Heart Rhythm. 2011;8:1608–14.

Part II

The Autonomic Regulation and Dis-regulation of the Heart: Pathophysiology in Heart Failure

"The Autonomic Nervous System Symphony Orchestra": Pathophysiology of Autonomic Nervous System and Analysis of Activity Frequencies

5

Nicola Montano and Eleonora Tobaldini

5.1   Introduction

Autonomic nervous system (ANS) can be considered as the interface between external and internal stimuli, central nervous system (CNS), and effective responses, in order to maintain the homeostatic state of body functions reacting upon environmental challenges. Sympathetic and parasympathetic autonomic branches are essential for the control and regulation of different biological functions, such as cardiovascular, gastrointestinal, pulmonary, skin, and genitourinary systems.

Neural control of cardiovascular functions represents one of the most interesting and complex pathway of autonomic regulation of body functions [24] for several reasons. First, despite the definition of "autonomic," SNA seems to be not "autonomous" at all, considering that several evidences sustain the theory of a complex and integrated control mechanisms operating at different levels; for instance, animal studies have shown that insular and infralimbic cortex have been involved as potential sites where cardiovascular autonomic responses are generated [2]. Moreover, electrical stimulation of prefrontal cortex using transcranial magnetic stimulation elicited autonomic responses in healthy subjects, namely, an increase of parasympathetic control, with no changes in sympathetic modulation [11].

Neural control of cardiovascular function is determined by the reciprocal interaction between sympathetic and parasympathetic control acting as a balance: in fact, in most of the physiological conditions, an increase of sympathetic activity is associated with a decreased vagal control and vice versa; however, it has been shown that coactivation of both sympathetic and parasympathetic occurs during several

N. Montano, MD, PhD (✉) • E. Tobaldini, MD
Department of Internal Medicine, IRCSS Ca' Granda Foundation,
Ospedale Maggiore Policlinico, Milan, Italy
e-mail: nicola.montano@unimi.it

Department of Biomedical and Clinical Sciences "L. Sacco", University of Milan,
Milan, Italy

© Springer International Publishing Switzerland 2016
E. Gronda et al. (eds.), *Heart Failure Management: The Neural Pathways*,
DOI 10.1007/978-3-319-24993-3_5

conditions. For instance, in response to exercise, as well as to peripheral chemoreflex activation, such as that occurring during apneas or hypovolemic shock, heart rate decreases while sympathetic peripheral activation increases peripheral vascular resistance and contractility [30].

In addition, recent evidences show that ANS plays a key role in the control of pathways other than vegetative functions: ANS can indeed modulate and regulate immune system, inflammation [10, 33, 34], and metabolic pathways [3].

In summary, ANS regulation of cardiac function is complex and integrated at different levels; several cardiovascular (hypertension, heart failure, myocardial infarction) and non cardiovascular (diabetes, depression) diseases are associated with altered autonomic control, characterized by reduction of total variability and sympathetic overactivity [12, 17, 27]. In fact, conditions characterized by increased sympathetic and decreased parasympathetic modulation are at increased risk for cardiovascular events, while, on the contrary, increased parasympathetic modulation is protective for cardiovascular system. Therefore, all treatments, pharmacologic and non-pharmacologic, which reduce sympathetic activity and increase vagal modulation (i.e. beta-blocker therapy in congestive heart failure and ischemic heart disease) are indeed effective. Thus, the evaluation of ANS seems to be crucial not only to investigate the pathophysiological mechanisms subserving cardiovascular diseases but also as new possible targets for pharmacological and non-pharmacological therapy [24] (see Fig. 5.1).

5.2 Methodologies

5.2.1 General Considerations

The appreciation that the technique for the assessment of autonomic cardiovascular control needs to be reliable, reproducible, and noninvasive has led to the development of several different tools during the last decades. Generally, we can classify three groups of techniques: (1) assessment of sympathetic activity by measuring plasmatic catecholamines, (2) direct recording of sympathetic nerve activity (e.g., muscle sympathetic nerve activity, MSNA, using a microneurographic techniques), and (3) the analysis of sympathetic and parasympathetic oscillations embedded in heart period and arterial pressure time series.

Plasmatic catecholamines are less reproducible even within the same patient and are an unreliable index of sympathetic activity as their levels are influenced by several factors, thus supporting the idea that this measure must not be considered a consistent and reproducible tool. The direct measure of sympathetic nerve activity is a reliable and reproducible tool to evaluate sympathetic nerve activity in health and diseases [6, 24]; however, its invasivity, although mild, could be a possible limiting factor for this tool specifically when large populations are involved. On the opposite, the analysis of cardiovascular oscillatory components related to sympathetic and parasympathetic controls to sinus node and vascular tree is able to assess autonomic regulation in health and pathologies being a noninvasive, reliable, and reproducible tool called heart rate variability (HRV) [24].

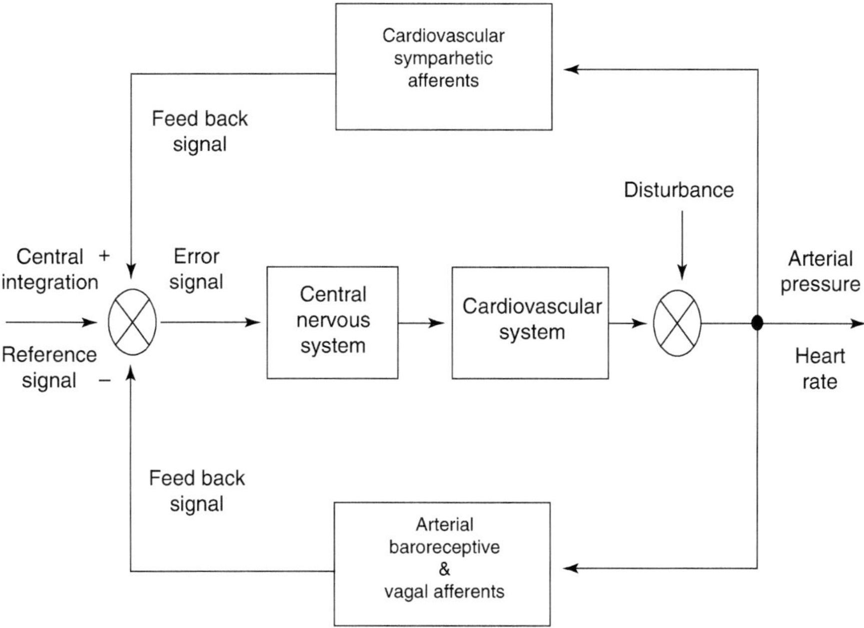

Fig. 5.1 In physiological conditions, different opposing positive and negative feedback mechanisms, such as baroreceptors and vagal and sympathetic afferents, in addition to central integration, promote neural control of the cardiovascular system

5.2.2   Muscle Sympathetic Nerve Activity (MSNA)

Neural pathways convey biological information coded simultaneously based on two different modalities, i.e., intensity, which represent the amplitude of the signal, or tonic activity, and oscillatory discharge pattern, i.e., modulation [7].

The direct recording of muscle sympathetic nerve activity (MSNA) allows the evaluation of both intensity and modulation of sympathetic neural discharge. In fact, absolute values of MSNA can provide information on sympathetic tonic activity when considering the dynamic responses to stressor stimuli (i.e., orthostatic challenge, pharmacological stimulation), because MSNA signal fluctuates depending on amplification and filters, electrode position, and the number of single units [23]. MSNA variability contains two main rhythmic oscillatory components, low-frequency (LF) and high-frequency (HF) rhythms [5], which are coherent with the corresponding heart period and blood spectral components.

Parasympathetic activation, induced by the pressure response to phenylephrine infusion, is characterized by a predominant HF component in heart period, blood pressure, and MSNA variability, while, on the contrary, sympathetic activation induced by nitroprusside infusion is associated with LF component [29], thus suggesting that these oscillations are index of neural excitation (LF) and inhibition (HF). Gravitational stimulus (i.e., tilt test maneuver) induced similar MSNA responses, showing that orthostatism was able to induce a significant increase of LF and a decrease of HF component of MSNA [6].

Interestingly, it has been shown that acute beta-blockade affected cardiovascular and MSNA spectral profile in healthy subjects: in fact, atenolol infusion caused an increase in R-R intervals, as expected, and an increased power of MSNA in the HF band and a higher coherence between HF component of MSNA and respiration, suggesting an increased cardiorespiratory coupling [4].

However, in addition to sympathetic neural recording, direct recording of renal sympathetic nerve activity in animals (RSNA) and skin (SSNA) has provided interesting information on autonomic reflexes in different situations (orthostatism, exercise, cardiovascular diseases) [26, 37].

In summary, MSNA can be considered a reliable tool able to provide important information on the sympathetic neural discharge in terms of tonic activity and rhythmic oscillations. However, MSNA provides information only on sympathetic neural discharge, while no information is provided on the vagal branch; in addition, MSNA is a relatively invasive technique, thus rendering this tool unsuited to researches on large scales [23, 24].

5.2.3　Heart Rate Variability

Five decades ago, pioneer studies reported that changes in RR intervals could have been used for an early identification of fetal distress before heart rate modifications were detected 16. The same was then reported for detection of diabetic neuropathy [25] and for the quantification of respiratory sinus arrhythmia (RSA) in post-myocardial infarction (i.e., reduced RSA associated with an increased mortality) [39].

These studies supported the hypothesis that heart rate and blood pressure rhythmically oscillate around their mean values and that these oscillations are due to the sympathetic and vagal modulation of sinus node function and vascular tree. Since each biological time series, including heart period and blood pressure time series, are the sum of several oscillatory components, characterized by a certain frequency and amplitude, the analysis of cardiovascular oscillations can provide reliable information on sympathetic and parasympathetic control of cardiovascular functions in physiological conditions as well as in cardiac and noncardiac diseases [1, 22, 23]. Thus, the analysis of these rhythmical components can be considered a window over cardiovascular autonomic control, i.e., heart rate and blood pressure variability (HRV and BPV) [28].

In the seventies, the idea was introduced that a computational analysis of heart rate and blood pressure variability (HRV and BPV, respectively) could have been a reliable method to investigate cardiovascular autonomic modulation. The important clinical relevance of this technique has later been demonstrated by the fact that HRV possesses a strong prognostic value in cardiac diseases. For instance, Kleiger et al. were the first to demonstrate that a reduction of HRV parameters following acute myocardial infarction was an independent predictor of mortality [15, 18]. In the last years, a growing interest has been focused on the complex interaction between sympathetic and parasympathetic afferent and efferent pathways, the sympatho-sympathetic excitatory reflexes [20], and the reciprocal and non-reciprocal changes of the sympathovagal balance in health and diseases.

5.2.3.1 Linear Analysis

Frequency domain analysis is based on the evaluation of different rhythmic oscillatory components embedded in cardiovascular time series. Several different techniques have been validated in the past years for HRV analysis, usually categorized into parametric and nonparametric methods. Parametric approaches, such as autoregressive models, can identify spectral components independently of preselected frequency bands and they can provide accurate evaluation of spectra on small samples. Nonparametric methods use a simple algorithm, such as Fast Fourier Transform, and are characterized by higher process speed (Task Force of the European Society of Cardiology the North American Society of Pacing Electrophysiology [32]).

Spectral analysis of HRV assesses rhythmical oscillations embedded in cardiovascular time series. By using an autoregressive model, the algorithm can identify three main oscillatory components which are embedded in heart period and blood pressure time series:

- Very low-frequency component (VLF), frequency band below 0.04 Hz
- Low-frequency component (LF), frequency band bounded between 0.04 and 0.15 Hz
- High-frequency component (HF), frequency band bounded between 0.15 and 0.4 Hz, synchronous with respiration

Experimental studies showed that VLF can be considered a marker of very slow oscillations such as hormonal changes, circadian rhythms, etc.; LF component is a marker of sympathetic heart rate modulation, while HF component is a marker of vagal heart rate modulation. The sum of VLF, LF, and HF represents the area under the curve, also called al total power (TP), or total variability; TP is a global marker of autonomic cardiovascular variability, representing the capability of the autonomic control to respond to stressors stimuli. Aging and diseases are associated with gradual decrease of TP, suggesting a loss of autonomic control to reliably counteract exogenous and endogenous stimuli [24].

Each oscillation can be described in terms of both frequency, expressed in Hz, and amplitude, which can be expressed both in absolute units (ms^2 and $mmHg^2$ for heart period and blood pressure time series, respectively) and normalized units (nu). Nu represent the relative value of LF and HF components with respect to the total power, and they are calculated dividing the component by total power to which VLF have been subtracted, i.e., LF nu = [LF absolute units / (total power − VLF power)] and the HF nu = [HF absolute units / (total power-VLF)]. The ratio between LF and HF power can be calculated and it is considered marker of the sympathovagal balance (see Figs. 5.2).

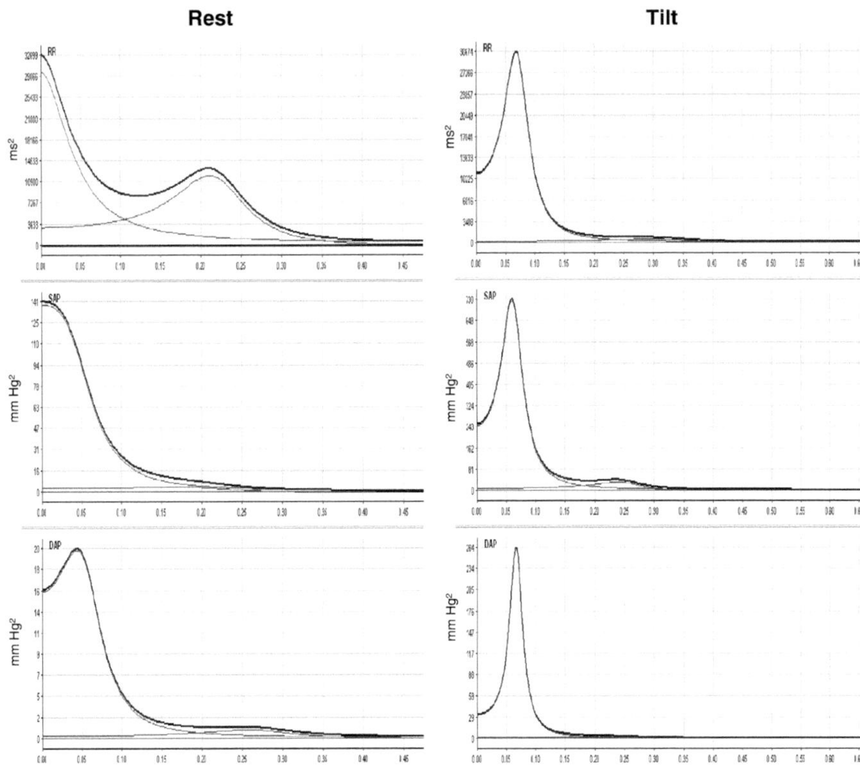

Fig. 5.2 Spectral analysis of heart rate and systolic and diastolic blood pressure during Rest (*left column*) and during Tilt (*right column*). During Tilt, LF component, marker of sympathetic modulation, significantly increases in both heart period and blood pressure time series compared to rest

5.2.3.2 Nonlinear Analysis

Nonlinear analysis of HRV can be considered complementary to spectral analysis for autonomic cardiovascular assessment. It has been hypothesized, and then demonstrated, that most of the biological system functions, including the cardiovascular one, are nonlinear, at least in specific situations. Therefore, the development of new techniques able to assess autonomic control in situations of nonlinearity became necessary for a reliable assessment of sympathetic and parasympathetic evaluation in health and diseases. In addition, we have to underline that ANS regulation is based on the interaction of subsystems at different time and space scales, acting in coordination and collaboration in order to control a certain variable, in the case that matters here, heart rate and blood pressure variations. This situation, which represents a physiological state, is characterized by a higher complexity, meaning that the system has good chances and flexibility to adapt itself to various stressors. On the contrary, when one of these systems becomes predominant on the others, meaning that this becomes the only system responsible for the regulation of that variable, the complexity of the system declines and the system becomes more rigid and less able to respond to stressor stimuli [8, 9, 14, 18, 31, 36].

It has been proposed that, among a biological signal, complexity and nonlinearity can be related to three main components: first, there are several subsystems which act, with feedback controls, in order to properly react and adapt to stressor stimuli; second, subsystems must adapt when conditions change, for instance, due to a pathological condition; third, in case one of the subsystem fails in control, other subsystems should act in order to compensate it.

Due to this conceptual important background, several different methods have been developed in order to assess nonlinear autonomic control in health and diseases and to evaluate the complexity of autonomic cardiovascular control using ad hoc algorithms. Namely, nonlinear analysis can be grouped into three families: fractal measure, such as power-law correlation and detrended fluctuation analysis, symbolic analysis, and, finally, complexity measures (such as Sample Entropy, Approximate Entropy, Multiscale Entropy, Shannon Entropy, Conditional Entropy, and Corrected Conditional Entropy). Although a mathematical description of these methods is beyond the scope of this chapter, we will briefly describe symbolic analysis, which can now be considered a complementary tool to linear spectral analysis in assessing autonomic cardiovascular control in health and diseases.

5.2.3.3 Symbolic Analysis

Several kinds of symbolic analysis (SA) have been recently proposed and validated for autonomic assessment in physiological and pathological states [13, 31]. Conceptually, compared to classical linear spectral tools, SA has three important advantages: first, it is independent of the a priori frequency band identification of the heart period and blood pressure oscillations. Secondly, SA is reliable in detecting autonomic changes in cases characterized by very low total variability, where classical spectral tools can fail, such as in end-stage congestive heart failure. Finally, while most of the time autonomic control acts as a balance (the so-called sympathovagal balance), it is well known that there are situations that are characterized by a coactivation of the two autonomic branches (such as exercise, diving reflex, specific pathological conditions, etc.) [31].

SA is based on the conversion of a series into sequence of symbols, which are suitable for the identification of sympathetic and parasympathetic control, based on the transformation of time series into a sequence of symbols and then the construction of patterns (i.e., words). The application of different mathematical methods to the distribution of the words allows the identification of complexity of the time series [35, 38, 31]. Porta et al. proposed an SA characterized by three steps, transformation of a time series into short patterns, their classification, and the evaluation of their occurrence. In fact, this SA spreads the full range of sequences over six levels and then constructs short patterns of three beats length. All patterns are then classified by grouping them into four families: 0V family (patterns with no variations), 1V family (patterns with one variation), 2LV family (patterns with two like variations), and 2UV family (patterns with two unlike variations) [31]. The percentage of their rate of occurrence is then calculated.

Experimental data in healthy subjects who underwent different pharmacological and non-pharmacological tests demonstrated that family family 0V is a marker of sympathetic modulation, while 2LV and 2UV families are marker of vagal modulation. Porta and colleagues demonstrated that SA is able to track gradual increase of sympathetic modulation in healthy subjects during graded head-up tilt test and better than classical spectral tools. In addition, in a clinical study, Guzzetti et al. showed that SA is reliable tool to assess autonomic control preceeding sudden cardiac events, such as major arrhythmias in patients with implantable cardioverter defibrillator [13]. Finally, SA was able to identify high-risk patients after acute myocardial infarction [35] and to predict the incidence of major arrhythmias in post-myocardial infarction patients.

Take-Home Messages Autonomic nervous system can be considered as the interface between external and internal stimuli, central nervous system, and effective responses.

- Neural control of cardiovascular function is determined by the reciprocal interaction between sympathetic and parasympathetic control acting as a balance; however, the coactivation of both sympathetic and parasympathetic branches occurs during several conditions.
- Several techniques have been validated for the assessment of autonomic cardiovascular control: (1) urinary and plasmatic catecholamines, (2) direct recording of sympathetic nerve activity using microneurography, and (3) heart rate variability (HRV).
- HRV is a noninvasive, reliable, and reproducible technique able to provide information on autonomic cardiovascular control in health and diseases.
- Frequency domain analysis, such as spectral analysis of HRV, is based on the hypothesis that heart rate and blood pressure rhythmically oscillate around their mean values and that these oscillations are due to the sympathetic and vagal modulation of sinus node function and vascular tree.
- Recently, new nonlinear methods, such as symbolic analysis and entropy-derived measures, have been proposed as tools able to provide complementary information on autonomic control in health and disease.

References

1. Akselrod S, Gordon D, Ubel FA, et al. Power spectrum analysis of heart rate fluctuation: a quantitative probe of beat-to-beat cardiovascular control. Science. 1981;213(4504):220–2.
2. Cechetto DF. Forebrain control of healthy and diseased hearts. In: Armour JA, Aradell JL, editors. Basic and clinical neurocardiology. New York: Oxford University Press; 2004. p. 220–2.
3. Coats AJ, Cruickshank JM. Hypertensive subjects with type-2 diabetes, the sympathetic nervous system, and treatment implications. Int J Cardiol. 2014;174(3):702–9. doi:10.1016/j.ijcard.2014.04.204.
4. Cogliati C, Colombo S, Ruscone TG, et al. Acute beta-blockade increases muscle sympathetic activity and modifies its frequency distribution. Circulation. 2004;110(18):2786–91.
5. Eckberg DL, Nerhed C, Wallin BG. Respiratory modulation of muscle sympathetic and vagal cardiac outflow in man. J Physiol. 1985;365:181–96.

6. Furlan R, Porta A, Costa F, et al. Oscillatory patterns in sympathetic neural discharge and cardiovascular variables during orthostatic stimulus. Circulation. 2000;101(8):886–92.
7. Gerstner W, Kreiter AK, Markram H, et al. Neural codes: firing rates and beyond. Proc Natl Acad Sci U S A. 1997;94(24):12740–1. Review.
8. Goldberger AL, West BJ. Applications of nonlinear dynamics to clinical cardiology. Ann N Y Acad Sci. 1987;504:195–213.
9. Goldberger AL, Rigney DR, Mietus J, et al. Nonlinear dynamics in sudden cardiac death syndrome: heart rate oscillations and bifurcations. Experientia. 1988;44(11–12):983–7.
10. Grassi G, Quarti-Trevano F, Seravalle G, et al. Cardiovascular risk and adrenergic overdrive in the metabolic syndrome. Nutr Metab Cardiovasc Dis. 2007;17(6):473–81. Review.
11. Gulli G, Tarperi C, Cevese A, et al. Effects of prefrontal repetitive transcranial magnetic stimulation on the autonomic regulation of cardiovascular function. Exp Brain Res. 2013;226(2):265–71.
12. Guzzetti S, Piccaluga E, Casati R, et al. Sympathetic predominance in essential hypertension: a study employing spectral analysis of heart rate variability. J Hypertens. 1988;6(9):711–7.
13. Guzzetti S, Borroni E, Garbelli PE, et al. Symbolic dynamics of heart rate variability: a probe to investigate cardiac autonomic modulation. Circulation. 2005;112(4):465–70.
14. Huikuri HV, Exner DV, Kavanagh KM, et al. Attenuated recovery of heart rate turbulence early after myocardial infarction identifies patients at high risk for fatal or near-fatal arrhythmic events. Heart Rhythm. 2010;7(2):229–35.
15. Kleiger RE, Miller JP, Bigger Jr JT, et al. Decreased heart rate variability and its association with increased mortality after acute myocardial infarction. Am J Cardiol. 1987;59(4):256–62.
16. Lee St, Hon Eh. Unusual Variations In The Qrs Complex During Labor. The Fetal Electrocardiogram. IV. Am J Obstet Gynecol. 1965;15(92):1140–8.
17. Lombardi F. Acute myocardial ischemia, neural reflexes and ventricular arrhythmias. Eur Heart J. 1986;7(Suppl A):91–7.
18. Maestri R, Pinna GD, Accardo A, et al. Nonlinear indices of heart rate variability in chronic heart failure patients: redundancy and comparative clinical value. J Cardiovasc Electrophysiol. 2007;18(4):425–33.
19. Malik M, Farrell T, Cripps T, et al. Heart rate variability in relation to prognosis after myocardial infarction: selection of optimal processing techniques. Eur Heart J. 1989;12:1060–74.
20. Malliani A, Montano N. Heart rate variability as a clinical tool. Ital Heart J. 2002;3(8):439–45. Review.
21. Malliani A, Montano N. Emerging excitatory role of cardiovascular sympathetic afferents in pathophysiological conditions. Hypertension. 2002;39(1):63–8.
22. Malliani A, Pagani M, Lombardi F, et al. Cardiovascular neural regulation explored in the frequency domain. Circulation. 1991;84(2):482–92. Review.
23. Montano N, Furlan R, Guzzetti S, et al. Analysis of sympathetic neural discharge in rats and humans. Philos Trans A Math Phys Eng Sci. 2009;367(1892):1265–82.
24. Montano N, Porta A, Cogliati C, et al. Heart rate variability explored in the frequency domain: a tool to investigate the link between heart and behavior. Neurosci Biobehav Rev. 2009;33(2):71–80. doi:10.1016/j.neubiorev.2008.07.006. Epub 2008 Jul 30. Review.
25. Murray A, Ewing DJ, Campbell IW, et al. RR interval variations in young male diabetics. Br Heart J. 1975;37(8):882–5.
26. Narkiewicz K, Somers VK. Sympathetic nerve activity in obstructive sleep apnoea. Acta Physiol Scand. 2003;177(3):385–90. Review.
27. Pagani M, Lucini D. Autonomic dysregulation in essential hypertension: insight from heart rate and arterial pressure variability. Auton Neurosci. 2001;90(1–2):76–82. Review.
28. Pagani M, Lombardi F, Guzzetti S, et al. Power spectral analysis of heart rate and arterial pressure variabilities as a marker of sympatho-vagal interaction in man and conscious dog. Circ Res. 1986;59(2):178–93.
29. Pagani M, Montano N, Porta A, et al. Relationship between spectral components of cardiovascular variabilities and direct measures of muscle sympathetic nerve activity in humans. Circulation. 1997;95(6):1441–8.

30. Paton JF, Nalivaiko E, Boscan P. Reflexly evoked coactivation of cardiac vagal and sympathetic motor outflows: observations and functional implications. Clin Exp Pharmacol Physiol. 2006;33(12):1245–50.
31. Porta A, Gnecchi-Ruscone T, Tobaldini E, et al. Progressive decrease of heart period variability entropy-based complexity during graded head-up tilt. J Appl Physiol. 2007;103(4):1143–9.
32. Task Force of the European Society of Cardiology and the North American Society of Pacing and Electrophysiology. Heart rate variability: standards of measurement, physiological interpretation and clinical use. Circulation. 1996;93(5):1043–65.
33. Thayer JF, Sternberg E. Beyond heart rate variability: vagal regulation of allostatic systems. Ann N Y Acad Sci. 2006;1088:361–72.
34. Tracey KJ. The inflammatory reflex. Nature. 2002;19–26;420(6917):853–9. Review.
35. Voss A, Kurths J, Kleiner HJ, et al. Improved analysis of heart rate variability by methods of nonlinear dynamics. J Electrocardiol. 1995;28(Suppl):81–8.
36. Voss A, Schulz S, Schroeder R, et al. Methods derived from nonlinear dynamics for analysing heart rate variability. Philos Trans A Math Phys Eng Sci. 2009;367(1887):277–96. doi:10.1098/rsta.2008.0232. Review.
37. Wallin BG, Charkoudian N. Sympathetic neural control of integrated cardiovascular function: insights from measurement of human sympathetic nerve activity. Muscle Nerve. 2007;6(5):595–614. Review.
38. Wessel N, Schirdewan A, Malik M, et al. Symbolic dynamics- an independent method for detecting nonlinear phenomena of heart rate regulation. Biomed Tech (Berl). 1998;43(Suppl):510–1.
39. Wolf MM, Varigos GA, Hunt D, et al. Sinus arrhythmia in acute myocardial infarction. Med J Aust. 1978;2(2):52–3.

Autonomic Pathophysiology After Myocardial Infarction Falling into Heart Failure

6

Emilia D'Elia, Paolo Ferrero, Marco Mongillo, and Emilio Vanoli

6.1　Introduction

Why shall we, once more, bother about the pathophysiology of HF? Why shall we wonder if there is anything more that we need to know? Well: shall we wonder why for 30 years we treated HF patients with inotropic agents including beta-adrenergic receptor agonists, increasing mortality, and nowadays, we use beta-blockers? Shall we wonder why we treat the cardiac pandemic with drugs 50 years old? Shall we wonder why in the same time frame needed to go from the first trans-Atlantic flight to the moon landing we have not been able to go beyond the end-organ response to the autonomic storm without even approaching the core of the storm? So many questions are still waiting for an answer!

The mechanisms and pathways of cardiac neurons response to an ischemic insult were described in the 1970s, with direct neural recording, by leading investigators in the field who established specific milestones. Such knowledge was then,

E. D'Elia (✉)
Department of Internal Medicine, University of Pavia, Pavia, Italy
e-mail: edelia@hpg23.it

Department of Cardiology, Papa Giovanni XXIII Hospital, Bergamo, Italy

P. Ferrero
Department of Cardiology, Papa Giovanni XXIII Hospital, Bergamo, Italy

M. Mongillo
Department of Biomedical Science, University of Padova, Padova, Italy

Venetian Institute of Molecular Medicine, University of Padova, Padova, Italy

E. Vanoli
Department of Molecular Medicine, University of Pavia, Pavia, Italy

IRCCS MultiMedica, Sesto S Giovanni, Italy

© Springer International Publishing Switzerland 2016
E. Gronda et al. (eds.), *Heart Failure Management: The Neural Pathways*,
DOI 10.1007/978-3-319-24993-3_6

somehow, neglected and the common perception in the scientific and medical community was that the right intervention to restore the deranged autonomic balance, typical of heart failure, was the restoration of the mechanical function of the heart, with the consequent restoration of the baroreceptorial signal. In other words, the general belief was that, regardless of the incredible neural network innervating the heart at the level of the single myocyte, the key element controlling autonomic balance was some few receptors, outside of the heart! The ATRAMI trial and its precedent experimental background set the stage documenting the baroreceptorial activity was a *marker* and NOT a *mechanism* of the autonomic imbalance accompanying the ischemic heart disease since the very first few seconds of its first manifestation even not perceived by the patient. The central network has then the nucleus of the tractus solitarius (NTS) as a primary relay of the integration and distribution to other centers of the afferent neural information.

Here after a brief summary of the mechanisms often described and reappraised in review articles and chapters will be recalled. After that, novel understanding at the level of the gene control of cardiac innervation and at the level of the neuromuscular junction will be extensively presented.

6.2 The History

The study of the activity of single vagal and sympathetic fibers directed to the heart has clearly described the pathophysiology of this sympathovagal interaction and its implication for arrhythmogenesis [1, 2]. Sympathetic nerves, through β-adrenoceptors, and vagal parasympathetic nerves, through muscarinic acetylcholine (ACh) receptors, are the main regulators of heart rate (HR), with a positive and negative chronotropic effect, respectively [3]. There are regional differences between right and left cardiac nerves [4].

Large experimental evidence describes the facilitatory effects of tonic sympathetic activity on spontaneous ventricular ectopy, and stimulation of the left stellate ganglion (LSG) enhances lethal cardiac arrhythmogenesis during acute myocardial ischemia [5, 6]. A clear sequence of events following coronary occlusion was documented by Heusch et al. in 23 anesthetized dogs [7]: ischemia produced by experimental coronary stenosis increased the activity of sympathetic nerves, leading in turn to poststenotic vasoconstriction and aggravation of ischemia. On the other hand, a bulk of evidence documented over the last decades the potent protective effect of vagal activation on the ischemic heart. High cardiac vagal activity has indeed been shown to be associated with a lower risk for lethal arrhythmia, both in experimental and clinical studies [8, 9]. Neural remodeling process begins in a few minutes/hours after acute coronary occlusion and may lead to denervation, nerve sprouting, and sympathetic hyperinnervation [10]. The first consequence of a transmural myocardial infarction is indeed sympathetic denervation of the surviving tissue distal to the necrotic area [11]. This area might be specifically arrhythmogenic as it displays electrophysiologic super sensitivity resulting in exaggerated refractoriness shortening when exposed to catecholamine perfusion. The postmyocardial infarction (MI) sympathetic re-innervation possibly reflects the neural, structural, and electrophysiologic remodeling after an ischemic insult, and the understanding of the pathophysiology of an MI requires a thorough comprehension of such a mechanism. A critical aspect of this understanding involves the role of autonomic reflexes within seconds of an acute coronary artery occlusion. Such reflexes reflect intrinsic individual characteristics of cardiac innervation and can be predicted by the analysis of the autonomic control of the heart. Furthermore, this individual autonomic profile can affect arrhythmic risk from the first manifestation of the ischemic heart disease [12] through the entire progression of the disease till end-stage heart failure [13].

The neural regeneration process after an ischemic cardiac insult is mainly directed by neurotrophins, among which nerve growth factor (NGF) is the most important. Experimental data in conscious dogs documented that NGF infusion in the LSG induces a significant nerve sprouting (evaluated by the analysis of the tyrosine hydroxylase (TH) and the growth-associated protein 43 (GAP43) markers), leading to excessive expression of cardiac innervations, ventricular fibrillation (VF), and sudden cardiac death (SCD) [14].

An alternative understanding of NGF activation in the ischemic heart has been portrayed by new clinical studies on ischemic heart. They documented that (a) NGF is produced by cardiac myocytes and specific receptors for this neurotrophin, namely, TrkA, have been discovered on the myocytes membrane, (b) NGF has a pleiotropic effect favoring neoangiogenesis and giving protection to the ill myocardium [15]. These observations suggest that the process of cardiac nerve regeneration following a heart attack is useful both to sustain the failing cardiac contractility but, in the meantime, can lead to a higher risk of life-threatening arrhythmias just in the acute phase of the events.

6.3   Physiopathology of the Sympathetic Activation

Sympathetic–parasympathetic interaction plays a major role in the evolution and outcome of many cardiovascular disorders: the study of the activity of single vagal and sympathetic fibers directed to the heart described the main expression of this interaction some 40 years ago. The nerve regeneration process is mainly activated by neurotrophins, among which nerve growth factor (NGF) has a major role. In the setting of myocardial infarction, myocytes die in the ischemic heart region and sympathetic neurons start a sort of regeneration process called nerve sprouting, able to increase innervation density around the damaged area. In this framework, it is reasonable to assume that NGF arises after a heart attack and its increase drives a regeneration process of the sympathetic nerves [16]. Moreover, experimental data in conscious dogs documented that NGF infusion in the left stellate ganglion (LSG) induces significant nerve regeneration, as shown by increased tyrosine hydroxylase (TH) and GAP 13 protein, a marker of nerve sprouting [17, 18]. The most important observation from these studies is the evidence that this excessive expression of cardiac innervation is directly associated to ventricular fibrillation (VF) and sudden cardiac death (SCD). Consequently, the sympathetic hyperactivity generated by a heart attack could be due not only to an increase in nerve firing but also to an anatomic increase of the sympathetic nerve fiber density induced by the ischemia-dependent NGF expression.

6.4 Nerve Sprouting After Myocardial Injury

The role of autonomic responses to cardiac insults had been firstly investigated in experimental models of myocardial ischemia (MI), documenting the antiarrhythmic effect of sympathetic denervation. After experimental coronary occlusion, survival mostly depended on the predominance of the profibrillatory action of sympathetic activity or the protective action of vagal activation [19]. Functional and anatomical autonomic remodeling after MI has impact both on the cardiac remodeling (CR) causing left ventricle (LV) dysfunction and on the cardiac arrhythmic circuits causing potential fatal events. CR after a heart attack is accompanied by a sprouting of cardiac nerves under the stimulus of NGF. NGF exists mainly in peripheral sympathetic and sensory nerves and in tissues receiving innervation from those nerves, including the cardiac atrium, ventricles, and coronary arteries. NGF is necessary for the survival of sympathetic ganglionic neurons, including the ones innervating the heart. Experimental evidence documents elevated tissue and plasma NGF levels early after an MI. On the other hand, the nerve density of the failing heart tends to progressively decrease with heart dysfunction worsening, and this is a potential consequence of NGF inhibition by high catecholamine levels [20].

6.5 NGF Changes following an Ischemic Injury: From Short-Term to Long-Term Events

As mentioned, NGF is expressed in the heart and other sympathetic targets and its presence correlates with the density of sympathetic innervation. The amount of NGF may affect the sympathetic nerve survival and synaptic transmission between neurons and cardiac myocytes [21]. In line with this concept, it was initially documented that NGF was able to enhance cardiac reinnervation of surgically denervated canine heart. Later on, in a dog model of MI, it was found that both NGF protein and mRNA levels increased at the infarcted site and at the non-infarcted LV free wall. Specifically, this increase occurred earlier and was more pronounced at the infarcted site, where NGF protein was significantly higher after 3.5 h, while NGF mRNA rose within 3 days of MI induction. Interestingly, transcardiac NGF concentration (difference in NGF concentration between coronary sinus and aorta) increased immediately after MI, before a detectable elevation of cardiac NGF mRNA. This suggests that there is a prompt NGF transcardiac peak as the result of a cardiac release, probably from damaged cells, which is followed by a local NGF production. Overall, data obtained from both mouse and canine models of MI point out that MI causes, within a short time, a diffuse upregulation of NGF in the myocardium that is more pronounced in the area adjacent to the injury.

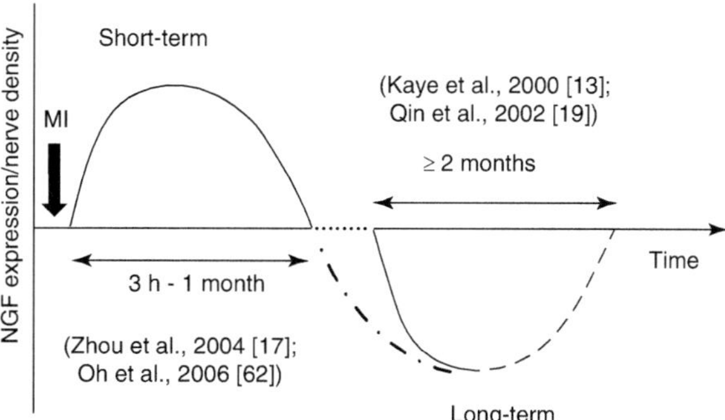

Fig. 6.1 A scheme of short- and long-term changes in NGF expression and nerve density in animal models of myocardial injury (Reproduced with permission from Govoni et al. [16])

It should be emphasized that the observed increase in NGF expression occurs within a short time following MI, while afterward its levels decline progressively. In fact, Kaye et al. [15] documented a significant reduction in NGF production 8 weeks after the induction of heart failure by coronary artery ligation in Sprague–Dawley rats. Similar to these results, another study demonstrated that dogs infused for 8 weeks with noradrenaline showed a decrease in NGF and TrKA both at mRNA and protein levels [22]. Thereby, the decrease in NGF expression may represent an adaptive response to prolonged exposure to a high sympathetic tone, finally entailing a reduction in sympathetic innervation density. This presumption may help to explain the paradoxical observation of a diminished sympathetic innervation density in the failing heart, despite an increased catecholamine overflow (Fig. 6.1).

6.6   From Acute Myocardial Injury to Chronic Heart Failure through Cardiac Remodeling

As already reported before, experimental evidence demonstrated a progressive decrease of NGF plasma level in rats 8 weeks after a coronary occlusion, following a prolonged catecholamine effect in an advanced heart failure [23]. Similarly, prolonged infusion of noradrenaline in rats is associated to a reduction of NGF and of its receptor TrkA, following a decrease in mRNA transcription [24] (Fig. 6.2). It seems that sympathetic cardiac innervation is firmly regulated by NGF expression and prolonged exposure to high catecholamines, as it happen in advanced heart failure (HF), may induce a reduction of NGF and a consequent decrease in sympathetic fibers density. Several studies also demonstrated that high catecholamine levels reduce metaiodobenzylguanidine (MIBG) uptake in HF, according to two possible mechanisms [25]. The former one implies a competitive reaction between high noradrenaline and MIGB reuptake. The latter one, much more reliable, implies a real cardiac denervation as a cause of a reduced MIGB reuptake. It is reasonable to hypothesize that sympathetic functional denervation comes along with anatomic denervation, which can be seen only in an advanced HF stage after a prolonged catecholamine expression. The negative prognostic value of a depressed MIBG reuptake in patients

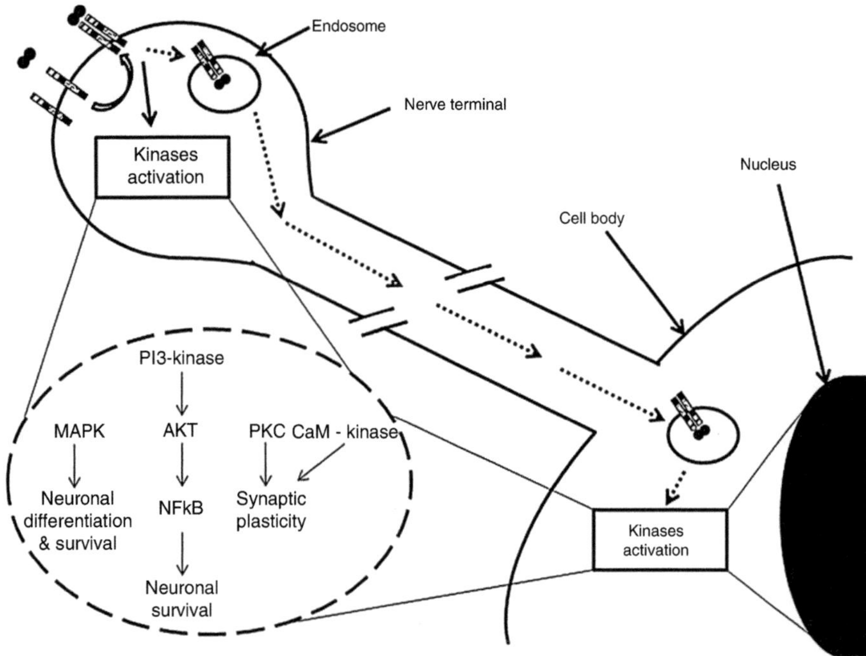

Fig. 6.2 Molecular events following NGF interaction with TrkA receptor in nerve terminals, possibly leading to neuronal remodeling (Reproduced with permission from Govoni et al. [16])

with HF has been clearly documented by the ADMIRE HF study [26]. In this study indeed a depressed MIBG reuptake identified patients at higher arrhythmic risk and/or at higher risk of an unfavorable progression of the disease.

Recent studies stressed the evidence of NGF expression on cardiac myocytes. Meloni et al. [16] observed NGF and TrkA expression on hearts affected by a recent fatal myocardial infarction: NGF was found in cardiomyocytes, and both cardiomyocytes and endothelial cell express TrkA. In the same experimental research, antibodies anti-NGF used in infarcted rats' hearts cause a lower angiogenesis, an increased apoptosis, and a worsened cardiac function. On the contrary, genetic NGF stimulation improved endothelial cell survival rate and promoted angiogenesis, ameliorating cardiac function 14 days after a heart attack.

In the complex system of neurohormonal interactions discussed above, NGF seems to have a protective role on the ischemic and failing heart, causing maybe also a paradox dangerous effect by increasing too much sympathetic innervation. The key factor to understand this process might involve heterogeneous NGF expression leading to adjacent areas of hyper and hyposympathetic innervation. This anatomical heterogeneity would result and in a marked increase in electrical inhomogeneity at the time of a sudden rise in sympathetic discharge to the heart.

To this last regard, we can speculate that molecules able to positively modulate NGF expression, as already described for other genes, may represent a novel pharmacological strategy that can contribute to counteract some of the negative effects associated with NGF decline and potentially favor cardiac repair after an acute ischemic insult. Conversely, molecules able to reduce NGF expression might be useful to prevent the nerve-sprouting phenomenon, occurring just after MI, which seems involved in the genesis of arrhythmias [27].

6.7   Molecular Pathophysiology of Cardiac Sympathetic Innervation

The extent of myocardial innervation by autonomic neurons is often overlooked when discussing the role of the adrenergic system in cardiac biology or pathology. As discussed above, both the atria and ventricles are densely innervated by sympathetic and parasympathetic autonomic neurons; in the normal heart, sympathetic neurons spread throughout the different regions of the heart with a well-defined distribution pattern. Myocardial innervation depends on a number of factors released by cardiomyocytes, cardiac fibroblasts, and endothelial cells that include neurotrophins such as NGF, neurotrophin-3, and endothelin-1 (ET-1) [28–30]. In addition to such molecules sustaining neuron growth and viability, chemorepulsive factors of the semaphorin family, like Sema3, are secreted by cardiac cells and participate to the guidance of sympathetic axons throughout the myocardium [31]. In the mouse heart, a transmural distribution pattern is established with higher neuronal density in the subepicardial than in the subendocardial areas, and in Sema3a-knockout mice, the failure to develop the correct innervation pattern increased arrhythmic propensity [32]. The balance between neuron-attractant and neuron-repellent factors released by myocardial cells finely shapes the density of sympathetic innervation throughout the cardiac walls. As described above, remodeling of cardiac sympathetic innervation is determinant in the pathogenesis of heart failure following ischemic damage. The neurotrophic factor GDNF (glial cell line-derived neurotrophic factor) was able to increase cardiac innervation in vivo in rats after cardiac cryoinjury and counteracted the progress to HF [33]. This extends the observations of earlier work, in which direct NGF injection into the stellate ganglia neurons was able to increase the function of sympathetic innervation, NE reuptake, and improve cardiac function in an animal model of HF [34], and conversely, genetic knockdown of the NGF gene leads to worsened prognosis after myocardial infarction, due to reduced sympathetic innervation and angiogenesis [35].

The fine architecture of the cardiac neuronal network was recently described using 3-D reconstruction of the distribution of GFP+ cardiac neurons in the intact heart of DBH-GFP mice [36]. When observed at high resolution with methods highlighting adrenergic neurons, axonal "varicosities" can be observed with regular distribution along the neuronal processes (Mongillo M 2015, unpublished). These structures, which represent neuronal sites enriched in secretory vesicles containing noradrenaline and other sympathetic neurotransmitters [37], are found close to the cardiomyocyte sarcolemma, with variable frequency in the different heart regions (Mongillo M 2015, unpublished). Evidence from in vitro models based on sympathetic neurons and cardiomyocyte cocultures demonstrates that direct interaction of the two cell types occurs at specific contact sites and is accompanied by specialization in the cardiomyocyte "postsynaptic" membrane in which β-adrenergic receptors (ARs), together with adaptor/scaffold proteins and intercellular contact proteins, are all specifically enriched [38]. Although with much less definition from the morphological and biochemical standpoint, the interaction site between sympathetic neurons and cardiomyocytes shares features of the well-known neuromuscular junction [39]. The hypothesis of cardiac synapses has been proposed by many authors in the last four decades. It has been suggested that such specific junctions would increase the efficiency of activation of cardiomyocyte b-AR by neuronally released noradrenaline, a requisite for the rapid activation of the cardiac inotropic and chronotropic effects of the *fight-or-flight* response [40].

Although the details on molecular signaling by beta-adrenergic receptors have been obtained using isolated or cultured cardiomyocytes, it is worth considering them in the context of the cell–cell interaction between sympathetic neurons and cardiomyocytes.

The adrenergic receptor system mediates cardiac responses to the release of catecholamines by the sympathetic neurons. Cardiomyocyte β-1 and β-2 adrenergic receptors (βARs) couple to the activation of cyclic adenosine monophosphate (cAMP) that, mainly through activation of protein kinase A and EPAC [41], operate the increase in rate and force of contraction of the heart. Studies performed in isolated cardiac myocytes showed that the subtype-specific stimulation of the two b-AR isoforms activates a distinct pattern of intracellular downstream targets, with different effects on cardiomyocyte function [42]. While β-1 selective activation exerts potent inotropic and lusitropic effects, β-2 AR have only a minor effect on contractility and fail to enhance relaxation [43]. Furthermore, chronic β-1 AR stimulation caused cardiomyocyte apoptosis [44], and its overexpression in transgenic mice leads to progressive hypertrophy and heart failure [45], while β2AR stimulation showed anti-apoptotic effect [46]. Although both b1 and b2 AR lead to cAMP synthesis, their singular effect has mostly been attributed to partitioning of the receptors on the cell membrane and to the restriction of cAMP diffusion in distinct intracellular compartments [47, 48], where the target effector proteins (e.g., ion channels, SERCa pumps, ryanodine receptors) are localized [49, 15].

Interestingly, direct intercellular contact might also be involved in retrograde cardiomyocyte-to-neuron signaling mediated by neurotrophins. Reduced efficiency of neurocardiac communication, due to alterations in the specific contact structures, would therefore result in decreased activation of b-AR, noradrenaline spillover in the myocardial interstitium, and depletion of noradrenaline stores, all of which are features commonly appreciated in failing hearts [50]. In addition, it would decrease the trophic input to cardiac neurons, which may result, with time, in denervation, also commonly observed in failing hearts [51].

In addition to the role in the acute control over heart rate and contractility, cardiac sympathetic neurons have a role in the regulation of fundamental homeostatic mechanisms in cardiomyocytes. The expression level of the major cardiac ubiquitin ligases, namely, MuRF1 and Atrogin-1 [52], key mediators of the cardiomyocyte ubiquitin–proteasome system, is negatively controlled by b2-AR activation, through PI3K/Akt modulation of the FOXO family of transcription factors [53, 54]. Consistently, selective stimulation of b2-AR causes cardiac hypertrophy, while its inhibition by either receptor antagonists or removal of neuronal input with cardiac sympathetic denervation leads to atrophic remodeling in rodent and rabbit hearts [55]. Interestingly, UPS targets directly regulated by adrenergic receptors including signaling elements involved in the degradation of cAMP, like phosphodiesterases [56] as well as cardiac proteins determinant for cellular coupling and electrophysiology, including Connexin43 [57].

In addition to the pharmacological inhibition of beta-AR, direct modulation of cardiac autonomic nerves has also received considerable attention. Experimental therapies aimed at the shift in autonomic balance toward reduced sympathetic drive and increased vagal activity have been obtained in several ways including pharmacological approaches [58, 59] and direct electrical stimulation. In rats, electrical stimulation of the ear endings and the brainstem exerts an antiarrhythmic effect. Similar results were obtained with electrical stimulation of carotid baroreceptors, which also leads to sympathetic inhibition; chronic vagal stimulation, as elicited by a surgically implantable stimulator [60], has been shown to produce a significant drop in systemic pressure and is currently in clinical trials in drug-resistant hypertension [61]. Given the abundance of data demonstrating the arrhythmogenic potential of sympathetic activity, it seems obvious that the prevention of life-threatening events in patients at high risk of developing VT/VF may represent another clinical application of cardiac sympathetic nerve modulation. To date, however, experimental studies have not adequately addressed this issue.

Conclusions

The autonomic nervous system responds within seconds to any even minimal cardiac insult. The level of autonomic response might be, in several instances, exaggerated with detrimental consequences of cardiac negative remodeling during and after acute myocardial ischemia. The key issue here is that *autonomic responses are the cause* and not the consequence of the negative cardiac remodeling (Fig. 6.3). The understanding of the autonomic pathophysiology had eventually critical clinical consequences when, after 25 years of denial toward the use of them, beta-blockers became first-line therapy in heart failure. This understanding needs to be fully appreciated at time like today when the available therapy seems to be unable to further meet the growing challenge of heart failure and direct nerve modulation represents the new hope for such a challenge.

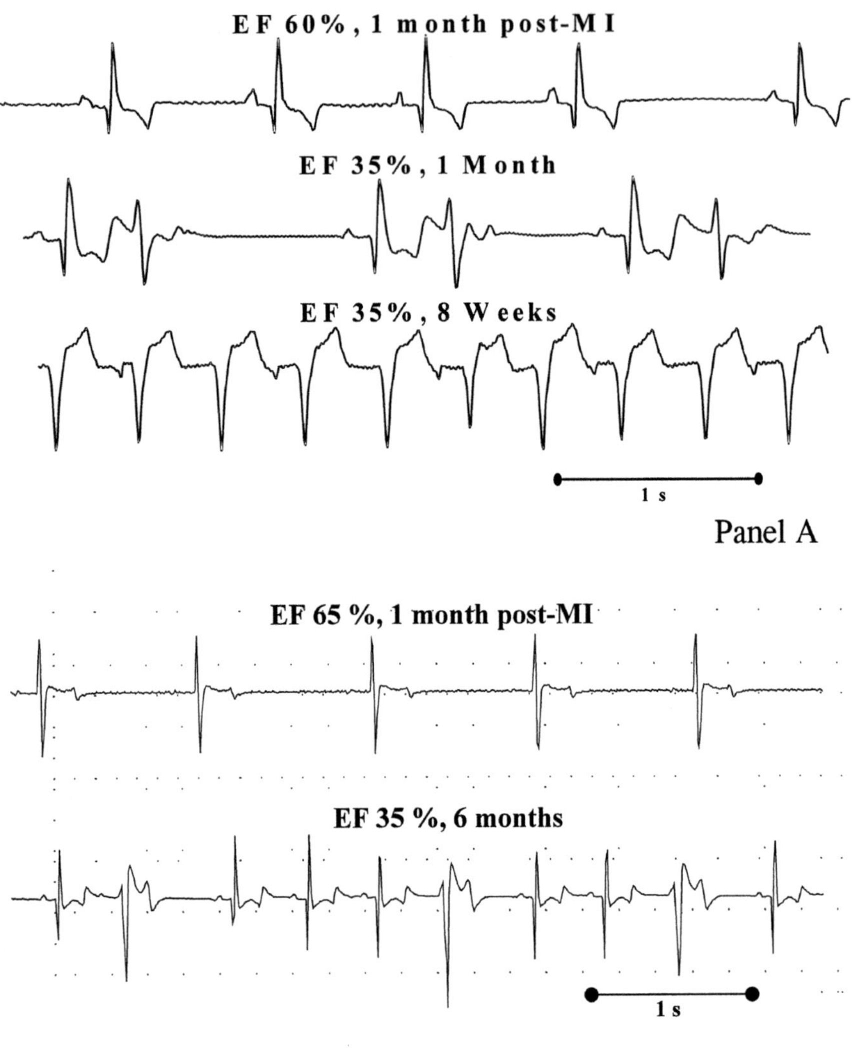

Fig. 6.3 Spontaneous arrhythmias in conscious dogs with a healed anterior MI and circumflex ischemia-dependent progression of left ventricular dysfunction at high and low risk for sudden death. In panel (**a**) the rapid occurrence of a fatal ventricular tachyarrhythmia in dogs with a depressed vagal control of heart rate is shown. In panel (**b**) the arrhythmia pattern in a dog with analogous cardiac damage but with preserved vagal reflexes is shown. The level of reflex vagal control determines the fatal or nonfatal consequence of a chronic ischemic LV dysfunction (Reproduced with permission from Adamson and Vanoli [13])

References

1. Schwartz PJ, De Ferrari GM. Sympathetic-parasympathetic interaction in health and disease: abnormalities and relevance in heart failure. Heart Fail Rev. 2011;16:101–7.
2. Fukuda K, Kanazawa H, Aizawa Y, Ardell JF, Shivkumar K. Cardiac innervation and sudden cardiac death. Circ Res. 2015;116:2005–19.
3. Berg T, Jensen J. Simultaneous parasympathetic and sympathetic activation reveals altered autonomic control of heart rate, vascular tension, and epinephrine release in anesthetized hypertensive rats. Front Neurol. 2011;2:71.
4. Zaza A, Malfatto G, Schwartz PJ. Sympathetic modulation of the relation between ventricular repolarization and cycle length. Circ Res. 1991;68:1191–203.
5. Harris AS. Delayed development of ventricular ectopic rhythms following experimental coronary occlusion. Circulation. 1950;1:1318–28.
6. Schwartz PJ, La Rovere MT, Vanoli E. Autonomic nervous system and sudden cardiac death. Experimental basis and clinical observations for post-myocardial infarction risk stratification. Circulation. 1992;85:I77–91.
7. Heusch G, Deussen A, Thamer V. Cardiac sympathetic nerve activity and progressive vasoconstriction distal to coronary stenoses: feed-back aggravation of myocardial ischemia. J Auton Nerv Syst. 1985;13:311–26.
8. Vanoli E, De Ferrari GM, Stramba Badiale M, et al. Vagal stimulation and prevention of sudden death in conscious dogs with a healed myocardial infarction. Circ Res. 1991;68:1471–81.
9. La Rovere MT, Bigger Jr JT, Marcus FI, et al. Baroreflex sensitivity and heart-rate variability in prediction of total cardiac mortality after myocardial infarction. ATRAMI (Autonomic Tone and Reflexes After Myocardial Infarction) Investigators. Lancet. 1998;351:478–84.
10. Chen PS, Chen LS, Cao JM, et al. Sympathetic nerve sprouting, electrical remodeling and the mechanisms of sudden cardiac death. Cardiovasc Res. 2001;50:409–16.
11. Barber MJ, Mueller TM, Henry DP, et al. Transmural myocardial infarction in the dog produces sympathectomy in noninfarcted myocardium. Circulation. 1983;67:787–96.
12. Vanoli E, Adamson PB, Hull Jr SS, et al. Prediction of unexpected sudden death among healthy dogs by a novel marker of autonomic neural activity. Heart Rhythm. 2008;5:300–5.
13. Adamson PB, Vanoli E. Early autonomic and repolarization abnormalities contribute to lethal arrhythmias in chronic ischemic heart failure: characteristics of a novel heart failure model in dogs with postmyocardial infarction left ventricular dysfunction. J Am Coll Cardiol. 2001;17:1471–8.
14. Kaye DM, Vaddadi G, Gruskin SL, et al. Reduced myocardial nerve growth factor expression in human and experimental heart failure. Circ Res. 2000;86:80–8.
15. Meloni M, Caporali A, Graiani G, et al. Nerve growth factor promotes repair following myocardial infarction. Circ Res. 2010;106:1275–84.
16. Govoni S, Pascale A, Amadio ML, et al. NGF and heart: is there a role in heart disease? Pharmacol Res. 2011;4:266–77.
17. Stramba-Badiale M, Vanoli E, De Ferrari GM, et al. Sympathetic-parasympathetic interaction and accentuated antagonism in conscious dogs. Am J Physiol. 1991;260:335–40.
18. Zhou S, Chen LS, Miyauchi Y, et al. Mechanisms of cardiac nerve sprouting after myocardial infarction in dogs. Circ Res. 2004;95:76–83.
19. Schwartz PJ, Billmann GE, Stone HL. Autonomic mechanisms in ventricular fibrillation induced by myocardial ischemia during exercise in dogs with a healed myocardial infarction. An experimental preparation for sudden cardiac death. Circulation. 1964;69:790–800.
20. Qin F, Vulapalli RS, Stevens SY, et al. Loss of cardiac sympathetic neurotransmitters in heart failure and NE infusion is associated with reduced NGF. Am J Physiol Heart Circ Physiol. 2002;282:363–71.
21. Lockhart ST, Turrigiano GG, Birren SJ. Nerve growth factor modulates synaptic transmission between sympathetic neurons and cardiac myocytes. J Neurosci. 1997;17:573–82.
22. Cao JM, Chen LS, KenKnight BH. Nerve sprouting and sudden cardiac death. Circ Res. 2000;86:816–21.

23. Kimura K, Kanazawa H, Ieda M. Norepinephrine-induced nerve growth factor depletion causes cardiac sympathetic denervation in severe heart failure. Auton Neurosci. 2010;156:27–35.
24. Hasan W, Smith PG. Decreased adrenoceptor stimulation in heart failure rats reduces NGF expression by cardiac parasympathetic neurons. Auton Neurosci. 2014;181:13–20.
25. Haider N, Bailiga RR, Chandrashekhar Y, et al. Adrenergic excess, hNET1 down-regulation, and compromised mIBG uptake in heart failure poverty in the presence of plenty. J Am Coll Cardiol. 2010;3:71–5.
26. Jacobson HF, Senior R, Cerquiera MD, et al. Myocardial iodine-123 meta-iodobenzylguanidine imaging and cardiac events in heart failure. Results of the prospective ADMIRE-HF (AdreView Myocardial Imaging for Risk Evaluation in Heart Failure) study. J Am Coll Cardiol. 2010;55:212–21.
27. D'Elia E, Pascale A, Marchesi N, et al. Novel approaches to the post-myocardial infarction/heart failure neural remodeling. Heart Fail Rev. 2014;19:611–9.
28. Glebova NO, Ginty DD. Heterogeneous requirement of NGF for sympathetic target innervation in vivo. J Neurosci. 2004;24:743–51.
29. Francis N, Farinas I, Brennan T, et al. NT-3, like NGF, is required for survival of sympathetic neurons, but not their precursors. Dev Biol. 1999;210:411–27.
30. Lehmann LH, Stanmore DA, Backs J. The role of endothelin-1 in the sympathetic nervous system in the heart. Life Sci. 2014;118:165–72.
31. Ieda M, Kanazawa H, Ieda Y, et al. Nerve growth factor is critical for cardiac sensory innervation and rescues neuropathy in diabetic hearts. Circulation. 2006;114:2351–63.
32. Ieda M, Kanazawa H, Kimura K, et al. Sema3a maintains normal heart rhythm through sympathetic innervation patterning. Nat Med. 2007;13:604–12.
33. Miwa K, Lee JK, Takagishi Y, et al. Axon guidance of sympathetic neurons to cardiomyocytes by glial cell line-derived neurotrophic factor (GDNF). PLos One. 2013;8:e65202.
34. Kreusser MM, Haass M, Buss SJ, et al. Injection of nerve growth factor into stellate ganglia improves norepinephrine reuptake into failing hearts. Hypertension. 2006;47:209–14.
35. Hu H, Xuan Y, Wang Y, et al. Targeted NGF siRNA delivery attenuates sympathetic nerve sprouting and deteriorates cardiac dysfunction in rats with myocardial infarction. PLoS One. 2014;9, e95106.
36. Freeman J, Vladimirov N, Kawashima T. Mapping brain activity at scale with cluster computing. J Neurosci Methods. 2014;11:941–50.
37. Landis SC. Rat sympathetic neurons and cardiac myocytes developing in microcultures: correlation of the fine structure of endings with neurotransmitter function in single neurons. Proc Natl Acad Sci U S A. 1976;73:4220–4.
38. Shcherbakova OG, Hurt CM, Xiang Y, et al. Organization of beta-adrenoceptor signaling compartments by sympathetic innervation of cardiac myocytes. J Cell Biol. 2007;176:521–33.
39. Ohlendieck K, Ervast JM, Matsumura K, et al. Dystrophin-related protein is localized to neuromuscular junctions of adult skeletal muscle. Neuron. 1991;7:499–508.
40. Gorelik J, Wright PT, Lyon AR, et al. Spatial control of the βAR system in heart failure: the transverse tubule and beyond. Circ Res. 2013;98:213–24.
41. Kuschel M, Zhou YY, Cheng H. G(i) protein-mediated functional compartmentalization of cardiac beta(2)-adrenergic signaling. J Biol Chem. 1999;274:22048–52.
42. Rohrer DK, Chruscinski A, Schauble EH, et al. Cardiovascular and metabolic alterations in mice lacking both beta1- and beta2-adrenergic receptors. J Biol Chem. 1999;274:16701–8.
43. Communal C, Singh K, Sawer DB, et al. Opposing effects of beta(1)- and beta(2)-adrenergic receptors on cardiac myocyte apoptosis : role of a pertussis toxin-sensitive G protein. Circulation. 1999;100:2210–2.
44. Engelhardt S, Hein L, Wiesmann F. Progressive hypertrophy and heart failure in beta1-adrenergic receptor transgenic mice. Proc Natl Acad Sci U S A. 1999;96:7059–64.
45. Zhu WZ, Zheng M, Koch WJ, et al. Dual modulation of cell survival and cell death by beta(2)-adrenergic signaling in adult mouse cardiac myocytes. Proc Natl Acad Sci U S A. 2001;98:1607–12.

46. Buxton IL, Brunton LL. Compartments of cyclic AMP and protein kinase in mammalian cardiomyocytes. J Biol Chem. 1983;258:10233–9.
47. Jurevicious J, Fischmeister R. cAMP compartmentation is responsible for a local activation of cardiac Ca2+ channels by beta-adrenergic agonists. Proc Natl Acad Sci U S A. 1996;93: 295–9.
48. Nikolaev VO, Bünemann M, Schmitteckert E, et al. Cyclic AMP imaging in adult cardiac myocytes reveals far-reaching beta1-adrenergic but locally confined beta2-adrenergic receptor-mediated signaling. Circ Res. 2006;99:1084–91.
49. Zaccolo M, Pozzan T. Discrete microdomains with high concentration of cAMP in stimulated rat neonatal cardiac myocytes. Science. 2002;295:1711–5.
50. Centner T, Yano J, Kimura E, et al. Identification of muscle specific ring finger proteins as potential regulators of the titin kinase domain. J Mol Biol. 2001;306:717–26.
51. Bodine SC, Latres E, Baumhueter S, et al. Identification of ubiquitin ligases required for skeletal muscle atrophy. Science. 2001;294:1704–8.
52. Sandri M, Sandri C, Gilbert A, et al. Foxo transcription factors induce the atrophy-related ubiquitin ligase atrogin-1 and cause skeletal muscle atrophy. Cell. 2004;117:399–412.
53. Zhang W, Yano N, Deng M, et al. β-Adrenergic receptor-PI3K signaling crosstalk in mouse heart: elucidation of immediate downstream signaling cascades. PLoS One. 2001;6:e26581.
54. Zaglia T, Milan G, Franzoso M, et al. Cardiac sympathetic neurons provide trophic signal to the heart via β2-adrenoceptor-dependent regulation of proteolysis. Cardiovasc Res. 2013;97:240–50.
55. Li X, Baillie GS, Houslay MD. Mdm2 directs the ubiquitination of beta-arrestin-sequestered cAMP phosphodiesterase-4D5. J Biol Chem. 2009;284:16170–82.
56. Mollerup S, Hofgaard JP, Braunstein TH, et al. Norepinephrine inhibits intercellular coupling in rat cardiomyocytes by ubiquitination of connexin43 gap junctions. Cell Commun Adhes. 2011;18:57–65.
57. La Rovere MT, Pinna GD, Maestri R, et al. Prognostic implications of baroreflex sensitivity in heart failure patients in the beta-blocking era. J Am Coll Cardiol. 2009;53:193–9.
58. La Rovere MT, De Ferrari GM. New potential uses for transdermal scopolamine (hyoscine). Drugs. 1995;50:769–76.
59. Tordoir JH, Scheffers I, Schmidli J, et al. An implantable carotid sinus baroreflex activating system: surgical technique and short-term outcome from a multi-center feasibility trial for the treatment of resistant hypertension. Eur J Endovasc Surg. 2007;33:414–21.
60. Lohmeier TE, Irwin ED, Rossing MA, et al. Prolonged activation of the baroreflex produces sustained hypotension. Hypertension. 2004;43:306–11.
61. Scheffers IJ, Kroon AA, Schmidli J, et al. Novel baroreflex activation therapy in resistant hypertension: results of a European multi-center feasibility study. J Am Coll Cardiol. 2010;56:1254–8.
62. Oh YS, Jong AY, Kim DT et al. Spatial distribution of nerve sprouting after myocardial infarction in mice. Heart Rhythm 2006;3:728–36

Cardiovascular Serenade: Listening to the Heart

Philip B. Adamson and Emilia D'Elia

7.1 Introduction

Cardiovascular control systems are designed to maintain systemic perfusion of vital organs to ensure survival, adapting to remarkable challenges with instantaneous changes in response to external and internal stimuli. Human survival relies on the heart and vasculature to provide blood flow to key body systems to quickly escape, exercise, or sleep. Cardiovascular control is mediated through a series of complex interactive neural and hormonal events that respond to sensed needs of the body. Understanding cardiovascular physiology from the control system's perspective is hypothesized to be a window into the clinical status of the human being [1]. Predictable control system changes occur when disease chronically or acutely changes any of the organ systems, such as heart failure (HF) [2–7].

In the advent of implantable electronic devices designed to treat certain cardiac rhythm disorders or "correct" conduction system disease, the concept emerged that collecting information sensed by implanted devices may provide a means to either continuously or frequently monitor control systems activity, thus providing potentially important clinical information. This concept was first tested using measurements of heart rate variability (HRV) measured from an implanted cardiac resynchronization device (CRT) in the Multicenter InSync Randomized Clinical Evaluation (MIRACLE) trial [8] and, subsequently, in the InSync II trials. These

P.B. Adamson, MD, MSc, FACC (✉)
Department of Physiology, University of Oklahoma Health Sciences Center,
Oklahoma City, OK, USA

Global Research and Development, St. Jude Medical, Inc.,
6300 Bee Cave Road, Austin, TX 78738, USA
e-mail: PAdamson02@sjm.com

E. D'Elia, MD
Cardiovascular Department, Hospital Papa Giovanni XXIII, Bergamo, Italy

Internal Medicine Department, Pavia University, Pavia, Italy

© Springer International Publishing Switzerland 2016
E. Gronda et al. (eds.), *Heart Failure Management: The Neural Pathways*,
DOI 10.1007/978-3-319-24993-3_7

studies demonstrated that continuously measured HRV reflected a shift in cardiac neural control toward increased vagal and decreased sympathetic influence with the application of CRT [9]. Patients with chronically low values or declining HRV, suggesting cardiac autonomic shifts toward sympathetic dominance and vagal withdrawal, were at high risk for impending hospitalization [10].

Subsequent studies demonstrated value in measuring a variety of cardiac parameters including atrial fibrillation burden, episodes of ventricular arrhythmia, percentage of ventricular or atrial pacing, activity, or intrathoracic impedance [11]. The theoretical advantage to these measurements is that they are continuously measured and can be remotely monitored, allowing the clinician to monitor patients in their own environment, supplementing face-to-face encounters.

The purpose of this review is to outline the physiologic information available for remote monitoring of patients with heart disease, in particular patients with HF who represent the most studied group with implanted electronic devices. The evolution of this concept led to development of permanently implanted sensors that provide actionable information used to remotely guide clinical decision making. The future of such technology is significant with applications that may incorporate typical commercial devices, such as "smart" phones or other monitors commonly used in modern society. An exciting ongoing story can be heard when listening to the heart transcends simple auscultation.

7.2 Heart Rate Variability

Inter-beat variability of heart rate is determined predominately by parasympathetic efferent activity synchronized with respiration rate [12, 13]. Increased parasympathetic activity slows the spontaneous depolarization rate characteristic of the pacemaker current (I_f) in the sinoatrial (SA) node, thus increasing the interval between atrial depolarizations and slowing heart rate. The parasympathetic nervous system influences heart rate at a relatively high frequency intending to alter filling and output in concert with respiration rates. Low-frequency variability (0.1–0.25 Hz) is mostly mediated through neural and hormonal sympathetic effect [12]. Other influences on HRV include ultralow-frequency events, mostly mediated by body temperature and other basal metabolic inputs. Overall HRV is the result of interactions between all these influences resulting in a finely tuned regulated cardiovascular system. More variability in SA nodal depolarization reflects stronger parasympathetic effect, while less variability heart rates usually arise from vagal withdrawal. Concomitant increases in sympathetic end-organ effect are usually associated with lower HRV values. Low HRV sometimes can be associated with "saturation" in conditions in which cardiac vagal effect is very strong, such as in distance trained athletes.

Traditionally, HRV was calculated from surface ECG signals using RR intervals to calculate variability in both "time domain" and "frequency domain" [12]. This approach required sophisticated extraction and concatenation formulae intended to exclude beats that were not generated by SA nodal depolarization, such as premature atrial or ventricular beats. These ectopic beats are thought not to reflect cardiac autonomic control and were excluded from analysis. RR interval measurements of

HRV were also limited by signal acquisition time, usually 24–48 h. Another limitation of RR interval variability measurements was that it only considered electrical events that passed the AV node causing ventricular depolarization. Finally, HRV is not informative in patients with chronic or persistent atrial fibrillation. In fact, most algorithms require at least 25 % of the sensed time to be sinus rhythm. Therefore, HRV measurements in patients with very frequent atrial or ventricular ectopy are usually invalid.

Some of these limitations were addressed in patients with implanted electronic devices such as pacemakers, biventricular pacemakers, or implantable cardioverter defibrillators (ICD) by using electrical signals sensed by the atrial lead. This approach has the advantage of continuous monitoring which dramatically increases the sample size of the sensed signals which minimizes the impact of ectopic beats [12].

The first device-based HRV calculation used the median heart rate sensed from 5-min bins of heart rate [9]. The median atrial-atrial (a-a) depolarization intervals from the 5-min bins were then used to calculate standard deviation of the median a-a interval over the entire 24 h (from midnight to midnight). The daily HRV measurement was then assessed as the standard deviation of the a-a interval (SDAAM) and expressed in ms. This HRV measurement was compared in the MIRACLE trial between patients randomized to CRT on vs. those with CRT off. HRV values were not different at baseline between the groups, but were significantly higher in the CRT-on group after 6 months of therapy. Tthis led to the conclusion that correction of interventricular conduction delay in patients with advanced HF syndromes improved cardiac autonomic control by reducing sympathetic input and improving parasympathetic effect.

The second major study of HRV from implanted devices asked two specific questions [10]. First, do basal HRV levels reflect clinical stability/instability in patients with HF receiving CRT and thereby predict long-term event rate, such as hospitalizations? The second hypothesis tested was that both vagal withdrawal and sympathetic activation should occur (i.e., declining HRV value) as HF patients decline in clinical status leading to a decompensated state and hospitalization. Both hypotheses were retrospectively evaluated in a prospectively obtained database from the InSync III registry involving 288 patients with information available for analysis. Patients with persistently low SDAAM measurements (<50 ms) were at 3.2 times higher risk for mortality ($p=0.02$) and had higher hospitalization rates compared to those with higher HRV values (Fig. 7.1). Furthermore, SDAAM measurements declined significantly as patients progressed toward hospitalization confirming the expected autonomic reaction to progressive congestion and hospitalization [10].

Subsequently, several novel HRV methods were introduced into device-based diagnostic packages, each demonstrating prognostic value of remote monitoring of patients with HF [14]. The limitations of HRV measurements are important to understand. The measurement cannot provide direct guidance for medication changes intended to maintain clinical stability and, as such, can only provide a remotely available "early warning system" that identifies either patients who chronically are at high risk for hospitalization (basal HRV) or are in the process of decompensation (dynamic HRV). Additionally, HRV cannot be measured in patients with atrial fibrillation or with >75 % of sensed heart beats as "non-sinus" initiated [9].

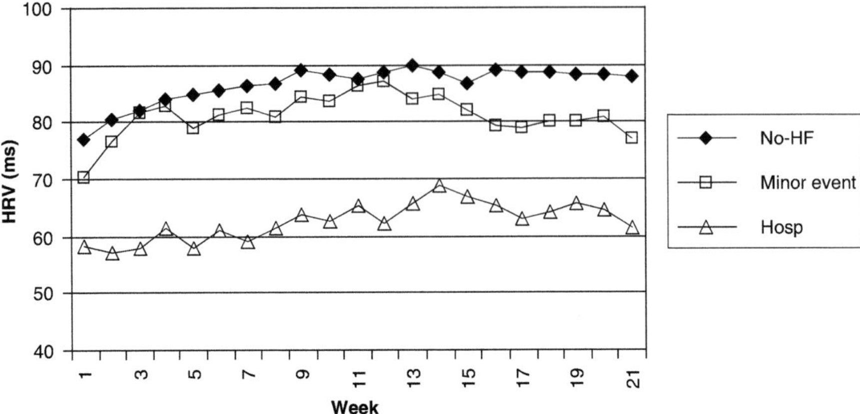

Fig. 7.1 Heart rate variability levels in patients with subsequent heart failure events (With permission from Ref. [10])

This crucial first step, however, was important in stimulating the development of monitoring systems designed to remotely enable practitioners to improve surveillance of patients with symptomatic HF. The search continued for a clearer signal that could provide remotely obtainable information concerning the pathophysiology of decompensation with congestion in HF patients. The ideal signal would appropriately follow progressive changes in body volume, which are typically associated with decompensation and hospitalization, inform clinical decision making by guiding changes in medication dosing, and allow confirmation of successful treatment with the goal of maintaining stability rather than reacting to the consequences of severe decompensation.

7.3 Intrathoracic Impedance Measurement

Measuring intrathoracic impedance with an implanted device was the next step in pursuit of a more direct marker of lung fluid and excess volume in HF patients at risk for decompensation. The concept was based on a very simple calculation of electrical impedance of a subthreshold impulse as it traversed the thorax from the right ventricular (RV) lead of an implanted electronic device to the pulse generator [5]. The theoretical advantage to this approach was that the vector distance between the RV and the pulse generator was fixed, which led to the hypothesis that a change in impedance would only occur in the presence of a change in lung fluid composition. Early studies in small numbers of HF patients demonstrated that intrathoracic impedance measurements correlated well to pulmonary capillary wedge pressure and the amount of fluid removed from acutely decompensated patients. Subsequent small trials suggested that meaningful changes in intrathoracic impedance measurements were apparent up to 14 days prior to hospitalization in decompensating patients. When coupled with other device-based diagnostics, such as HRV, activity, or nighttime heart rate, intrathoracic impedance changes were associated with increased hospitalization risk in the near term.

Unfortunately, this measurement was unable to guide medical therapy in hopes of maintaining stability in patients with HF. In an early terminated prospective randomized trial called DOT-HF performed at multiple European sites, changes in intrathoracic impedance were tied to a patient alert system generated by the implanted device [15]. The intent of the trial was to act on patient alerts by intensifying diuretic therapy and averting decompensation leading to hospitalization. The lack of clear understanding of false-positive and false-negative rates led to confusion which resulting in increased rate of hospitalizations in the monitored group compared to standard of care [15]. This disappointing result led to early termination of the PRECEDE-HF trial, which was a US-based investigation of the impact of intrathoracic impedance on HF outcomes.

The collective experience with implanted device-based intrathoracic impedance measurements remains unclear. Predictive statistical evaluation may help clarify what other events, such as pneumonia, COPD exacerbation, non-critical volume shifts, or device abnormalities, change the impedance signal without an excess in body volume. A large multicenter randomized trial is ongoing in Europe to further evaluate the value of intrathoracic impedance and guide its use in remote monitoring of patients with HF [16], but preliminary reports in an abstract presentation found no benefit of intrathoracic impedance in reducing hospitalizations in 1,002 patients followed for over 12 months [late breaking clinical trials, European Society of Cardiology, London, 2015].

7.4 Implantable Hemodynamic Monitoring

Traditional history and physical examination monitoring of patients with HF in clinical settings are designed to estimate body volume and organ perfusion. As over 90 % of hospitalizations involve excesses in body volume resulting in signs and symptoms of congestion, monitoring body volume is the key element of frequent assessment of high-risk patients [17]. HF disease management strategies typically involve frequent physical assessment by HF specialists with the hopes of early detection of volume accumulation that may lead to changes in diuretics or maximization of neurohormonal interventions.

The obvious limitation of these expert evaluations is that the examination and assessment cannot be done frequently or remotely. Patients are typically instructed to weigh themselves daily as a surrogate of body volume with the hypothesis that sudden increases in body weight would lead to medication changes in time to avoid acute decompensation and hospitalization. The common theme of all these clinical tools is to estimate cardiac filling pressures to guide medical management. Unfortunately, each maneuver, including physical examination and daily weights, is insensitive for detecting significant changes in filling pressures. In one study the sensitivity of a 2 kg body weight change in 72 h for predicting impending hospitalization was measured at 9 % [18–22]. Therefore, traditional clinical tools, even when remotely available as with body weight, are insensitive for assessing cardiac filling pressures which rise predictably as patients progress to decompensated state.

In fact, other typical parameters monitored in patients with HF, such as intrathoracic impedance and serial BNP measurements, were validated as surrogates of cardiac filling pressures (PCWP) [23]. Until recently, sensor technology suitable for the hostile environment of the human body was not available. However, in the mid-1990s Steinhaus and colleagues tested the first fully implantable hemodynamic monitoring system, which included a pressure transducer and oxygen saturation probe implanted in the right ventricular outflow tract (RVOT) in patients with HF [24]. This feasibility study found that the oxygen saturation sensor failed at a fairly high rate leading to removal of this component in subsequent designs. The Chronicle device was then developed using the basic framework of a pacemaker with a single lead housing the transducer implanted in the RVOT using a passive tine tip that also measured the local electrogram. The lead and transducer were then attached to a battery and memory system housed in a pulse generator that was implanted subcutaneously [25–27]. The implantation of this device was associated with typical complications of single lead pacemakers such as lead dislodgement, pocket infection, and system failure. Ultimately, the polyurethane lead design of the sensor was found to have an unacceptably high rate of single-source failure after 4 years of follow-up, and the system development was abandoned [28]. The clinical trials associated with this device, however, provided a rich database that described HF pathophysiology in a manner that was never seen before. A summary of clinical investigation using implantable hemodynamic monitoring systems and outcomes is shown in Table 7.1.

The Chronicle device measured right ventricular systolic, diastolic, and mean pressures and had an algorithm to estimate pulmonary artery (PA) diastolic pressure

Table 7.1 Summary of clinical investigation using implantable hemodynamic monitoring devices

Trial	Level of evidence	Mean duration of follow-up	Annualized reduction in HF hospitalization rates	Patient population
COMPASS Feasibility [26]	Historic control	17 months	57 % ($p<0.01$)	NYHA classes III–IV HFrEF $n=32$
COMPASS-HF [29]	Randomized prospective single blinded	6 months	21 % All HF events ($p=0.33$) 36 % time to first ($p<0.01$)	NYHA classes III–IV Any EF $n=274$
REDUCEhf [28]	Uncompleted randomized single blinded	12 months	N/A	NYHA classes II–III ICD indication $N=400$
CHAMPION Trial [35, 36]	Randomized prospective single blinded	6 months primary 17 months supplemental	28 % ($p<0.001$) 37 % ($p<0.0001$)	NYHA class III Any EF $N=550$

HFrEF heart failure with reduced ejection fraction, *ICD* implantable cardioverter defibrillator, *EF* ejection fraction

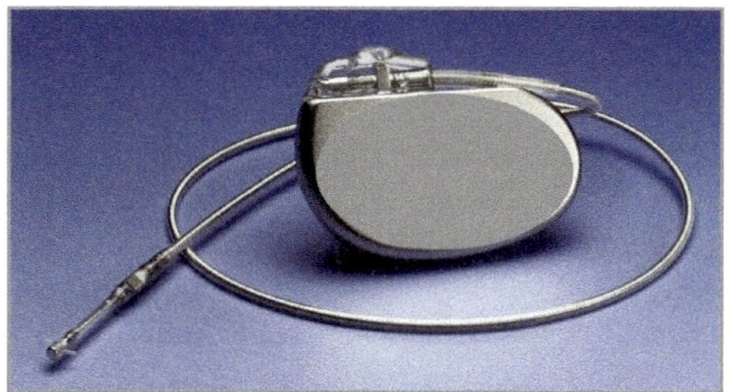

Fig. 7.2 Implantable hemodynamic monitoring system used in the COMPASS-HF trial (Adapted from Ref. [29])

(Fig. 7.2). PA diastolic pressure estimate was the pressure in the RVOT at the time of maximum dP/dt, which corresponded to the opening of the pulmonary valve. Heart rate and other derivatives of the pressure signal were recorded beat to beat, averaged, and stored in a user-defined time bin. Hemodynamic information was sent by a radio-frequency (RF) uplink to a bedside device that transmitted the information to a secured website for investigator and provider review. The first clinical experience with this device proved it to be precise and accurate over time [25]. In addition, it became clear that pressures increased as patients decompensated and returned to baseline with successful treatment of decompensated HF [26]. Significant hospitalization reductions, using historic control analysis, were observed in the feasibility patients when pressures were validated and then used to guide medications. This supported the hypothesis that implantable hemodynamic monitoring may be a superior means to manage high-risk patients with persistently symptomatic HF.

The first prospective, randomized, single-blinded, implanted control trial evaluating the strategy of hemodynamic guided HF care was called COMPASS-HF, which enrolled 274 patients with NYHA class III or IV HF symptoms and a hospitalization in the previous 6 months [29]. The primary end point of the trial was a composite of HF-related events that included emergency department visits requiring intravenous HF care, intravenous medication interventions in the office, and HF-related hospitalizations evaluated after 6 months of hemodynamic-guided care in the treatment group vs. standard of care in the control group. The trial was designed with 80 % power to detect a 30 % reduction in all primary end points assuming a control group rate of 1.2 events/6 months. These assumptions were quite ambitious and led to a grossly underpowered study unable to adequately test the hypothesis. In contrast to the predicted event rates, the COMPASS-HF control group did very well with 0.85 events/6 months, which rendered the treatment group's 21 % reduction in all events (0.67 events/6 months) nonsignificant [29]. A retrospective time-to-first-event analysis revealed a significant 36 % reduction in the primary end point. Additionally, approximately 17 % of the patients had NYHA class IV symptoms at enrollment. These patients seemed to have an increased event rate in the treatment group. Ambulatory NYHA class III patients seemed to benefit from hemodynamic monitoring, but this was a retrospective subgroup analysis in a trial that did not statistically meet its primary end point. The findings, then, supported the hypothesis, but did not provide sufficient evidence for benefit to outweigh the risks associated with implantation of the device.

The COMPASS-HF trial provided a unique and never-before-seen perspective into cardiovascular pathophysiology. These significant contributions illustrate the value of "listening to the heart." Continuous hemodynamic evaluation of ambulatory HF patients demonstrated that elevated cardiac filling pressures were common and elevations had prognostic value [30]. Very importantly, the COMPASS-HF experience found that there were two components to hemodynamic-guided care and both must be addressed for ultimate clinical success. Whereas it was clear that pressures progressively and predictably increased from baseline as patients decompensated [3, 4, 6, 7], only reacting to changes was not complete. Stevenson and colleagues reported that pressure levels were clearly related to subsequent risks for HF events [30]. Their retrospective analysis from COMPASS-HF found that patients entering the trial with elevated pressures who had their pressures treated and lowered were among those with the lowest event rates. Patients entering the trial with high pressures that persisted throughout the trial had the highest event rates, which were equal to patients who entered with lower pressures that experienced persistent increases over time. The final group, patients with pressures that stayed low from implant to the end of follow-up, were also at low risk. This concept led to a better understanding of the clinical relationship between filling pressures and perfusion. Although perfusion is important to monitor, most patients with chronic HF do not require high pressures to maintain cardiac output. In fact, the evidence is clear that higher filling pressures are detrimental and lead to high risk for decompensation [30]. The retrospective data by Stevenson and colleagues developed a significant hypothesis that was to form an important component of the CHAMPION Trial protocol.

Further insight into the pathophysiology of HF was provided by Zile and colleagues who demonstrated that the hemodynamic characteristics of patients with HF and reduced ejection fraction (HFrEF) were similar to those patients with HF and preserved ejection fraction (HFpEF) [3]. This was an important point as the only consensus agreement about therapy for HFpEF patients was control of volume (i.e., filling pressures). Albeit pressures tended to change with a steeper pressure/time relationship in HFpEF patients, they still significantly increased 17–21 days before decompensating patients were hospitalized. This further supported the general hypothesis that this important and underserved group of HF patients may benefit from hemodynamic-guided HF management.

Further development of the Chronicle device included adding a single-chamber defibrillator to the circuitry to evaluate the impact of hemodynamic-guided HF management in patients with an indication for ICD therapy. The REDUCEhf trial was then designed to evaluate up to 1200 HF patients followed for 12 months with a similar end point of HF events used in COMPASS-HF [27]. Unfortunately, the lead failure problem in the Chronicle system was discovered after 400 patients were enrolled in the REDUCEhf trial, but the trial did discover that patients with NYHA class II HF following a previous hospitalization had a much different event rate in the year following implantation of the monitor. Event rates in the NYHA class II patients were very low after implantation (0.24 events/patient/year) suggesting that hemodynamic monitoring in these patients, if the goal was to reduce hospitalization rates, may not be effective [28]. Additionally, patients with treated arrhythmias tended to have higher filling pressures, although a high-resolution view of pressures temporally associated with ventricular arrhythmias was difficult to establish with the technology [31].

Therefore, previous hemodynamic monitoring trials produced a very important database to further understand the hemodynamic pathophysiology of HF. Appropriate patient populations most likely to respond to the therapeutic approach were identified, and a general understanding of the appropriate medical interventions needed to control chronically measured filling pressures was learned. This typical learning curve associated with completely novel approaches to management is understandable and served to develop the appropriate assumptions, patient selection, and protocol developed in the CHAMPION Trial.

7.5 CHAMPION Trial

The CHAMPION Trial utilized a novel technology to acquire hemodynamic information that had a much different risk profile compared to previous monitoring systems [32]. The MEMS-based sensor did not require a lead or battery and was empowered by radio-frequency interrogation by an external antenna [32, 33]. The sensor consists of a coil and a pressure-sensitive capacitor encased in a hermetically sealed silica capsule covered by silicone. The coil and capacitor form an electrical circuit that resonates at a specific frequency. Pressure on the sensor deflects the pressure-sensitive surface which, in turn, results in a characteristic shift in the resonant frequency. The sensor is empowered by interrogation from an external antenna held against the patient's body. Once electromagnetic coupling is achieved, the interrogating device continuously measures the sensor's resonant frequency at a very high sampling rate, converting the resonant frequency into pressure waveform. The interrogating device has an atmospheric barometer which automatically subtracts the ambient pressure from that measured from the implanted sensor. Calibration of the sensor is accomplished using simultaneous pressures from a fluid-filled catheter at the time of implantation. The sensor wafer has nitinol loops placed on the ends to anchor the sensor in the pulmonary artery branch serving also to automatically size the device to the vessel caliber (Fig. 7.3a, b).

After the long-term accuracy and precision of the sensor was established [32–34], the CHAMPION Trial was designed as a prospective, randomized, single-blinded, controlled trial testing the hypothesis that active medical management of

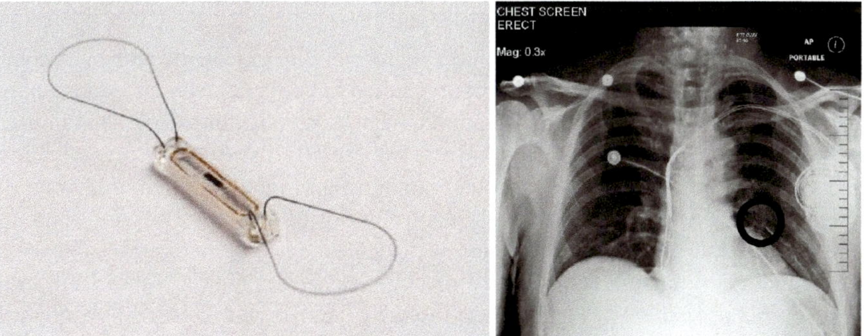

Fig. 7.3 (**a**) Implantable MEMS-based sensor used in the CHAMPION Trial (Adapted from Ref. [33]). (**b**) Anteroposterior chest X-ray in a patient with a CardioMems Implantable Hemodynamic sensor placed in the left pulmonary artery (*circle*)

PA pressures in patients with persistent NYHA class III HF symptoms following a previous hospitalization would maintain stability and prevent future rehospitalizations [33]. Five-hundred fifty HF patients, regardless of ejection fraction, were enrolled and implanted with the sensor during right heart catheterization. Hemodynamic information was available for medical decision making in all patients at the time of sensor implantation, and patients were then randomized to a treatment group that received standard HF disease management in addition to ongoing access to daily uploaded PA pressures. The control group received standard HF disease management, but uploaded pressures were not accessible to the investigators.

After implantation, patients were instructed how to use the bedside interrogation unit that incorporated the external antenna into a pillow for the patients to recline against. This was done for ease of use and to standardize body position during PA pressure acquisition. Patients uploaded pressures daily, and investigators were asked to review treatment group pressures weekly. Suggested pressure-guided medication changes were outlined in the protocol and, in general, set pressure target ranges (PA diastolic 8–20 mmHg and PA mean 10–25 mmHg) and first considered elevations from target pressures to be due to excess body volume. Diuretic intensification was the first medical intervention followed by addition of vasodilators as long as perfusion was adequate.

The primary end point of the CHAMPION Trial was rate of hospitalizations compared between the treatment and control group after 6 months of management. All patients remained in their original randomized group until the last patient finished 6-month follow-up allowing supplementary analyses examining the duration of a potential treatment effect. Further follow-up of an additional 13 months of the strategy was reported at the US Food and Drug Administration (USFDA) Advisory Panel. The final 13-month follow-up period examined the experience of the control group transitioning into hemodynamic-guided care. This period of time was considered free from limitations of a single-blinded trial and examined a more "real-world" experience with hemodynamic monitoring [35].

7.6   CHAMPION Trial Results: Benefits of Listening to Central Hemodynamic Data

The CHAMPION Trial proved that maintaining stability in patients with symptomatic HF using hemodynamic-guided care resulted in both clinically and statistically important reduction in decompensation requiring hospitalization [36]. This impact on hospitalizations was above and beyond intense HF disease management using signs and symptoms, daily weights, and monitoring of other device and laboratory diagnostics, which were operant in the control group of the trial. The control group in CHAMPION received excellent care as evidenced by an event rate of 0.44 events per patient per 6 months, which was almost ½ that seen in the COMPASS-HF trial (0.85 events per patient per 6 months) (Table 7.1). In fact, the CHAMPION control group had one of the lowest annualized event rates seen in hemodynamic monitoring trials which were substantially lower than used in the power calculations designing the trial's enrollment. The magnitude of hospitalization rate reduction in CHAMPION is even more profound when one considers how well the control group was treated in the trial [36].

Several subsequent analyses from the CHAMPION Trial provide further insight into hemodynamic monitoring in patients with HF. For example, patients with HFpEF, defined as LVEF $\geq$ 40 %, were a predetermined subgroup analysis in CHAMPION [37]. Hospitalization rates after the entire randomized follow-up period were 50 % lower in HFpEF treatment patients compared to control. Hospitalization rates in the HFpEF group with LVEF $\geq$ 50 % were 70 % lower in the treatment group compared to control. Hemodynamic-guided care of patients with HFpEF is the first successful treatment strategy in this important and underserved group. This is important as over ½ of hospitalized patients in the ADERE registry had preserved EF, but currently there is no consensus about successful treatment strategies [38].

HF patients almost always have multiple comorbidities, many of which produce shortness of breath, exercise intolerance, and fatigue. Patients with the comorbidity of chronic obstructive pulmonary disease (COPD), for example, may have worsening dyspnea because of bronchitis or HF. In the CHAMPION Trial, patients with COPD and HF had better outcomes in the treatment group compared to control both for HF and respiratory hospitalizations [39]. This may illustrate that having PA pressures in this population of patients provides clarity of diagnosis leading to early intervention of the appropriate illness cause symptoms. Other patient groups, such as those with severe World Health Organization (WHO) group II secondary pulmonary hypertension, were at higher risk for hospitalization, but the treatment group fared better in the follow-up period [40]. The transpulmonary gradient found at implantation, in fact, was helpful in differentiating the extent to which volume vs. resistance contributed to the elevated pressures.

Hospitalizations in patients with HF are thought to contribute to progression of cardiac failure and dysfunction, thus decreasing the patient's expected life span [41]. This is underscored by the observation that few if any clinical trials treating the already decompensated patient have shown positive results. As a result more and more prospective clinical trials examining new interventions include hospitalization as the target end point or, at least, part of the primary end point. However, the direct link between hospitalization prevention and mortality is ill defined. A retrospective analysis of patients in the CHAMPION Trial already receiving maximal guideline-directed medical and device therapies appropriate for their disease state supports the link between hospitalization and mortality. In CHAMPION, approximately 75 % of the patients with reduced ejection fraction were on angiotensin intervention with ACE inhibitor therapy or ARB along with beta-blocker therapy. The baseline dosing was in line with targets set in the clinical trials that defined their use. These patients were also receiving ICD and CRT device therapies as well. Over the 17 months of hemodynamic-guided care in the randomization phase of CHAMPION, those on guideline-directed medical therapy had 42 % less hospitalizations and mortality, adjusted for baseline demographic differences, was 50 % less in the treatment group compared to control [42]. This effect was even more profound in patients receiving

CRT, whose adjusted mortality reduction was 61 % [43]. With the limitation of retrospective analysis and nonrandomized subgroup analysis, these data strongly support the hypothesis that the goal of HF management should be to maintain stability, but not just to prevent costly hospitalizations, but also to prolong life.

Conclusions

The "Cardiac Serenade" contains a very beautiful song that provides rich insight into how the body perceives the human condition. The design of such complex and interactive control systems not only ensures survival but recognizes change and anticipates needs to provide humans with perfusion on demand, even when the system is diseased. With the advent of implantable technology capable of recording physiologic signals either continuously or frequently, the clinician's job of providing effective care has become much more streamlined and clear. The end result is a noticeable paradigm change, at least for the management of HF: maintaining stability by tapping into the data stream produced by the body's control system prevents decompensation, reduces the need for hospitalization, and improves survival along with improving overall quality of life.

References

1. Adamson PB. Pathophysiology of the transition from chronic compensated and acute decompensated heart failure: New insights from continuous monitoring devices. Curr Heart Fail Rep. 2009;6:287–92.
2. Adamson PB. Using cardiac resynchronization therapy diagnostics for monitoring heart failure patients. Heart Fail Clin. 2009;5:249–60.
3. Zile MR, Bennett TD, Sutton M, et al. Transition from chronic compensated to acute decompensated heart failure: pathophysiological insights obtained from continuous monitoring of intracardiac pressures. Circulation. 2008;118:1433–41.
4. Adamson PB, Zile MR, Cho YK, et al. Hemodynamic factors associated with acute decompensated heart failure: part 2 – use in automated detection. J Card Fail. 2011;17:366–73.
5. Yu CM, Wang L, Chau E, et al. Intrathoracic impedance monitoring in patients with heart failure: correlation with fluid status and feasibility of early warning preceding hospitalization. Circulation. 2005;112:841–88.
6. Zile MR, Bourge RC, Bennett TD, et al. Application of implantable hemodynamic monitoring in the management of patients with diastolic heart failure: a subgroup analysis of the COMPASS-HF Trial. J Card Fail. 2008;14:816–23.
7. Zile MR, Adamson PB, Cho YK, et al. Hemodynamic factors associated with acute decompensated heart failure: part 1 – insights into pathophysiology. J Card Fail. 2011;17:282–91.
8. Abraham WT, Fisher WG, Smith AL, et al. Cardiac resynchronization therapy in chronic heart failure. N Engl J Med. 2002;346:1845–53.
9. Adamson PB, Kleckner K, VanHout WL, Srinivasan S, Abraham WT. Cardiac resynchronization therapy improves heart rate variability in patients with symptomatic heart failure. Circulation. 2003;108:266–9.
10. Adamson PB, Smith AL, Abraham WT, et al. Continuous autonomic assessment in patients with symptomatic heart failure: prognostic value of heart rate variability measured by an implanted cardiac resynchronization device. Circulation. 2004;110:2389–94.
11. Sharma V, Rathman LD, Small RS, et al. Stratifying patients at the risk of heart failure hospitalization using existing device diagnostic thresholds. Heart Lung. 2015;44:129–36.
12. Hedman AE, Poloniecki JD, Camm AJ, Malik M. Relation of mean heart rate and heart rate variability in patients with left ventricular dysfunction. Am J Cardiol. 1999;84:225–8.

13. Adamson PB. Continuous heart rate variability from and implanted device: a practical guide for clinical use. Congest Heart Fail. 2005;11:327–30.
14. Gilliam 3rd FR, Singh JP, Mullin CM, McGuire M, Chase KJ. Prognostic value of heart rate variability footprint and standard deviation of average 5-minute intrinsic R-R intervals for mortality in cardiac resynchronization therapy patients. J Electrocardiol. 2007;40:336–42.
15. Van Veldhuisen DJ, Braunschweig F, Conraads V, et al. Intrathoracic impedance monitoring audible patient alerts and outcome in patients with heart failure. Circulation. 2011;124:1719–26.
16. Brachmann J, Bohm M, Rybak K, et al. Fluid status monitoring with a wireless network to reduce cardiovascular-related hospitalizations and mortality in heart failure: rationale and design of the OptiLink HF Study (Optimization of Heart Failure Management using OptiVol Fluid Status Monitoring and CareLink). Eur J Heart Fail. 2011;13:796–804.
17. Adams Jr KF, Fonarow GC, Emerman CL, et al. Characteristics and outcomes of patients hospitalized for heart failure in the United States: rationale, design and preliminary observations from the first 100,000 cases in the Acute Decompensated Heart Failure National Registry (ADHERE). Am Heart J. 2005;1(49):209–16.
18. Stevenson LW, Perloff JK. The limited reliability of physical signs for estimating hemodynamics in chronic heart failure. JAMA. 1989;261:884–8.
19. Capomolla S, Cersa M, Pinna GD, et al. Echo-Doppler and clinical evaluations to define hemodynamic profile in patients with chronic heart failure: accuracy and influence on therapeutic management. Eur J Heart Fail. 2005;7:624–30.
20. Chaudhry SI, Wang Y, Concato J, Gill TM, Krumholz HM. Patterns of weight change preceding hospitalization for heart failure. Circulation. 2007;116:1549–54.
21. Lewin J, Ledwidge M, O'Loughlin C, McNally C, McDonald K. Clinical deterioration in established heart failure: what is the value of BNP and weight gain in aiding diagnosis? Eur J Heart Fail. 2005;7:953–7.
22. Abraham WT, Compton S, Haas G, et al. Intrathoracic impedance vs daily weight monitoring for predicting worsening heart failure events: results of the Fluid Accumulation Status Trial (FAST). Congest Heart Fail. 2011;17:51–5.
23. Daniels LB, Maisel AS. Natriuretic peptides. J Am Coll Cardiol. 2007;50:2357–68.
24. Steinhaus D, Lemery R, Bresnahan J, et al. Initial experience with an implantable hemodynamic monitor. Circulation. 1996;93:745–52.
25. Magalski A, Adamson PB, Linde C, et al. Continuous ambulatory right heart pressure measurements with an implantable hemodynamic monitor: 12-month follow-up in a multi-center trial of chronic heart failure patients. J Cardiac Fail. 2002;8:63–70.
26. Adamson PB, Magalski A, Braunschweig F, et al. Ongoing right ventricular hemodynamics heart failure: clinical value of measurements derived from an implantable monitoring system. J Am Coll Cardiol. 2003;41:563–7.
27. Adamson PB, Conti JB, Smith AL, et al. Reducing events in patients with chronic heart failure (REDUCEhf) study design: continuous hemodynamic monitoring with an implantable defibrillator. Clin Cardiol. 2007;30:567–75.
28. Adamson PB, Gold MR, Bennett T, et al. Continuous hemodynamic monitoring in patients with mild to moderate heart failure: results of the Reducing Decompensation Events Utilizing Intracardiac Pressures in Patients with chronic heart failure (REDUCEhf) Trial. Congest Heart Fail. 2011;17:248–54.
29. Bourge RE, Abraham WT, Adamson PB, et al. COMPASS-HF Study Group: randomized controlled trial of an implantable continuous hemodynamic monitor in patients with advanced heart failure: the COMPASS-HF study. J Am Coll Cardiol. 2008;51:1073–9.
30. Stevenson LW, Zile M, Bennett TD, et al. Chronic ambulatory intracardiac pressures and future heart failure events. Circ Heart Fail. 2010;3:580–7.
31. Reiter MJ, Stromberg KD, Adamson PB, Whitman T, Benditt DG, Gold MR. Influence of intracardiac pressure on spontaneous ventricular arrhythmias in patients with systolic heart failure: insights from the REDUCEhf Trial. Circ Electrophysiol. 2013;6:272–8.
32. Verdejo HE, Castro PF, Concepcion R, et al. Comparison of a radiofrequency-based wireless pressure sensor to Swan-Ganz catheter and echocardiography for ambulatory assessment of pulmonary artery pressure in heart failure. J Am Coll Cardiol. 2007;50:2375–82.

33. Adamson PB, Abraham WT, Aaron M, et al. CHAMPION Trial Rationale and design: the long-term safety and clinical efficacy of a wireless pulmonary artery pressure monitoring system. J Card Fail. 2010;17:3–10.
34. Abraham WT, Adamson PB, Hasan A, et al. Safety and accuracy of a wireless pulmonary artery pressure monitoring system in patients with heart failure. Am Heart J. 2011;161:558–66.
35. Abraham WT, Stevenson LW, Bourge RC, et al. Sustained efficacy of pulmonary artery pressure to guide adjustment of chronic heart failure therapy: Complete follow-up from the CHAMPION Randomised Trial. The Lancet, in press, November 8, 2015, http://dx.doi.org/10.1016/S0140-6736(15)00723-0.
36. Abraham WT, Adamson PB, Bourge RC, et al. for the CHAMPION Trial Study Group: wireless pulmonary artery hemodynamic monitoring in chronic heart failure. Lancet. 2011;377:658–66.
37. Adamson PB, Abraham WT, Costanzo MR, et al. Wireless pulmonary artery pressure monitoring guides management to reduce decompensation in heart failure with preserved ejection fraction. Circ Heart Fail. 2014;7:935–44.
38. Yancy CW, Jessup M, Bozkurt B, et al. 2013 ACCF/AHA guideline for the management of heart failure: a report of the American College of Cardiology Foundation/American Heart Association Task Force on Practice Guidelines. J Am Coll Cardiol. 2013;62:e147–239.
39. Krahnke JS, Abraham WT, Adamson PB, et al. Heart failure and respiratory hospitalizations are reduced in heart failure subjects with chronic obstructive pulmonary disease using an implantable pulmonary artery pressure monitoring device. J Card Fail. 2015;21:240–9.
40. Benza RL, Raina A, Abraham WT, et al. Pulmonary hypertension related to left heart disease: insight from a wireless implantable hemodynamic monitor. J Heart Lung Transplant. 2014;34:329–37.
41. Gheorghiade M, De Luca L, Fonarow GC, et al. Pathophysiologic targets in the early phase of acute heart failure syndromes. Am J Cardiol. 2005;96:11G–7.
42. Abraham WT, Adamson PB, Stevenson LW, et al. Pulmonary artery pressure management in heart failure patients with reduced ejection fraction significantly reduces heart failure hospitalizations and mortality above and beyond background guideline-directed medical therapy. J Am Coll Cardiol. 2015;(abstract).
43. Abraham WT, Adamson PB, Stevenson LW, et al. Pulmonary artery pressure management in heart failure patients with cardiac resynchronization therapy or implantable cardioverter defibrillator devices significantly reduces hospitalizations and mortality above and beyond background guideline-directed medical therapy. Heart Rhythm. 2015;(abstract).

Whispering During Sleep: Autonomic Signaling During Sleep, Sleep Apnea, and Sudden Death

8

Maria Teresa La Rovere and Gian Domenico Pinna

Sleep is an orchestrated neurochemical process involving different biological systems. Many theories have attempted to explain the biological meaning of sleep including a primary restorative function, a central role in reinforcement, and consolidation of memory, and an important place for thermoregulatory processes. Despite the lack of a general consensus on its purposes, the brain mechanisms controlling sleep and wakefulness as well as the associated changes in cardiovascular and respiratory function are largely known. The autonomic nervous system is of paramount importance in the regulation of the cardiovascular function during sleep, and it can also mediate cardiovascular events occurring during sleep as a result of cardiovascular diseases or primary sleep disorders such as sleep-disordered breathing.

The aim of this chapter is to review the autonomic effects of normal sleep and of sleep-related breathing abnormalities, the relationship of the autonomic nervous system to arrhythmogenesis and sudden death, and the role of the autonomic nervous system in mediating cardiovascular consequences of sleep apnea in heart failure.

8.1 The Cardiovascular System and Sleep Architecture

Polysomnography is the standard tool used to study the overall sleep process and diagnose sleep disorders. It involves the recording of the electroencephalogram (EEG), the electro-oculogram (EOG), and the electromyogram (EMG). Based on these signals, sleep is divided into two strikingly distinct states: non-rapid eye movement (NREM) sleep and rapid eye movement (REM) sleep. NREM sleep is subdivided further into

M.T. La Rovere, MD (✉)
Division of Cardiology, Istituto Scientifico di Montescano, Montescano, Pavia, Italy
e-mail: mariateresa.larovere@fsm.it

G.D. Pinna, MS
Biomedical Engineering, Fondazione "Salvatore Maugeri", IRCCS, Istituto Scientifico di Montescano, Montescano, Pavia, Italy

© Springer International Publishing Switzerland 2016
E. Gronda et al. (eds.), *Heart Failure Management: The Neural Pathways*,
DOI 10.1007/978-3-319-24993-3_8

light sleep (NREM1 and NREM2 or N1 and N2) and deep sleep (NREM3 or N3, sometimes referred to as slow wave sleep). NREM and REM occur in a cycle that is repeated four to six times every night, each cycle lasting approximately 90–110 min.

A normal sleep cycle begins with light N1 sleep, during which the theta waves (4–7 Hz) replace the alpha rhythm (8–13 Hz) of wakefulness. As sleep approaches, muscle activity, which is highest during wakefulness, starts to decrease. With transition to N2, sleep spindles and K complexes appear in the EEG, thus signaling the increasing depth of sleep. Sleep spindles are bursts of rapid, rhythmic brain wave activity in the range 12–15 Hz, while K complexes are slow (>4 Hz), large waves that stand out from the background with a negative than a positive deflection. In N3, the EEG pattern is characterized by synchronized high-amplitude (>75 μV), slow (0.5–3 Hz) delta waves. Slow wave sleep is associated with no eye movements and with a higher arousal threshold and a further decline in muscle tone than during lighter sleep. In contrast with the synchronized activity of NREM sleep, REM sleep is characterized by a very intense and desynchronized EEG activity (similar to wakefulness) coupled with a complete loss of muscle tone, bursts of rapid eye movements, and irregularities in respiration and heart rate.

It has to be underscored, however, that this sequence of sleep stages (N1, N2, N3, REM) undergoes some changes as sleep progresses from cycle to cycle. In the first cycle, sleep begins in N1 and progresses into N2 and N3. Afterward, N2 sleep is repeated before entering REM sleep. Once REM sleep is over, there is usually a return to N2 sleep. Thus, N1 sleep accounts for <5 % of total sleep as it usually occurs at sleep onset and as a transitional state across the night. N2 sleep occurs constantly through the night and represents about 45–55 % of sleep. N3 sleep, which represents about 15–25 % of total sleep time, is predominant in the first half of the night. The first cycle of REM sleep usually lasts only a short amount of time and becomes progressively longer at each new sleep cycle. REM sleep can last up to an hour as sleep progresses, amounting to 20–25 % of total sleep time [1].

Substantial changes in cardiovascular function occur during sleep being mediated by the autonomic nervous system. However, it has to be emphasized that cardiovascular activity during sleep may not only be a consequence of sleep mechanisms, but may also reflect the influence of the circadian system [2]. Under normal circumstances, there is a fall in blood pressure and heart rate during NREM sleep as compared to relaxed wakefulness [3]. Blood pressure and heart rate may also be lower in slow wave sleep than stage 2 [4, 5]. During REM sleep, blood pressure undergoes frequent marked oscillations and heart rate becomes very variable. This behavior has led to contradictory results in the literature whenever mean values have been reported. Actually, both blood pressure and heart rate can further decrease during tonic REM sleep as compared to NREM, while they transiently increase to levels similar to wakefulness in association with phasic REM events [6].

8.2 The Autonomic Nervous System During Sleep

The autonomic nervous system with its two branches, the sympathetic and the parasympathetic systems, working in a delicately tuned, yet opposing fashion, provides adaptation of the cardiovascular system to the various activities of daily life. While the sympathetic system increases heart rate, myocardial contractility, and peripheral resistance, the parasympathetic system slows heart rate with a limited effect on cardiac contractility. It is worth noting that not only the sinus node but also the electrophysiological properties of the entire heart are modulated by these antagonistic influences [7]. The autonomic outflow to the heart and the peripheral circulation is regulated by cardiovascular reflexes, among which the arterial baroreflexes represent the primary mechanism for homeostatic control of arterial pressure and the maintenance of the optimal perfusion of critical organs. The baroreflex control of circulatory homeostasis occurs on a negative feedback basis. Generally, an increase in the loading condition of the baroreceptors by a rise in systemic arterial pressure increases their discharge to the cardiovascular control center in the brainstem that initiates appropriate compensatory responses, including an increase in the vagal outflow and a decrease in the sympathetic outflow to the heart and blood vessels. Conversely, an opposite response is elicited when the arterial baroreceptors are unloaded by a decrease in systemic arterial pressure.

It is worth to underscore that high brain centers continuously modulate baroreceptor responses and cardiovascular reflexes according to behavioral and physiological conditions. In particular, the sleep-dependent changes in cardiovascular function result from the integration between cardiovascular reflexes and central command that are specific to each sleep stage [8].

The first description that sleep alters the function of the arterial baroreceptors (i.e., that during sleep the baroreceptors do not follow the operating logic of wakefulness) dates back to 1969 when Smyth et al. [9] reported the occurrence of a nocturnal reduction of heart rate and arterial pressure as well as an increased gain of the reflex arc in the majority of subjects under study (Fig. 8.1), thereby suggesting that "fluctuations in the level of arousal might in turn alter the activity of baroreceptor reflexes and of other autonomic mechanisms."

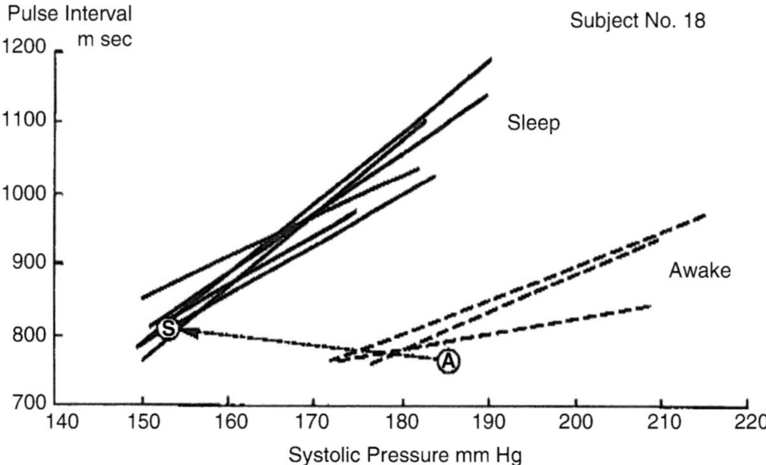

Fig. 8.1 Baroreflex changes with sleep in one subject. Each line represents one baroreflex sensitivity estimation. *A* average systolic pressure awake, both before and after sleep, *S* average systolic pressure during slow wave sleep (Reproduced with permission from Ref. [12])

Although the neural mechanisms involved in the complex integration between sleep stages and cardiovascular reflexes are not completely known, the available evidence indicates that NREM sleep is characterized by a progressive decrease in neural sympathetic nerve activity [10] with an accompanying parasympathetic predominance [6, 11], and a downward resetting of the arterial baroreceptor reflex [12, 13]. The relative autonomic stability of NREM sleep is, however, interrupted by those burst of sympathetic nerve activity that are observed on the occurrence of arousals [10]. The resulting phasic increase in arterial pressure does not evoke the bradycardic response which would be expected due to the arterial baroreflex, but rather an increase in heart rate.

A marked sympathetic activation and instability in blood pressure and heart rate, likely of central origin, also characterize phasic REM sleep, during which sudden bursts of sympathetic nerve traffic, about twice the level seen during wakefulness, are documented [10]. As these increases in sympathetic activity are interspersed between the predominantly parasympathetic activity of tonic REM periods, this sleep stage as a whole appears to induce complex fluctuations in autonomic function.

In light of the lengthening of REM cycles as sleep progresses, it has been hypothesized that REM sleep represents a vulnerable state for the cardiovascular system that can set the stage for nocturnal arrhythmias and cardiovascular events [10, 14, 15]. The fluctuations in autonomic activity across sleep stages and their impact on arrhythmia susceptibility may become particularly dangerous in the context of underlying cardiovascular diseases that are often associated with a deranged sympatho-vagal balance [16]. It has been described that after myocardial infarction, the loss in the capability of the vagal activity to physiologically increase during sleep results in a condition of relative sympathetic dominance even during NREM sleep, normally described as a condition at low risk for lethal events [17]. However, it is the sympathetic surge of the normal morning transition from sleep to wakefulness that has been more consistently implicated in the early morning peak in the occurrence of sudden death and implanted defibrillator discharges [18, 19].

8.3 The Respiratory System During Sleep and Sleep Apnea

Falling asleep removes postural muscle tone, voluntary respiratory control, and the wakefulness stimulus for breathing, leaving metabolic demand as the primary determinant of minute ventilation [20].

The sensors for chemical stimuli include the central and peripheral chemoreceptors. With increasing hypoxemia and hypercapnia, the carotid bodies send afferent impulses to the medullary centers to increase ventilation. Similarly, with hypercapnia, linear changes in ventilation occur in response to central chemoreceptor stimulation. The control of ventilation is organized as a negative feedback system to maintain the $PaCO_2$ at approximately 40 mmHg during wakefulness. Three main factors determine the stability of this control system [21, 22]:

controller gain (the ventilatory response to changes in arterial blood gas tensions), plant gain (the responsiveness of changes in arterial blood gases to changes in ventilation), and system delays (the combined effect of circulation time from the lungs to chemoreceptors and of phase shifts resulting from mixing and diffusion processes in the lungs, heart, vasculature, and brain tissues). In general, both the hypoxic and hypercapnic ventilatory responses – that represent the important elements of the controller gain in the respiratory control loop – decline during NREM sleep and decline further with REM sleep [23]. Thus, the transition from wakefulness to NREM sleep is accompanied by a decrease in ventilation (largely through a decrease in tidal volume) associated with an increase in upper airway resistance. As a result, the sleep eupneic $PaCO_2$ increases by 2–7 mmHg, and oxygen saturation decreases by 1–3 %. While reductions in $PaCO_2$ during wakefulness have no or limited effects on the breathing pattern, in NREM sleep small transient reductions in $PaCO_2$ (even only to the waking levels) result in significant apnea [24]. Breathing during REM sleep is characteristically more rapid than during NREM sleep (despite muscle atonia) as a consequence of an excitatory drive to breath. Periods of hyperventilation are interspersed with period of more regular respiration and apneas of varying length.

In most healthy subjects of any age, the loss of wakefulness influences on neurochemical control of breathing and airway patency during sleep is of minor physiological consequences. In some other healthy subjects, and even more in individuals with cardiac abnormalities, these changes predispose to respiratory abnormalities during sleep, generally referred to as sleep-disordered breathing. Commonly, sleep-disordered breathing is divided into "central," denoting an absence or marked reduction in central motor drive to respiratory muscle and "obstructive" events which are comprised of respiratory efforts against a narrowed or closed upper airway.

8.4 Sleep Apnea in Heart Failure

Both obstructive sleep apnea (OSA) and central sleep apnea (CSA) are a common comorbidity in patients with heart failure (independently of reduced or preserved left ventricular function) (Figs. 8.2 and 8.3), occurring approximately in half of them despite optimal pharmacological therapy [25–27].

Irrespective of their origin, central or obstructive, such disorders typically manifest as a cyclic waxing and waning of tidal volume [28, 29], a pattern commonly referred to as periodic breathing [28].

Using an apnea-hypopnea index (AHI, the number of apneas or hypopneas per hour of sleep) ≥15/h as a diagnostic threshold, the prevalence of OSA and CSA in patients with chronic stable heart failure and reduced ejection fraction ranges from 15 % to 26 % [25–27] and from 21 % to 38 % [25–27], respectively.

As for the relative distribution of OSA and CSA, data from previous investigations range from 28 % vs. 72 % [25, 26, 30] to 55 % vs. 45 % [27], respectively. However, it has to be underscored that many of these patients experience during the

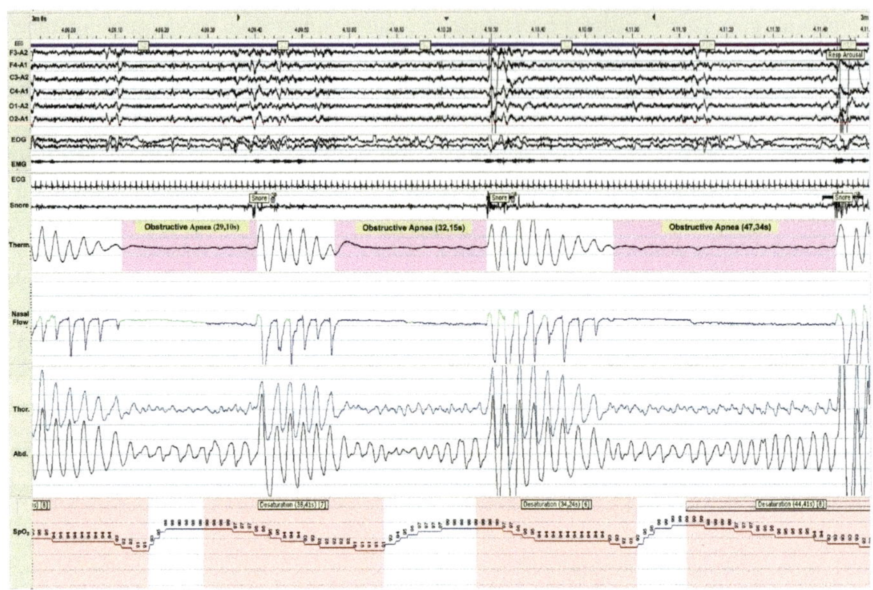

Fig. 8.2 A 3-min polysomnogram of a patient with heart failure revealing three obstructive apneas during stage 2 NREM sleep and REM sleep. Note the futile respiratory efforts associated with hypoxemia (min SpO$_2$, 87 %) terminated by an abrupt arousal. Abbreviations: F3-A2, F4-A1, C3-A2, C4-A1, O1-A2, O2-A1, electroencephalograms, *EOG* electro-oculogram, *EMG* chin electromyogram, *ECG* electrocardiogram, *Therm* thermistor, *Thor* thorax, *Abd* abdomen

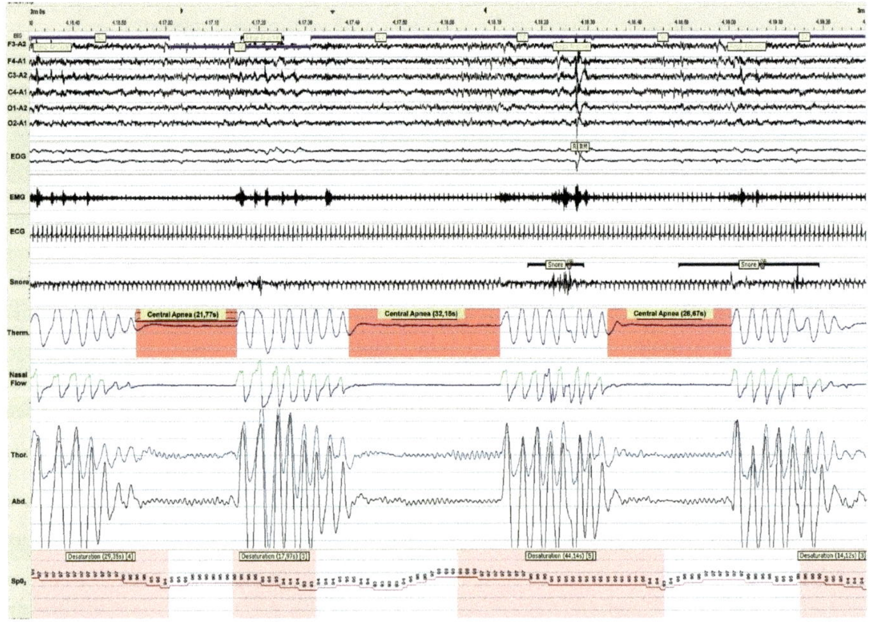

Fig. 8.3 A 3-min polysomnogram of a patient with heart failure revealing three central apneas during stage 2 NREM sleep. Abbreviations as in Fig. 8.2

same night varying degrees of both central and obstructive sleep apneas [31]. Compared to patients without sleep apnea or OSA, patients with CSA have a worse hemodynamic profile and higher NYHA class [32].

It is recognized that heart failure contributes to the development of CSA and OSA by several mechanisms. First, in patients with heart failure, the ventilatory control system may become unstable and give rise to self-sustaining ventilatory oscillations owing to a long circulatory delay and an increased loop gain brought about, respectively, by impaired hemodynamics and augmented chemosensitivity [33, 34]. Second, the presence of a narrowed CO_2 reserve enhances the susceptibility to central apneas [35]. Third, overnight rostral fluid displacement from the legs may cause fluid accumulation in the neck and lungs, thereby predisposing to the occurrence of OSA (due to the increased collapsibility of upper airways) and CSA (due to an increase in pulmonary congestion leading to worsening of the lung function and to stimulation of pulmonary vagal receptors, both of which would promote ventilatory instability) [36, 37].

The hallmark of sleep-disordered breathing – being central or obstructive in nature – is the triggering of intermittent episodes of hypoxemia and hypercapnia and of arousals which cause fragmentation of physiological sleep [38]. These events take place in repetitive cycles during sleep and induce the activation of a number of pathophysiological consequences including sympathetic activation, endothelial dysfunction, oxidative stress, metabolic dysregulation, and inflammation [39, 40], which have been shown to impact on the clinical outcome [41, 42]. Interestingly, in heart failure patients, disordered breathing also occurs during day time, possibly contributing to poor prognosis [43].

8.5   Sleep Apnea and the Autonomic Nervous System in Heart Failure

Autonomic cardiovascular control may be importantly implicated as a potential link between sleep-disordered breathing and its pathophysiological consequences. Autonomic responses to apnea are complex and mainly involve chemoreflex and baroreflex regulation.

In OSA patients, several studies have demonstrated that recurrent nocturnal apneas are followed by sympathetic activation [44] and impaired baroreflex control [45] that persist during daytime wakefulness [44, 46], thus leading to a chronic dysfunction in autonomic balance (Fig. 8.4). Interestingly, the OSA-induced baroreflex dysfunction can be partly reversed following effective continuous positive airway (CPAP) treatment [47].

It is currently thought that in patients with heart failure, sleep-disordered breathing causes cyclical increases in sympathetic nerve activity which results from the complex interplay of several mechanisms, including: (i) the reflex cardiac response to cyclical stimulation of chemoreceptors by hypoxia and hypercapnia, (ii) central effects of the cyclical increase in inspiratory drive and of arousals from sleep on sympathetic outflow, and (iii) the elimination of reflex inhibition of sympathetic outflow by pulmonary stretch receptors during obstructive apneas [37, 48, 49].

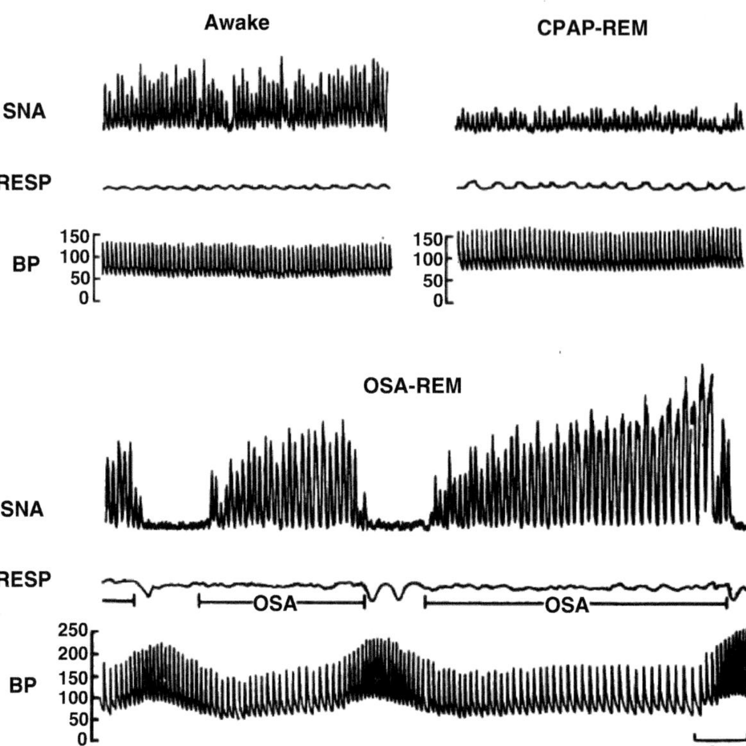

Fig. 8.4 Recording of sympathetic neural activity (*SNA*), respiration (*RESP*), and intra-arterial blood pressure (*BP*) in the same subject when awake, with obstructive sleep apnea during REM sleep and with elimination of obstructive apnea by CPAP therapy during REM sleep. SNA is very high during wakefulness, but increases even further secondary to obstructive sleep apnea during REM. Blood pressure increases from 130/65 when awake to 256/110 at the end of the apnea. Elimination of apneas by CPAP results in decreased nerve activity and prevents BP surges during REM sleep (Reproduced with permission from Ref. [44])

In patients with heart failure, the sympathetic activation that accompanies sleep-disordered breathing may significantly add to the already existing autonomic dysfunction that characterizes heart failure [50], thus contributing to the progression of the disease. Not only awake sympathetic activity – as assessed by microneurography – was significantly higher in patients with heart failure and either obstructive or central sleep apnea [51], but also baroreceptor sensitivity was found to be significantly more depressed when compared to patients with similar cardiac function but without breathing disorders [52].

8.6   Sleep Apnea and Sudden Death in Heart Failure

It has been previously shown how sleep apnea can be the cause of a derangement in autonomic cardiovascular control resulting in sympathetic overactivity [44, 45]. Moreover, the autonomic effects of arousals that can occur hundreds of times per night in patients with sleep-disordered breathing, also provide the milieu for an increased arrhythmia susceptibility. Clinical data support an increased risk for nocturnal arrhythmia and sudden death in patients with sleep-disordered breathing. In the Sleep Heart Health Study, not only the prevalence of nonsustained ventricular tachycardia was significantly higher in subjects with sleep-disordered breathing as compared to those without [53], but also the relative risk of the occurrence of an arrhythmia was markedly increased within 90 s after a respiratory disturbance in subjects with sleep-disordered breathing [54]. A retrospective analysis on death certificates of patients known to have OSA demonstrated a shift to nighttime (from midnight to 6 am) in the circadian distribution of sudden death as compared to the usual early morning peak of subjects without OSA in the general population [55]. In a large study on 10,701 consecutive adults undergoing a diagnostic polysomnogram who were followed up to 15 years, OSA predicted incident sudden cardiac death, and the magnitude of risk was predicted by multiple parameters characterizing OSA severity [56].

The role of the autonomic nervous system in triggering cardiac arrhythmias might be particularly relevant with regard to arrhythmic events taking place in patients with heart failure and sleep-disordered breathing. Several studies in patients with heart failure reported that the presence of both obstructive and central sleep apnea poses an independent risk factor for the occurrence of malignant arrhythmias documented by implantable cardioverter defibrillator therapies [57, 58]. In a study analyzing the circadian pattern, a striking increase in the incidence of ventricular arrhythmias occurring during the sleep period as opposed to periods of wakefulness was observed in patients with sleep-disordered breathing [59] (Fig. 8.5). Finally, a major impairment of the autonomic control has also been documented in patients with SDB and ventricular arrhythmias suggesting that sympathetic overactivity and vagal withdrawal are important contributing mechanisms [60].

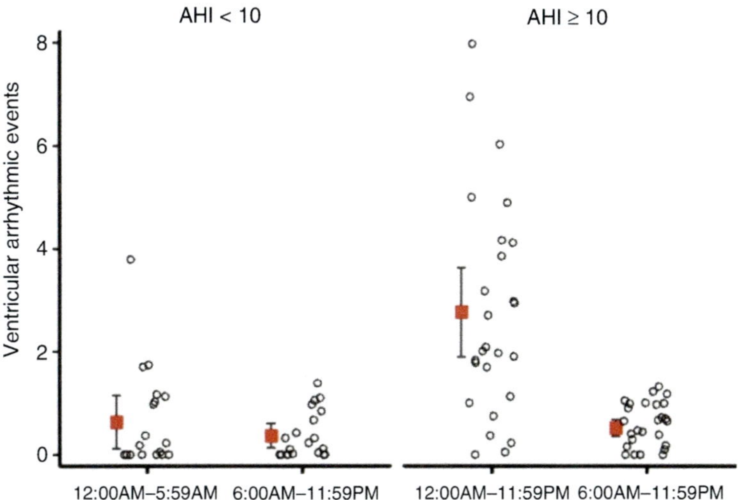

Fig. 8.5 Ventricular arrhythmias in patients with (*right*) and those without (*left*) sleep-disordered breathing according to the time of day. Error bars represent mean and 95 % confidence interval. Each circle represents the number of events in one patient. *AHI* apnea-hypopnea index (Reproduced with permission from Ref. [59])

Conclusions

The autonomic nervous system is deeply involved in the mechanisms mediating the cardiovascular effects of sleep within its different stages. Autonomic cardiac control during sleep is characterized by a vagal predominance for most of the time that is interrupted by bursts of sympathetic activity during arousals in NREM sleep and even more during the phasic REM sleep periods. The autonomic fluctuation during sleep associated with the lasting sympathetic activation that occurs in many cardiovascular diseases, particularly heart failure, sets the stage for an increased susceptibility to life-threatening arrhythmias. Sleep apneas, which are a common comorbidity in patients with heart failure, further complicate the picture of autonomic dysregulation and the risk of cardiac events in these subjects by eliciting a further sympathetic activation mostly due to the associated oxygen desaturation and recurrent arousals. Further understanding of the pathophysiological pathways linking sleep disorders to cardiac events is however important to improve clinical management and reduce cardiovascular risk.

References

1. Carskadon MA, Dement WC. Normal human sleep: an overview. In: Principle and practice of sleep medicine. 5th ed. St Louis: Elsevier Saunders; 2011. p. 17–26.
2. Trinder J, Waloszek J, Woods MJ, Jordan AS. Sleep and cardiovascular regulation. Pflugers Arch. 2012;463:161–8.
3. Coote JH. Respiratory and circulatory control during sleep. J Exp Biol. 1982;100:223–44.
4. George CF, Kryger MH. Sleep and control of heart rate. Clin Chest Med. 1985;6:595–601.
5. Carrington MJ, Barbieri R, Colrain IM, Crowley KE, Kim Y, Trinder J. Changes in cardiovascular function during the sleep onset period in young adults. J Appl Physiol. 2005;98:468–76.
6. Zemaityte D, Varoneckas G, Sokolov E. Heart rhythm control during sleep. Psychophysiology. 1984;21:279–89.
7. Shen MJ, Zipes DP. Role of the autonomic nervous system in modulating cardiac arrhythmias. Circ Res. 2014;114:1004–21.
8. Silvani A. Physiological sleep-dependent changes in arterial blood pressure: central autonomic commands and baroreflex control. Clin Exp Pharmacol Physiol. 2008;35:987–94.
9. Smyth HS, Sleight P, Pickering GW. Reflex regulation of arterial pressure during sleep in man. A quantitative method of assessing baroreflex sensitivity. Circ Res. 1969;24:109–21.
10. Somers VK, Dyken ME, Mark AL, Abboud FM. Sympathetic-nerve activity during sleep in normal subjects. N Engl J Med. 1993;328:303–7.
11. Furlan R, Guzzetti S, Crivellaro W, Dassi S, Tinelli M, Baselli G, Cerutti S, Lombardi F, Pagani M, Malliani A. Continuous 24-hour assessment of the neural regulation of systemic arterial pressure and RR variabilities in ambulant subjects. Circulation. 1990;81:537–47.
12. Bristow JD, Honour AJ, Pickering TG, Sleight P. Cardiovascular and respiratory changes during sleep in normal and hypertensive subjects. Cardiovasc Res. 1969;3:476–85.
13. Parati G, Di Rienzo M, Bertinieri G, Pomidossi G, Casadei R, Groppelli A, Pedotti A, Zanchetti A, Mancia G. Evaluation of the baroreceptor-heart rate reflex by 24-hour intra-arterial blood pressure monitoring in humans. Hypertension. 1988;12:214–22.
14. Mancia G. Autonomic modulation of the cardiovascular system during sleep. N Engl J Med. 1993;328:347–9.
15. Verrier RL, Josephson ME. Impact of sleep on arrhythmogenesis. Circ Arrhythm Electrophysiol. 2009;2:450–9.

16. La Rovere MT, Pinna GD, Hohnloser SH, Marcus FI, Mortara A, Nohara R, ATRAMI (Autonomic Tone and Reflexes After Myocardial Infarction) Investigators, et al. Baroreflex sensitivity and heart rate variability in the identification of patients at risk for life-threatening arrhythmias. Implications for clinical trials. Circulation. 2001;103:2072–7.
17. Vanoli E, Adamson PB, Ba-Lin, Pinna GD, Lazzara R, Orr WC. Heart rate variability during specific sleep stages. A comparison of healthy subjects with patients after myocardial infarction. Circulation. 1995;91:1918–22.
18. Willich SN, Goldberg RJ, Maclure M, Perriello L, Muller JE. Increased onset of sudden cardiac death in the first three hours after awakening. Am J Cardiol. 1992;70:65–8.
19. Englund A, Behrens S, Wegscheider K, Rowland E. Circadian variation of malignant ventricular arrhythmias in patients with ischemic and nonischemic heart disease after cardioverter defibrillator implantation. European 7219 Jewel Investigators. J Am Coll Cardiol. 1999;34:1560–8.
20. Sowho M, Amatoury J, Kirkness JP, Patil SP. Sleep and respiratory physiology in adults. Clin Chest Med. 2014;35:469–81.
21. Khoo MC, Kronauer RE, Strohl KP, Slutsky AS. Factors inducing periodic breathing in humans: a general model. J Appl Physiol. 1982;53:644–59.
22. Cherniack NS, Longobardo GS. Mathematical models of periodic breathing and their usefulness in understanding cardiovascular and respiratory disorders. Exp Physiol. 2006;91:295–305.
23. Kara T, Narkiewicz K, Somers VK. Chemoreflexes-physiology and clinical implications. Acta Physiol Scand. 2003;177:377–84.
24. Dempsey JA, Smith CA, Przybylowski T, Chenuel B, Xie A, Nakayama H, Skatrud JB. The ventilatory responsiveness to $CO(2)$ below eupnoea as a determinant of ventilatory stability in sleep. J Physiol. 2004;560(Pt 1):1–11.
25. Oldenburg O, Lamp B, Faber L, Teschler H, Horstkotte D, Topfer V. Sleep-disordered breathing in patients with symptomatic heart failure: a contemporary study of prevalence in and characteristics of 700 patients. Eur J Heart Fail. 2007;9:251–7.
26. Vazir A, Hastings PC, Dayer M, McIntyre HF, Henein MY, Poole-Wilson PA, Cowie MR, Morrell MJ, Simonds AK. A high prevalence of sleep disordered breathing in men with mild symptomatic chronic heart failure due to left ventricular systolic dysfunction. Eur J Heart Fail. 2007;9:243–50.
27. Yumino D, Wang H, Floras JS, Newton GE, Mak S, Ruttanaumpawan P, Parker JD, Bradley TD. Prevalence and physiological predictors of sleep apnea in patients with heart failure and systolic dysfunction. J Card Fail. 2009;15:279–85.
28. Cherniack NS. Apnea and periodic breathing during sleep. N Engl J Med. 1999;341:985–7.
29. Ryan CM, Bradley TD. Periodicity of obstructive sleep apnea in patients with and without heart failure. Chest. 2005;127:536–42.
30. Pinna GD, Robbi E, Pizza F, Taurino AE, Pronzato C, La Rovere MT, Maestri R. Can cardio-respiratory polygraphy replace portable polysomnography in the assessment of sleep-disordered breathing in heart failure patients? Sleep Breath. 2014;18:475–82.
31. Tkacova R, Niroumand M, Lorenzi-Filho G, Bradley TD. Overnight shift from obstructive to central apneas in patients with heart failure: role of PCO2 and circulatory delay. Circulation. 2001;103:238–43.
32. Solin P, Bergin P, Richardson M, Kaye DM, Walters EH, Naughton MT. Influence of pulmonary capillary wedge pressure on central apnea in heart failure. Circulation. 1999;99:1574–9.
33. Pinna GD, Maestri R, Mortara A, La Rovere MT, Fanfulla F, Sleight P. Periodic breathing in heart failure patients: testing the hypothesis of instability of the chemoreflex loop. J Appl Physiol. 2000;89:2147–57.
34. Solin P, Roebuck T, Johns DP, Walters EH, Naughton MT. Peripheral and central ventilatory responses in central sleep apnea with and without congestive heart failure. Am J Respir Crit Care Med. 2000;162:2194–200.
35. Xie A, Skatrud JB, Puleo DS, Rahko PS, Dempsey JA. Apnea-hypopnea threshold for CO2 in patients with congestive heart failure. Am J Respir Crit Care Med. 2002;165:1245–50.

36. Yumino D, Redolfi S, Ruttanaumpawan P, Su MC, Smith S, Newton GE, Mak S, Bradley TD. Nocturnal rostral fluid shift: a unifying concept for the pathogenesis of obstructive and central sleep apnea in men with heart failure. Circulation. 2010;121:1598–605.
37. Kasai T, Arcand J, Allard JP, Mak S, Azevedo ER, Newton GE, Bradley TD. Obstructive sleep apnea and heart failure: pathophysiologic and therapeutic implications. J Am Coll Cardiol. 2011;57:119–27.
38. Pinna GD, Robbi E, Pizza F, Caporotondi A, La Rovere MT, Maestri R. Sleep-wake fluctuations and respiratory events during Cheyne-Stokes respiration in patients with heart failure. J Sleep Res. 2014;23:347–57.
39. Sánchez-de-la-Torre M, Campos-Rodriguez F, Barbé F. Obstructive sleep apnoea and cardiovascular disease. Lancet Respir Med. 2013;1:61–72.
40. Floras JS. Sleep apnea and cardiovascular risk. J Cardiol. 2014;63:3–8.
41. Javaheri S, Shukla R, Zeigler H, Wexler L. Central sleep apnea, right ventricular dysfunction, and low diastolic blood pressure are predictors of mortality in systolic heart failure. J Am Coll Cardiol. 2007;49:2028–34.
42. Jilek C, Krenn M, Sebah D, Obermeier R, Braune A, Kehl V, Schroll S, Montalvan S, Riegger GA, Pfeifer M, Arzt M. Prognostic impact of sleep disordered breathing and its treatment in heart failure: an observational study. Eur J Heart Fail. 2011;13:68–75.
43. La Rovere MT, Pinna GD, Maestri R, Robbi E, Mortara A, Fanfulla F, Febo O, Sleight P. Clinical relevance of short-term day-time breathing disorders in chronic heart failure patients. Eur J Heart Fail. 2007;9:949–54.
44. Somers VK, Dyken ME, Clary MP, Abboud FM. Sympathetic neural mechanisms in obstructive sleep apnea. J Clin Invest. 1995;96:1897–904.
45. Parati G, Di Rienzo M, Bonsignore MR, Insalaco G, Marrone O, Castiglioni P, Bonsignore G, Mancia G. Autonomic cardiac regulation in obstructive sleep apnea syndrome: evidence from spontaneous baroreflex analysis during sleep. J Hypertens. 1997;15:1621–6.
46. Carlson JT, Hedner JA, Sellgren J, Elam M, Wallin BG. Depressed baroreflex sensitivity in patients with obstructive sleep apnea. Am J Respir Crit Care Med. 1996;154:1490–6.
47. Bonsignore MR, Parati G, Insalaco G, Marrone O, Castiglioni P, Romano S, Di Rienzo M, Mancia G, Bonsignore G. Continuous positive airway pressure treatment improves baroreflex control of heart rate during sleep in severe obstructive sleep apnea syndrome. Am J Respir Crit Care Med. 2002;166:279–86.
48. van de Borne P, Oren R, Abouassaly C, Anderson E, Somers VK. Effect of Cheyne-Stokes respiration on muscle sympathetic nerve activity in severe congestive heart failure secondary to ischemic or idiopathic dilated cardiomyopathy. Am J Cardiol. 1998;81:432–6.
49. Yumino D, Bradley TD. Central sleep apnea and Cheyne-Stokes respiration. Proc Am Thorac Soc. 2008;5:226–36.
50. La Rovere MT, Pinna GD, Maestri R, Robbi E, Caporotondi A, Guazzotti G, Sleight P. Prognostic implications of baroreflex sensitivity in heart failure patients in the beta-blocking era. J Am Coll Cardiol. 2009;53:193–9.
51. Spaak J, Egri ZJ, Kubo T, Yu E, Ando S, Kaneko Y, Usui K, Bradley TD, Floras JS. Muscle sympathetic nerve activity during wakefulness in heart failure patients with and without sleep apnea. Hypertension. 2005;46:1327–32.
52. Ueno LM, Drager LF, Rodrigues AC, Rondon MU, Mathias Jr W, Krieger EM, Júnior RF, Negrão CE, Lorenzi-Filho G. Day-night pattern of autonomic nervous system modulation in patients with heart failure with and without sleep apnea. Int J Cardiol. 2011;148:53–8.
53. Mehra R, Benjamin EJ, Shahar E, Gottlieb DJ, Nawabit R, Kirchner HL, Sahadevan J, Redline S. Sleep heart health study. Association of nocturnal arrhythmias with sleep-disordered breathing: the sleep heart health study. Am J Respir Crit Care Med. 2006;173:910–6.
54. Gami AS, Howard DE, Olson EJ, Somers VK. Day-night pattern of sudden death in obstructive sleep apnea. N Engl J Med. 2005;352:1206–14.
55. Gami AS, Olson EJ, Shen WK, Wright RS, Ballman KV, Hodge DO, Herges RM, Howard DE, Somers VK. Obstructive sleep apnea and the risk of sudden cardiac death: a longitudinal study of 10,701 adults. J Am Coll Cardiol. 2013;62:610–6.

56. Monahan K, Storfer-Isser A, Mehra R, Shahar E, Mittleman M, Rottman J, Punjabi N, Sanders M, Quan SF, Resnick H, Redline S. Triggering of nocturnal arrhythmias by sleep-disordered breathing events. J Am Coll Cardiol. 2009;54:1797–804.
57. Bitter T, Westerheide N, Prinz C, Hossain MS, Vogt J, Langer C, Horstkotte D, Oldenburg O. Cheyne-Stokes respiration and obstructive sleep apnoea are independent risk factors for malignant ventricular arrhythmias requiring appropriate cardioverter-defibrillator therapies in patients with congestive heart failure. Eur Heart J. 2011;32:61–74.
58. Kreuz J, Skowasch D, Horlbeck F, Atzinger C, Schrickel JW, Lorenzen H, Nickenig G, Schwab JO. Usefulness of sleep-disordered breathing to predict occurrence of appropriate and inappropriate implantable-cardioverter defibrillator therapy in patients with implantable cardioverter-defibrillator for primary prevention of sudden cardiac death. Am J Cardiol. 2013;111:1319–23.
59. Zeidan-Shwiri T, Aronson D, Atalla K, Blich M, Suleiman M, Marai I, Gepstein L, Lavie L, Lavie P, Boulos M. Circadian pattern of life-threatening ventricular arrhythmia in patients with sleep-disordered breathing and implantable cardioverter-defibrillators. Heart Rhythm. 2011;8:657–62.
60. Yamada S, Suzuki H, Kamioka M, Suzuki S, Kamiyama Y, Yoshihisa A, Saitoh S, Takeishi Y. Sleep-disordered breathing increases risk for fatal ventricular arrhythmias in patients with chronic heart failure. Circ J. 2013;77:1466–73.

Cerebral Aging: Implications for the Heart Autonomic Nervous System Regulation

Alessia Pascale and Stefano Govoni

The autonomic nervous system (ANS), including sympathetic and parasympathetic neuronal outflows, together with the afferent inputs and central control mechanisms, plays a key role in the maintenance of cardiovascular homeostasis. Preganglionic neurons of the sympathetic and parasympathetic systems are localized in the central nervous system, and their axons form synapses on postganglionic effector neurons in peripheral autonomic ganglia. Preganglionic neurons in the ANS utilize acetylcholine as a neurotransmitter, while postganglionic neurons typically employ either noradrenaline (sympathetic) or acetylcholine (parasympathetic).

There is now unequivocal evidence that progressive sympathetic activation occurs with aging. This sympathetic stimulation seems to implicate the sympathetic outflow to the heart, the skeletal muscle vasculature, and the gut and liver, but to exclude the kidneys [1]. Although the nature of the underlying disturbance in sympathetic control at central level remains largely unknown, the importance of better understanding the central mechanisms implicated in aging-induced sympathetic activation is stressed by the recognition that in a variety of cardiovascular disorders, including heart failure, whose incidence rises with age, the sympathetic nervous system (SNS) is causally involved [2].

9.1 Central Control of Sympathetic Outflow

Central sympathetic neuronal circuits regulate several components of the sympathetic nerve outflow, also including the sympathetic nerve discharge (SND). To this last regard, the forebrain, brain stem, and spinal neuronal circuits are specifically implicated in the control of SND in young and mature mammals (reviewed in [3]), thus indicating the existence of complex interactions at multiple levels. It is

A. Pascale • S. Govoni (✉)
Section of Pharmacology, Department of Drug Sciences, University of Pavia, Pavia, Italy
e-mail: alessia.pascale@unipv.it; govonis@unipv.it

© Springer International Publishing Switzerland 2016
E. Gronda et al. (eds.), *Heart Failure Management: The Neural Pathways*,
DOI 10.1007/978-3-319-24993-3_9

therefore presumable that age-associated alterations within the central sympathetic circuits may contribute to changes in SND regulation during senescence. Notably, as mentioned, the investigation of the effect of aging on the SNS is clinically pertinent because of the possible interconnection of age-dependent sympathetic nervous changes with cardiovascular disease development.

The *nucleus tractus solitarii* (NTS) is a brain stem nucleus which is an extremely important central integration site since it receives the majority of primary nerve endings of chemoreceptors, baroreceptors, and cardiopulmonary afferents. In turn, the NTS projects to several areas of the forebrain, brain stem, and spinal cord which are engaged in the control of SND [4–6]. Ito and Buñag [7] reported that, following the injection of serotonin directly into the NTS, the reduction in mean pressure, heart rate, and renal nerve firing were significantly smaller in 24-month-old than in 2-month-old rats, thus suggesting that the sensitivity of serotonergic mechanisms in the NTS to inhibit blood pressure, heart rate, and renal nerve activity decreases with senescence.

Excitatory sympathetic projections from the *locus coeruleus* and the A5 region of the brain stem to the hypothalamus and amygdala are relevant in the central control of sympathetic outflow [8, 9]. To this regard, Esler and collaborators [10] suggested, in humans, the possibility for age-related alterations in forebrain regulation of SND. In particular, they investigated the influence of senescence on brain noradrenaline turnover in young (20–30 years) and old (60–75 years) men by measuring the internal jugular venous overflow of noradrenaline and its lipophilic metabolites. They found that brain noradrenaline turnover is higher in older than in younger men and that this increase is confined to subcortical brain regions. The authors excluded the involvement of a central defect in neuronal noradrenaline reuptake since the relative patterns of metabolite overflow did not differ significantly between young and older subjects. Of interest, they also documented the existence of a statistically significant direct relationship between subcortical noradrenaline turnover and sympathetic tone in the cardiac sympathetic outflow.

Within this general context, an additional aspect that should be considered is that during senescence, neurons undergo morphological changes such as a reduction in the complexity of dendrite arborization and dendritic length. Taking into account the key role of dendrites in integrating and processing input signals, this event may impair neuronal communication. Moreover, a decrease in spine number has also been observed; notably, spines are the major sites for excitatory synapses; therefore, changes in their numbers could reflect an alteration in synaptic densities [11]. However, although these age-related morphological changes are evident in cortical neuronal circuits, the effect of aging on the total neuronal number of identified neurons involved in sympathetic circuits remains widely unknown [3].

9.2 Gangliar Level Control

Little is known about the age-dependent alterations at gangliar level. In animals, ganglionic long-term potentiation (gLTP) can be evoked by a brief period of high-frequency stimulation (20 Hz for 20 s) and has been reported in various autonomic ganglia from several animal species. In autonomic ganglia, gLTP is expected to increase tonic efferent impulses to a wide range of neuroeffector organs, including the heart and the blood vessels, thus affecting their functions. In old animals (28–32-month rats), changes in certain biochemical aspects found in cervical sympathetic ganglia (SCG) suggest an age-related enhancement in synaptic activity and may indicate the potentiation of ganglionic transmission [12]. Indeed, in the SCG from old rats, tyrosine hydroxylase activity is enhanced, and in reserpine-depleted ganglia, the recovery rate of catecholamines is slower. Specifically, this slow recovery rate has been ascribed to a higher secretion and not to a decreased catecholamine synthesis, thus indicating the presence of an enhanced neurotransmitter synthesis and release in aged rats ganglia [13] (Fig. 9.1). Considering that aging is often viewed as a progressive decline in physiological competence with a corresponding inability to adapt to stressful stimuli, it has been suggested that the increased activity of the SNS may be responsible for the development and/or aggravation of stress-induced hypertension (reviewed in [12]).

Concerning human subjects, structural changes in dendrites, axons, and synapses have been consistently identified in sympathetic ganglia of aged people, being the hallmark pathological alteration represented by neuroaxonal dystrophy. In particular, it has been reported that neuroaxonal dystrophy targets the presynaptic nerve terminal, thus critically altering neuron-to-neuron communication and also resulting in the typical distal axonopathy [14].

9.3   Nerve Ending Level: Presynaptic Control and Postsynaptic Signaling

Postganglionic sympathetic neurons which innervate the heart and resistance vessels contribute to the regulation of cardiac output, arterial blood pressure, and regional vascular conductance, thus ensuring the adequate perfusion of vital organs, being noradrenaline (NA) the key neurotransmitter. The stimulation of adrenaline release from the adrenal medulla significantly participates to the control of cardiovascular function as well as of energy metabolism.

Based on the concept that peripheral higher concentrations of NA would reflect an elevated sympathetic nerve firing rate (or vice versa), the initial experimental approaches were directed to measure NA levels in the urine (24-h collections) and in the plasma from arterial or venous blood samples [15]. To this regard, cross-sectional studies have reported a 10–15 % increase per decade of NA with respect to the adult age range [16–19], where the most consistent results have being obtained using arterial blood samples. However, the main limit of this approach is that it does not take into account the rate of NA metabolic clearance, which contributes to the final NA plasma levels [15]. Therefore, subsequent measurements were performed employing isotope dilution-based methods, where the rate of NA appearance (spillover) into the plasma was utilized to evaluate the activity of the SNS. Employing this strategy, plasma NA spillover rates have been documented to be higher in older subjects with respect to young adults [20–22] (Fig. 9.1). However, the differences

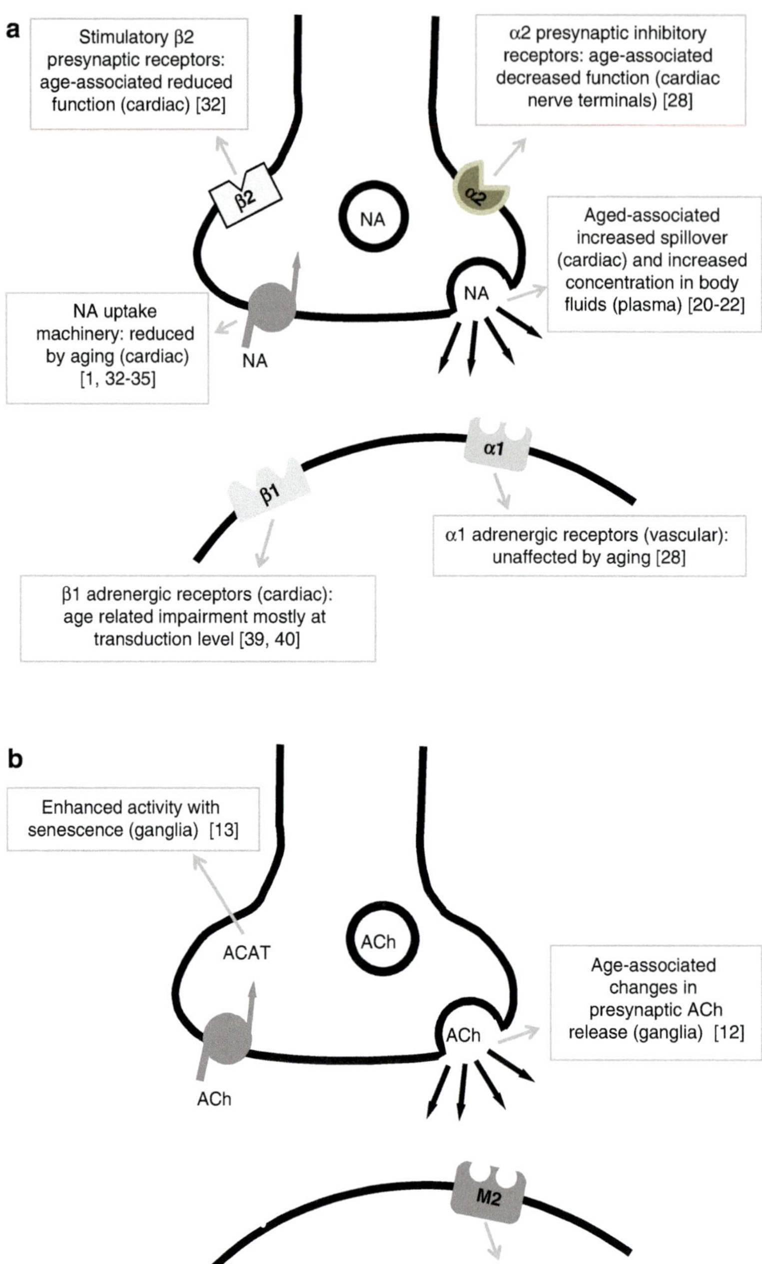

Fig. 9.1 Age-associated ANS and heart signaling changes at a glance. The figure reports the main effects on the noradrenergic (**a**) and cholinergic (**b**) signaling during senescence. In the ANS, preganglionic neurons employ acetylcholine as a neurotransmitter, while postganglionic neurons typically utilize either noradrenaline (sympathetic) or acetylcholine (parasympathetic). *ACAT* acetyl-CoA – acetyltransferase, *ACh* acetylcholine, *NA* noradrenaline. See text for more details

between young and old subjects were less strong in comparison to those found in the previous studies due to the fact that plasma NA clearance rates are often reduced with senescence [22–24]. Despite of an age-associated increase in plasma NA spillover, total adrenaline secretion has been reported to be approximately 40 % lower in older men at resting conditions. Moreover, in older men the release of adrenaline in response to mental stress, dynamic exercise, and isometric exercise is strongly impaired (between 33 and 44 %) with respect to the levels observed in younger subjects [25]. The lowered adrenaline secretion rate with aging, accompanied by SNS activation, emphasizes that the two elements of the "sympathoadrenal medullary system" do not always act in concert, so that a mismatching of sympathetic activity and adrenaline secretion rate can occur [10].

9.3.1 Presynaptic Control

Two important aspects which contribute to plasma NA spillover should be additionally considered: (a) the release of NA from sympathetic nerve endings is modulated at presynaptic level by adrenergic receptors and (b) active reuptake processes are implicated in getting back up to the 80–90 % of the released neurotransmitter. Therefore, age-dependent alterations within these mechanisms may considerably contribute to changes in plasma NA spillover (Fig. 9.1). To this regard, an age-related reduction of presynaptic $\alpha2$ receptors function has been reported in the rat [26–28] which may participate in elevating the amount of the released NA. In the rat heart, xylazine, an $\alpha2$ agonist, showed an age-associated reduced potency at inhibiting cardioacceleration to nerve stimulation [28]. In humans, the status of these receptors in the heart is not known; however, at peripheral level, it has been demonstrated that changes in $\alpha2$ adrenoceptor expression in the setting of heart failure do lead to altered NA spillover [29]. Presynaptic β-adrenoceptors have been documented on some noradrenergic nerve terminals, where they favor neurotransmitter release and are mainly represented by $\beta2$ adrenoceptors [30]. It has been hypothesized that they are targeted by circulating adrenaline, which manifests a much higher affinity than NA [31]. The $\beta2$ agonists procaterol and isoprenaline are significantly less able to enhance the stimulation-evoked release of NA in atria from old animals with respect to young rats [32], thus suggesting an age-related reduction of presynaptic β-adrenoceptors function. However, the precise role of these receptors in the regulation of neurotransmission and whether their aged-associated alterations are important still remain to be established.

Concerning reuptake mechanisms, a variety of studies, performed both in humans and animals, documented that in the heart, a reduction in NA reuptake is involved in the apparent age-dependent rise of NA release [33–35]. Indeed, a diminished NA reuptake has been implicated in the almost double increase of cardiac plasma NA spillover rate found in older healthy in comparison to young men [1]. The effectiveness of neuronal reuptake mechanisms can be examined employing cocaine, where a decline in these processes would correspond to a decreased capability of cocaine to improve neurotransmission. Indeed, in rat atria from old animals, cocaine has little effect in potentiating the stimulation-evoked release of NA in comparison to young rats [32]. Focusing on the heart, it has been postulated that the reduction in the efficacy of reuptake mechanisms is a cellular strategy useful to compensate the age-related decline in NA responsiveness, thus helping to preserve the contractile function.

9.3.2 Postsynaptic Signaling

Aging is associated with several changes involving noradrenergic transmission, resulting in a modified response to the transmitters (Fig. 9.1). Within this context, α-adrenoreceptor antagonists have been used to determine age-dependent modifications of blood pressure. No changes in hypotensive effects of α1-adrenoreceptors antagonists have been documented with senescence; indeed, in men, the hypotensive actions of prazosin and phentolamine have been reported unchanged by senescence [28].

Following catecholamine release, myocardial responses are mainly mediated by beta-adrenergic receptors, being β1 receptors significantly predominant. Therefore, β-adrenoceptor antagonists can be employed to evaluate age-dependent alterations in noradrenergic control of cardiac output and heart rate. To this regard, it has been found that β-antagonists are effective in lowering blood pressure in older subjects [36] and that, in the elderly, propranolol (a nonselective β-blocker) is as effective in decreasing heart rate and cardiac output during exercise [37], although causes larger falls in systolic blood pressure. Moreover, it has been demonstrated that isoproterenol (a β1-selective agonist) induces a reduced response in older subjects, thus suggesting a decline of cardiac β1-receptors during senescence [25, 38]. Although the issue regarding the age-associated decline of β1-receptors is still controversial, more consistent data support the existence of an impairment of post-receptor signaling during senescence [39]. Accordingly, Brodde et al. [40] demonstrated that in aged human atria, besides only a tendency of a reduction of β1-receptors, there is a significant impairment in the activation of the adenylyl cyclase by isoproterenol, terbutaline (a β2-selective agonist), and forskolin (an activator of adenylyl cyclase). However, it was reported that neither G protein-coupled receptor kinases nor inhibitory G proteins seem to contribute to the age-related decline of cardiac β-adrenergic receptors responsiveness [41]. Maximum exercise heart rate diminishes with senescence, thus potentially limiting the performance during acute exercise [42]. The intrinsic pacemaker rate of the heart, examined in the absence of outside influence (i.e., following blocking both sympathetic and vagal control via propranolol and atropine administration, respectively), also declines with aging [43], and this has been related to a reduced number of pacemaker cells [44]. Hence, a reduced intrinsic pacemaker rate coupled with a weakened responsiveness of pacemaker cells to β-receptor activation may account for the decreased maximal heart rate observed during senescence [32].

Concerning the parasympathetic branch, several studies have documented an age-associated decrease in the parasympathetic control of heart rate [45], although the underlying mechanisms are still uncertain. Within this context, it has been postulated that alterations in presynaptic control of acetylcholine release, a decline in muscarinic M2 receptor density, and changes in postsynaptic cholinergic signaling may all contribute to this dysfunction [46, 47]. In particular, in human atria, the reduction of M2 receptors was associated with a decreased capability of carbachol (a muscarinic agonist) to inhibit both the activation of adenylyl cyclase and the force of contraction mediated by forskolin [48]. Curiously, Liu et al. [49] found the presence of antibodies against M2 receptors in healthy subjects, reporting an increase of the frequency with increasing age. Taken together, these data indicate that in the human heart, the number and the functional responsiveness of M2 receptors are impaired with senescence.

9.4 The Baroreceptor Reflex

The baroreceptor reflexes, which act in a negative feedback manner, are key players in the maintenance of the circulatory homeostasis. Specifically, the baroreceptors represent the anatomical site where the baroreflex loop originates. The baroreceptors are highly specialized stretch-sensitive receptors which monitor changes in blood pressure and relay them to the brain stem. They are localized in several districts of the cardiovascular system; in particular those distributed in the aorta and in the carotid artery are sometimes named as *high-pressure* baroreceptors, while those placed in the cardiopulmonary regions are called *low-pressure* baroreceptors [50]. At the level of the central nervous system, the afferent impulses are integrated and the efferent arm of the baroreceptor reflex operates through the sympathetic and parasympathetic branches of the ANS. For example, following a transient decrease of the blood pressure (=reduced firing rate of the baroreceptors), the parasympathetic outflow is inhibited while the sympathetic one is stimulated, and vice versa.

The cardiac arm of the baroreceptor reflex is implicated in the regulation (shortening or prolongation) of the cardiac period (R-R) according to changes in the baroreceptor input, usually represented by blood pressure variations. Generally, a sigmoid curve describes the relation between the blood pressure and the cardiac period, where the linear portion of this curve reflects the cardiovagal (=cardiac response vagally mediated) baroreflex sensitivity. Experimental evidence indicates that this parameter may have a prognostic value in terms of sudden cardiac death risk, and, of interest, a decreased cardiovagal baroreflex sensitivity has been observed with senescence [50]. Indeed, cardiovagal baroreflex sensitivity has been shown to be inversely and linearly correlated with age [51, 52]. Concerning the underlying mechanisms, alterations in any component of the cardiac baroreflex arc, such as at the level of the afferent and the efferent arms or at the impulses integration, may be involved. To this regard, it should be taken into account that the ability to identify such age-associated changes in humans is very limited. However, data indicating a decrease in muscarinic receptors (M2) [46] and a reduced responsiveness of the heart to muscarinic activation [47] are consistent with a diminished vagal control in humans with senescence.

Within this general context, considering that arterial stretch is a fundamental determinant of baroreflex activation, it has been suggested that arterial stiffening may represent an important contributor to the age-dependent baroreflex dysfunction. Indeed, correlations at rest between cardiovagal baroreflex sensitivity and carotid arterial compliance across people of different age are consistent with this concept [52].

With reference to the sympathetic arm of the baroreflex, a reverse sigmoid curve describes the relation between blood pressure (stimulus) and the sympathetic outflow (response). Studinger and collaborators [53] documented that during senescence, the integrated baroreflex control of vascular sympathetic outflow displays a reduced sympathetic activation and a greater sympathoinhibition. Specifically, they observed that in older subjects, during pressure falls, the effects of carotid vascular stiffening cannot be counterbalanced by a stronger neural control of sympathetic outflow, thus resulting in an impaired sympathetic activity. Instead, during pressure rises, the presence of a more sensitive neural control allows to overcome the structural deficits, thus leading to an increased baroreflex-mediated sympathoinhibition. This finding may have a clinical value, since, for example, it may provide an explanation as to why hypotensive responses to some vasodilators augment with age, in spite of an unchanged local vascular response [54].

9.5 Plasticity of the Autonomic Nervous System, the Role of Neurotrophins

Neurotrophins (NTFs) are diffusible peptides secreted from neurons and neuron-supporting cells, being the most studied nerve growth factor (NGF) and brain-derived neurotrophic factor (BDNF) [55]. NTFs exert their effects by signaling through membrane receptors which, by means of their intrinsic tyrosine kinase activity, trigger several downstream cascades ultimately leading to transcriptional changes into the nucleus [56]. Neurotrophic factors regulate the differentiation, synaptogenesis, and survival of ANS neurons. NGF also induces the production of catecholamines in sympathetic neurons and stimulates neurite outgrowth in cultured parasympathetic neurons (see [57]). Of interest, NGF is produced by parasympathetic neurons where its expression can be modulated by sympathetic innervation [58]. Concerning BDNF, it is synthesized by both developing and mature sympathetic neurons, and preganglionic neurons express its specific receptor, namely, TrkB. In sympathetic neurons, BDNF overexpression results in the hypertrophy of preganglionic cell bodies and axons and in an enhancement in the number of synapses, while the opposite occurs when BDNF levels are reduced [59]. Increasing evidence indicates that, in the adult ANS, NTFs play a key role in the regulation of neurotransmitter signaling and neuronal remodeling (see [57]). For example, chick ciliary ganglion neurons express both BDNF and TrkB, and the activation of this pathway ultimately results in the upregulation of nicotinic acetylcholine receptors [60]. In humans, it has been documented that patients with mutations in TrkA (the NGF-specific receptor) exhibit impaired thermoregulation and deficits in sympathetic activation of the adrenal medulla [61].

At cardiovascular level, it has been shown that BDNF may modulate heart rate and blood pressure via ANS [62]. In particular, injection of BDNF, but not NGF, into the rostral ventrolateral medulla determines a decrease in blood pressure in rats [63]. Moreover, Yang et al. [64] documented that, when ANS neurons are cultured with cardiac myocytes, the neurons form synapses on the myocytes and the treatment with BDNF augments the release of acetylcholine from ANS neurons and reduces cardiac myocyte beat frequency. With reference to heart remodeling, literature evidence reports that NGF is upregulated following myocardial injury in animal models, and its rise is associated with the regeneration of cardiac sympathetic nerves and heterogeneous innervation [65]. Moreover, in dogs, it has been demonstrated that the infusion of NGF into the left stellate ganglion (LSG) induces a significant nerve sprouting [66]. Finally, pathological cardiac hyperinnervation and enlargement has been observed in transgenic mice which overexpress NGF selectively in the heart [67]. Indeed, it should be taken into account that an excessive nerve sprouting may also determine abnormal patterns in the heart innervation, thus leading to an augmented risk of arrhythmias [68]. In agreement with this concept, abnormal patterns of innervation have been observed in infarcted human hearts [69], and in explanted hearts of transplanted subjects a positive correlation has been described between nerve density and the clinical history of ventricular arrhythmia [70].

As previously mentioned, during senescence a shift of the cardiac autonomic nervous system toward an increase in sympathetic tone has been observed, which negatively affects all the age-related cardiovascular diseases. At cardiac level, NGF is the main neurotrophic factor which crucially controls the sympathetic tone of the mammalian heart, and it has been pointed as a key responsible for this age-dependent enhancement of sympathetic activity (Table 9.1). In particular, in rats, an increase of NGF expression has been found, at both mRNA and protein levels, from young to old animals in both the atria and ventricles. To this regard, considering that NGF also exerts antiapoptotic actions, the authors suggest that the observed NGF rise may represent a reflex mechanism to an increased degree of apoptosis in aging myocardium [71]. However, in agreement with the previously reported considerations, these findings also raise the possibility that an age-related increase of NGF levels may promote the development of sympathetic hyperinnervation in the aging heart, thus contributing to the changes in the autonomic tone identified in the elderly [71]. With regard to BDNF, Cai and colleagues [72] showed that, following permanent coronary occlusion, BDNF significantly augments the extent of myocardial injury in older rat hearts (Table 9.1), suggesting that age-related changes in BDNF cascade may predispose the senescent heart to increased injury after acute myocardial infarction and potentially contribute to the enhanced severity of cardiovascular disease in older individuals.

Table 9.1 Effect of senescence on neurotrophins in the heart

Neurotrophin/neurotrophin receptor	Anatomical site	Age-related change	Functional consequences
NGF	Atria and ventricles	↑ mRNA and protein	Sympathetic hyperinnervation
TrkA	Atria	↑ Expression	Antiapoptotic effects
BDNF	Heart	↑ Levels	Increased injury after myocardial infarction
TrkB	Heart	↑ Expression	Increased inflammatory response

NTFs signal through membrane receptors triggering several downstream cascades ultimately affecting gene expression [56]. The table reports the main age-related effects on NGF, BDNF, and their specific receptors at cardiac level and their functional consequences [71, 72]

References

1. Esler MD, Turner AG, Kaye DM, et al. Aging effects on human sympathetic neuronal function. Am J Physiol. 1995;268:R278–85.
2. Esler M, Kaye D. Sympathetic nervous system activation in essential hypertension, cardiac failure and psychosomatic heart disease. J Cardiovasc Pharmacol. 2000;35 Suppl 4:S1–7.
3. Kenney MJ. Animal aging and regulation of sympathetic nerve discharge. J Appl Physiol (1985). 2010;109(4):951–8.
4. Barman SM. Brainstem control of cardiovascular function. In: Klemm WR, Vertes RP, editors. Brainstem mechanisms of behavior. New York: Wiley; 1990. p. 353–81.
5. Sun MK. Central neural organization and control of sympathetic nervous system in mammals. Prog Neurobiol. 1995;47(3):157–233.
6. Dampney RA, Horiuchi J, Tagawa T, et al. Medullary and supramedullary mechanisms regulating sympathetic vasomotor tone. Acta Physiol Scand. 2003;177(3):209–18.
7. Itoh H, Buñag RD. Aging reduces cardiovascular and sympathetic responses to NTS injections of serotonin in rats. Exp Gerontol. 1992;27(3):309–20.
8. Huangfu DH, Koshiya N, Guyenet PG. A5 noradrenergic unit activity and sympathetic nerve discharge in rats. Am J Physiol Regul Integr Comp Physiol. 1991;261:R393–402.
9. Van Huysse JW, Bealer SL. Central nervous system norepinephrine release, hypotension and hyperosmolality in conscious rats. Am J Physiol Regul Integr Comp Physiol. 1991;260:R1071–6.
10. Esler M, Hastings J, Lambert G, et al. The influence of aging on the human sympathetic nervous system and brain norepinephrine turnover. Am J Physiol Regul Integr Comp Physiol. 2002;282(3):R909–16.
11. Dickstein DL, Kabaso D, Rocher AB, et al. Changes in the structural complexity of the aged brain. Aging Cell. 2007;6:275–84.
12. Alkadhi K, Alzoubi K. Role of long-term potentiation of sympathetic ganglia (gLTP) in hypertension. Clin Exp Hypertens. 2007;29(5):267–86.
13. Partanen M, Waller SB, London ED, et al. Indices of neurotransmitter synthesis and release in aging sympathetic nervous system. Neurobiol Aging. 1985;6:227–32.
14. Schmidt RE. Age-related sympathetic ganglionic neuropathology: human pathology and animal models. Auton Neurosci. 2002;96(1):63–72.
15. Seals DR, Esler MD. Human ageing and the sympathoadrenal system. J Physiol. 2000;528(Pt 3):407–17.

16. Ziegler MG, Lake CR, Kopin IJ. Plasma noradrenaline increases with age. Nature. 1976;261:333–5.
17. Jones DH, Hamilton CA, Reid JL. Plasma noradrenaline, age, and blood pressure: a population study. Clin Sci Mol Med Suppl. 1978;4:73s–5.
18. Goldstein DS, Lake CF, Chernow B, et al. Age-dependence of hypertensive-normotensive differences in plasma norepinephrine. Hypertension. 1983;5:100–4.
19. Padovani A, Govoni S, Battaini F, et al. Alcohol impairs age-dependent adaptation of human lymphocyte beta-adrenergic receptors. Eur J Clin Invest. 1987;17(6):511–4.
20. Rubin PC, Scott PJ, McLean K, et al. Noradrenaline release and clearance in relation to age and blood pressure in man. Eur J Clin Invest. 1982;12:121–5.
21. Schwartz RS, Jaeger LF, Veith RC. The importance of body composition to the increase in plasma norepinephrine appearance rate in elderly men. J Gerontol. 1987;42:546–51.
22. Marker JC, Cryer PE, Clutter WE. Simplified measurement of norepinephrine kinetics: application to studies of aging and exercise training. Am J Physiol. 1994;267:E380–7.
23. Esler M, Skews H, Leonard P, et al. Age-dependence of noradrenaline kinetics in normal subjects. Clin Sci (Lond). 1981;60:217–9.
24. Morrow LA, Linares OA, Hill TJ, et al. Age differences in the plasma clearance mechanisms for epinephrine and norepinephrine in humans. J Clin Endocrinol Metab. 1987;65:508–11.
25. Esler M, Kaye D, Thompson J, et al. Effects of aging on epinephrine secretion and regional release of epinephrine from the human heart. J Clin Endocrinol Metab. 1995;80:435–42.
26. Daly RN, Goldberg PB, Roberts J. The effect of age on presynaptic alpha 2 adrenoceptor autoregulation of norepinephrine release. J Gerontol. 1989;44:B59–66.
27. Buchholz J, Duckles SP. Effect of age on prejunctional modulation of norepinephrine release. J Pharmacol Exp Ther. 1990;252:159–64.
28. Docherty JR. Cardiovascular responses in ageing: a review. Pharmacol Rev. 1990;42(2):103–25.
29. Aggarwal A, Esler MD, Socratous F, et al. Evidence for functional presynaptic alpha-2 adrenoceptors and their down-regulation in human heart failure. J Am Coll Cardiol. 2001;37:1246–51.
30. Molderings G, Likungu J, Zerkowski HR, et al. Presynaptic β2-adrenoceptors on the sympathetic nerve fibres of the human saphenous vein: no evidence for involvement in adrenaline-mediated positive feedback loop regulating noradrenergic transmission. Naunyn-Schmiedeberg's Arch Pharmacol. 1988;337:408–14.
31. Starke K, Gothert M, Kilbinger H. Modulation of neurotransmitter release by presynaptic autoreceptors. Physiol Rev. 1989;69:864–989.
32. Docherty JR. Age-related changes in adrenergic neuroeffector transmission. Auton Neurosci. 2002;96(1):8–12.
33. Borton M, Docherty JR. The effects of ageing on neuronal uptake of noradrenaline in the rat. Naunyn Schmiedebergs Arch Pharmacol. 1989;340:139–43.
34. Li ST, Holmes C, Kopin IJ, et al. Aging-related changes in cardiac sympathetic function in humans, assessed by 6-18F-fluorodopamine PET scanning. J Nucl Med. 2003;44:1599–603.
35. Leenen FH, Coletta E, Fourney A, et al. Aging and cardiac responses to epinephrine in humans: role of neuronal uptake. Am J Physiol Heart Circ Physiol. 2005;288:H2498–503.
36. Klein C, Gerber JG, Gal J, et al. Beta-adrenergic receptors in the elderly are not less sensitive to timolol. Clin Pharmacol Ther. 1986;40(2):161–4.
37. Conway J, Wheeler R, Sannerstedt R. Sympathetic nervous activity during exercise in relation to age. Cardiovasc Res. 1971;5(4):577–81.
38. White M, Leenen FH. Aging and cardiovascular responsiveness to beta-agonist in humans: role of changes in beta-receptor responses versus baroreflex activity. Clin Pharmacol Ther. 1994;56:543–53.
39. Brodde OE, Leineweber K. Autonomic receptor systems in the failing and aging human heart: similarities and differences. Eur J Pharmacol. 2004;500(1–3):167–76.
40. Brodde OE, Zerkowski HR, Schranz D, et al. Age dependent changes in the beta-adrenoceptor–G-protein(s)–adenylyl cyclase system in human right atrium. J Cardiovasc Pharmacol. 1995;26:20–6.

41. Xiao RP, Tomhave ED, Wang DJ, et al. Age-associated reductions in cardiac beta1- and beta2-adrenergic responses without changes in inhibitory G proteins or receptor kinases. J Clin Invest. 1998;101(6):1273–82.
42. Kaye DM, Esler MD. Autonomic control of the aging heart. Neuromolecular Med. 2008;10(3):179–86.
43. Jose AD, Stitt F, Collison D. The effects of exercise and changes in body temperature on the intrinsic heart rate in man. Am Heart J. 1970;79(4):488–98.
44. Davies MJ. Pathology of the conducting system. In: Caird FL, Dall JLC, Kennedy RD, editors. Cardiology in old age. New York: Plenum; 1976. p. 57–9.
45. Masi CM, Hawkley LC, Rickett EM, et al. Respiratory sinus arrhythmia and diseases of aging: obesity, diabetes mellitus, and hypertension. Biol Psychol. 2007;74(2):212–23.
46. Brodde OE, Konschak U, Becker K, et al. Cardiac muscarinic receptors decrease with age. In vitro and in vivo studies. J Clin Invest. 1998;101(2):471–8.
47. Poller U, Nedelka G, Radke J, et al. Age-dependent changes in cardiac muscarinic receptor function in healthy volunteers. J Am Coll Cardiol. 1997;29(1):187–93.
48. Giessler C, Wangemann T, Zerkowski HR, et al. Age-dependent decrease in the negative inotropic effect of carbachol on isolated human right atrium. Eur J Pharmacol. 1998;357:199–202.
49. Liu HR, Zhao RR, Zhi JM, et al. Screening of serum autoantibodies to cardiac beta1-adrenoceptors and M2-muscarinic acetylcholine receptors in 408 subjects of varying ages. Autoimmunity. 1999;29:43–51.
50. Monahan KD. Effect of aging on baroreflex function in humans. Am J Physiol Regul Integr Comp Physiol. 2007;293(1):R3–12.
51. Laitinen T, Hartikainen J, Vanninen E, et al. Age and gender dependency of baroreflex sensitivity in healthy subjects. J Appl Physiol. 1998;84:576–83.
52. Monahan KD, Dinenno FA, Seals DR, et al. Age-associated changes in cardiovagal baroreflex sensitivity are related to central arterial compliance. Am J Physiol Heart Circ Physiol. 2001;281:H284–9.
53. Studinger P, Goldstein R, Taylor JA. Age- and fitness-related alterations in vascular sympathetic control. J Physiol. 2009;587(Pt 9):2049–57.
54. Monahan KD. A new answer to an old question: does ageing modify baroreflex control of vascular sympathetic outflow in humans? J Physiol. 2009;587(Pt 9):1857.
55. Lanni C, Stanga S, Racchi M, et al. The expanding universe of neurotrophic factors: therapeutic potential in aging and age-associated disorders. Curr Pharm Des. 2010;16(6):698–717.
56. Govoni S, Pascale A, Amadio M, et al. NGF and heart: is there a role in heart disease? Pharmacol Res. 2011;63(4):266–1277.
57. Mattson MP, Wan R. Neurotrophic factors in autonomic nervous system plasticity and dysfunction. Neuromolecular Med. 2008;10(3):157–68.
58. Hasan W, Smith PG. Nerve growth factor expression in parasympathetic neurons: regulation by sympathetic innervation. Eur J Neurosci. 2000;12:4391–7.
59. Causing CG, Gloster A, Aloyz R, et al. Synaptic innervation density is regulated by neuron-derived BDNF. Neuron. 1997;18:257–67.
60. Zhou X, Nai Q, Chen M, et al. Brain-derived neurotrophic factor and trkB signaling in parasympathetic neurons: relevance to regulating alpha7-containing nicotinic receptors and synaptic function. J Neurosci. 2004;24:4340–50.
61. Loewenthal N, Levy J, Schreiber R, et al. Nerve growth factor-tyrosine kinase A pathway is involved in thermoregulation and adaptation to stress: studies on patients with hereditary sensory and autonomic neuropathy type IV. Pediatr Res. 2005;57:587–90.
62. Wan R, Weigand LA, Bateman R, et al. Evidence that BDNF regulates heart rate by a mechanism involving increased brainstem parasympathetic neuron excitability. J Neurochem. 2014;129(4):573–80.
63. Wang H, Zhou XF. Injection of brain-derived neurotrophic factor in the rostral ventrolateral medulla increases arterial blood pressure in anaesthetized rats. Neuroscience. 2002;112:967–75.
64. Yang B, Slonimsky JD, Birren SJ. A rapid switch in sympathetic neurotransmitter release properties mediated by the p75 receptor. Nat Neurosci. 2002;5:539–45.

65. Zhou S, Chen LS, Miyauchi Y, et al. Mechanisms of cardiac nerve sprouting after myocardial infarction in dogs. Circ Res. 2004;95:76–83.
66. Cao JM, Chen LS, KenKnight BH, et al. Nerve sprouting and sudden cardiac death. Circ Res. 2000;86:816–21.
67. Hassankhani A, Steinhelper ME, Soonpaa MH, et al. Overexpression of NGF within the heart of transgenic mice causes hyperinnervation, cardiac enlargement, and hyperplasia of ectopic cells. Dev Biol. 1995;169:309–21.
68. Chen PS, Chen LS, Cao JM, et al. Sympathetic nerve sprouting, electrical remodeling and the mechanisms of sudden cardiac death. Cardiovasc Res. 2001;50:409–16.
69. Vracko R, Thorning D, Frederickson RG. Nerve fibers in human myocardial scars. Hum Pathol. 1991;22:138–46.
70. Cao JM, Fishbein MC, Han JB, et al. Relationship between regional cardiac hyperinnervation and ventricular arrhythmia. Circulation. 2000;101:1960–9.
71. Saygili E, Kluttig R, Rana OR, et al. Age-related regional differences in cardiac nerve growth factor expression. Age (Dordr). 2012;34(3):659–67.
72. Cai D, Holm JM, Duignan IJ, et al. BDNF-mediated enhancement of inflammation and injury in the aging heart. Physiol Genomics. 2006;24(3):191–7.

The Autonomic Cardiorenal Crosstalk: Pathophysiology and Implications for Heart Failure Management

Maria Rosa Costanzo and Edoardo Gronda

10.1 Introduction

The autonomic nervous system (ANS), which comprises the sympathetic and parasympathetic branches, has numerous essential physiologic functions, including modulation of blood pressure, heart rate, and body fluid volume [1]. It is now recognized that the ANS is organized to elicit organ-specific responses to maintain homeostasis in the face of external challenges [2].

An example of the differential organ effects of the ANS is the coordinated response to increase sodium concentration aimed at restoring normal plasma sodium concentration and volume. This process is especially relevant to the normal interactions between heart and kidney and to the understanding of their dysregulation in the settings of hypertension, heart failure (HF), and the cardiorenal syndrome (CRS) (Fig. 10.1). Experiments in conscious sheep have shown that increases in brain sodium concentration simultaneously augment cardiac sympathetic nerve activity (SNA) and arterial pressure and reduce renal SNA, promoting reduced renin secretion, renal vasodilatation, and renal sodium excretion [1]. Thus, inhibition of renal SNA is the logical homeostatic response to a sodium load, aimed at restoring normal plasma volume and sodium concentration. These organ-specific effects are mediated via a neural pathway that includes an angiotensinergic synapse, the lamina terminalis, and the paraventricular nucleus of the hypothalamus [3, 4]. In contrast to normal conditions, in experimental animal models of HF induced by rapid pacing, the

M.R. Costanzo, MD, FACC, FAHA (✉)
Medical Director, Midwest Heart Specialists-Advocate Medical Group Heart Failure and Pulmonary Arterial Hypertension Programs, Medical Director, Edward Hospital Center for Advanced Heart Failure Edward Heart Hospital, Naperville, Illinois 60566, USA
e-mail: Mariarosa.costanzo@advocatehealth.com

E. Gronda, MD
Cardiology and Heart Failure Research Unit, IRCCS MultiMedica - Sesto San Giovanni, Milan, Italy
e-mail: edoardo.gronda@multimedica.it

© Springer International Publishing Switzerland 2016
E. Gronda et al. (eds.), *Heart Failure Management: The Neural Pathways*,
DOI 10.1007/978-3-319-24993-3_10

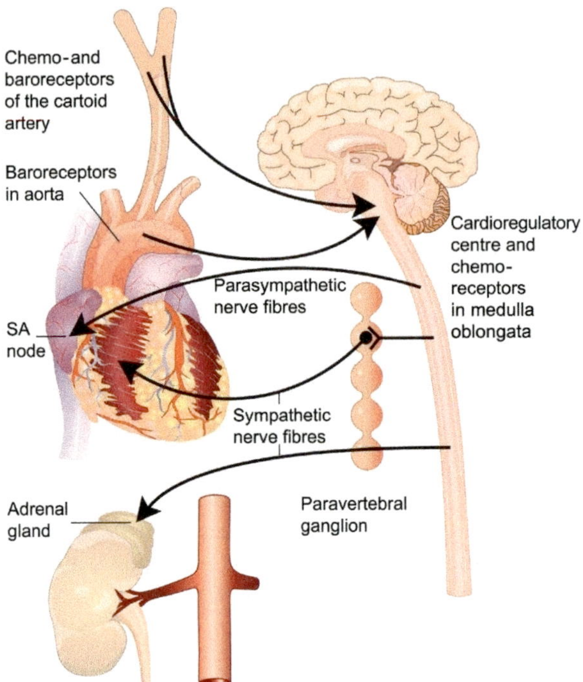

Fig. 10.1 Organization of the autonomic nervous system demonstrating the key interactions involving the brain, heart, and kidney. *SA* sino-atrial node (Reproduced with permission from Singh et al. [159])

cardiac and renal SNA activities increased to similar, almost maximal levels and the response of cardiac SNA to changes in blood volume was significantly attenuated [1, 5]. These data confirm many previous observations that in HF, a decreased arterial pressure reduces baroreflex inhibition of SNA, which, together with the lack of an inhibitory response to the increased volume and cardiac pressures, contributes to the heightened sympathetic activity typical of HF [1]. Excessive sympathetic drive is undoubtedly a major contributing factor to the pathogenesis of hypertension and to the progression of HF. Importantly, much of the excessive SNA in these conditions targets the kidney, where it leads to inappropriate sodium retention and renin stimulation and diminished renal function. In addition, the kidney itself is a source of increased SNA by way of the renal somatic afferent nerves. Therefore, in both hypertension and HF, the kidney is both the target and contributor to increased SNA [6].

10.2 Measurements of Autonomic Nervous System Activity

One important challenge to the understanding of the bidirectional autonomic interactions between the heart and the kidney is the ability to quantify individual regional SNA activity. For this purpose, sympathetic nerve recording techniques and radiotracer-derived measurements of norepinephrine (NE) spillover into the plasma from individual organs have been used. The limitations of each technique have led to the recommendation that they be used together [7]. Microneurography provides instantaneous multiunit or single-fiber recordings of electrical transmission in sympathetic nerves, but assessment may be skewed by interpreter's bias [8, 9].

The NE spillover method provides objective information on the release of this neurotransmitter from internal organs where microneurography is not feasible [10–12]. During infusion of titrated NE at a constant rate, output of endogenous NE from a given organ (NE "spillover") can be measured by isotope dilution according to the formula:

$$\text{Regional norepinephrine spillover} = \left[\left(C_V - C_A \right) + C_A E \right] \text{PF}$$

where C_V and C_A are the plasma concentrations of NE in the organ's venous and arterial plasma, E is the fractional extraction of titrated NE while the blood is flowing through the organ, and PF is the organ plasma flow [7].

Computer analysis of heart rate variability (HRV) predominantly reflects selective autonomic control of the heart. Vagal and sympathetic cardiac influences operate on the heart rate in different frequency bands. While vagal regulation has a relatively high cutoff frequency, modulating heart rate both at low and high frequencies (up to 1.0 Hz), sympathetic cardiac control operates only at <0.15 Hz [13–15]. Blood pressure variability is the result of complex interactions between cardiac and vascular neural regulation, mechanical influences of respiration, humoral and endothelial factors, large artery compliance, and genetic influence. Nevertheless, time or frequency domain analysis of either blood pressure or HRV can provide valuable information on autonomic cardiovascular regulation. While often lacking specificity, these measurements can be obtained in clinical practice and are not subject to interpreter's bias [16]. The ability of HRV and blood pressure fluctuations to reflect autonomic control of the cardiovascular system is improved by use of multivariate models for its assessment. The simplest ones consider the relationship between spontaneous fluctuations in blood pressure and heart rate, either in the time or frequency domain to assess baroreceptor sensitivity (BRS) and its modulation in daily life [17–20]. While spontaneous variations in blood pressure and heart rate clearly depend on autonomic mechanisms, caution is needed in considering them a quantitative measurement of efferent SNA to the heart and vasculature. In fact, in a variety of clinical situations, including HF, low-frequency heart rate spectral power has little or no relation to rates of NE spillover from the heart or sympathetic nerve firing measured by microneurography. Indeed, in HF, low-frequency heart rate spectral power is reduced, but cardiac NE spillover is markedly increased [21].

Cardiac SNA can also be noninvasively assessed by the use of ^{123}I-metaiodobenzylguanidine (MIBG), an analogue of NE, using semiquantitative analyses, namely, early heart-to-mediastinum ratio, late heart-to-mediastinum ratio, and myocardial washout [22]. Data from prospective studies and meta-analyses have shown that patients with decreased late heart-to-mediastinum ratio or increased myocardial ^{123}I-MIBG washout have a worse prognosis than those patients with normal semiquantitative myocardial MIBG parameters [23]. Furthermore, ^{123}I-MIBG has been found to independently predict sudden cardiac death regardless of left ventricular ejection fraction (LVEF) [24]. In addition, the ADMIRE-HF

(AdreView Myocardial Imaging for Risk Evaluation in Heart Failure) trial demonstrated that ^{123}I-MIBG cardiac imaging provides additional independent prognostic information for risk-stratifying HF patients on top of commonly used markers such as LVEF and B-type natriuretic peptide [25].

Thus, the clinical relevance of information on autonomic cardiac control is supported by the evidence that increased SNA is associated with increased mortality in myocardial infarction and HF patients, and with an increased risk of sudden arrhythmic death.

10.3 Sympathetic Innervation of the Kidney

The kidney is abundantly innervated with both efferent adrenergic and somatic afferent neurons [26, 27] (Fig. 10.2). The efferent neurons terminate at multiple sites within the nephron and independently influence tubular sodium reabsorption, renin secretion, and renal blood flow (RBF). Sodium reabsorption is enhanced at

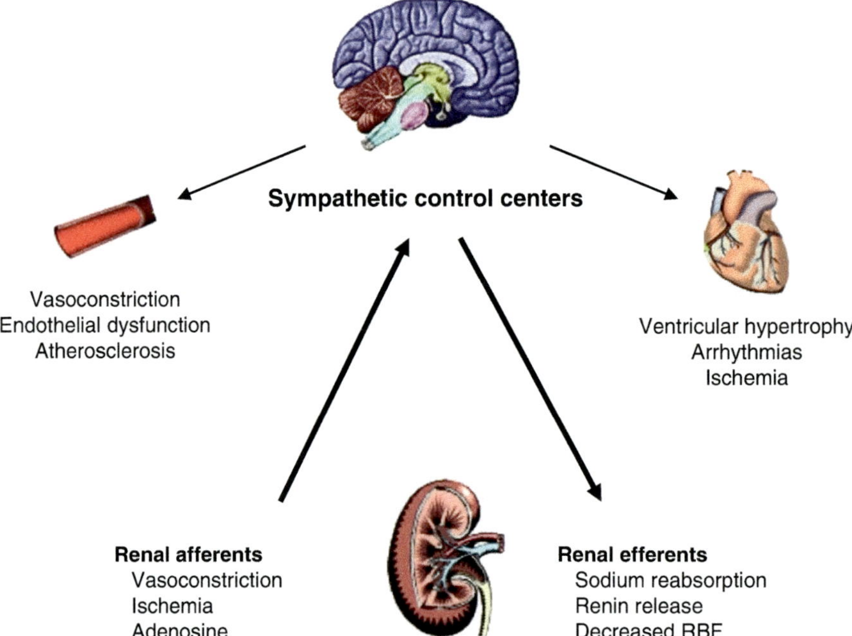

Fig. 10.2 Afferent sympathetic pathways travel from the kidney to the control centers for neuromodulation in the midbrain. Activation of these pathways increases global sympathetic traffic, which may adversely affect vascular tone and integrity, as well as lead to inappropriate myocardial hypertrophy, myocardial cell damage, and arrhythmias. Increased renal sympathetic signaling stimulates sodium retention, volume expansion, and renal vasoconstriction. The consequences of increased renal sympathetic efferent traffic may also lead to an increase in afferent traffic, thereby creating a positive feedback loop with many deleterious vascular, myocardial, and renal consequences. *RBF* renal blood flow (Reproduced with permission from Goldsmith et al. [39])

very low stimulation frequencies; higher stimulating frequencies increase renin secretion and lower RBF [28–30]. Thus, under conditions of mild sympathetic activation, sodium reabsorption increases and consequently plasma volume expands. With more intense sympathetic activation, sodium reabsorption is further augmented by the effects of angiotensin II (A II) and aldosterone and vasoconstriction occurs due to the combined vascular effects of NE and A II. Thus, increased efferent renal SNA produces simultaneously an increase in arterial pressure and blood volume and a decrease in RBF. When these compensatory responses to hypotension or hypovolemia become persistent and disproportionate to the cardiovascular abnormalities which initially trigger them, they become maladaptive and directly contribute to the progression of HF. These responses are particularly influential in the CRS where persistent vascular congestion and worsening renal function magnify the mutually detrimental effects of heart and kidney [31]. It should be noted that in addition to the effects of renal sympathetic efferent activation, somatic afferent nerves originating in the kidney act directly on the neural cardiovascular control centers in the midbrain [27]. The activity of these afferent nerves is stimulated by various factors including ischemia and adenosine release, both of which are the result of intense vasoconstriction. A direct neurological connection between the kidney and hypothalamus has been demonstrated in partially nephrectomized rats. In patients with end-stage renal disease (ESRD) and in renal transplant recipients, removal of the native kidney is associated with attenuated muscle SNA [32–35]. Because A II can directly stimulate central sympathetic drive, secretion of renin by the macula densa cells is another mechanism by which the kidney contributes to activation of SNA and of the renin-angiotensin-aldosterone system (RAAS) [36]. Increases in activation of either the afferent or the efferent loop of this "sympathorenal axis" may lead to a self-perpetuating cycle and sustained generalized SNA. However, it should be pointed out that many other reflexes and humoral substances, including natriuretic peptides (NP), can modify sympathetic tone, so that any contribution of the renal sympathetic afferent nerves to this self-perpetuating cycle can be modified by changes in activity of these other controllers [22].

10.4 The Sympathorenal Axis in Heart Failure

Increased plasma NE, muscle SNA, and total body, cardiac, and renal NE spillovers have been documented in patients with congestive HF [12, 37]. For more than three decades, plasma NE has been known to be a strong predictor of outcomes in HF patients [38]. The success of beta-blockers in decreasing mortality in HF patients convincingly supports the notion that excessive SNA directly contributes to HF progression [39].

However, the use in HF patients of moxonidine, an inhibitor of presynaptic NE release, was associated with increased mortality presumably due to hypotension caused by a precipitous fall in plasma NE levels [40]. Data are lacking on whether a more gradual reduction in NE levels would have produced different results in HF patients.

There is little doubt that renal NE spillover is, together with cardiac NE spillover, a major contributor to the total excess of sympathetic drive in HF patients [12]. Indeed, it has recently been shown that renal SNA, as measured by renal NE spillover, was highly predictive of outcomes despite concomitant therapy with antineurohormonal drugs [39]. In addition in an experimental myocardial infarction model, renal sympathetic denervation was associated with improved outcomes [41]. The enhanced efferent sympathetic signaling to the kidney seen in HF presumably has the same effects it has in hypertension (enhanced sodium retention, decreased RBF and activation of the RAAS). These effects are even more harmful in HF because volume expansion and increased arterial pressure will aggravate myocardial loading conditions and, together with the direct actions of NE, A II, and aldosterone, worsen myocardial remodeling. The SNA-related sodium avidity and renal hemodynamic abnormalities may be especially deleterious in the CRS, because persistent congestion may itself contribute to further deterioration of renal function [31]. Kidney dysfunction often occurs during intensive treatment with loop diuretics. This event is not surprisingly because loop diuretics are known to further stimulate SNA either directly or through activation of the RAAS [42]. Augmentation of afferent signaling from the kidney may then contribute to perpetuate the global sympathetic overdrive in HF, completing the sympathorenal loop [39] (Fig. 10.3).

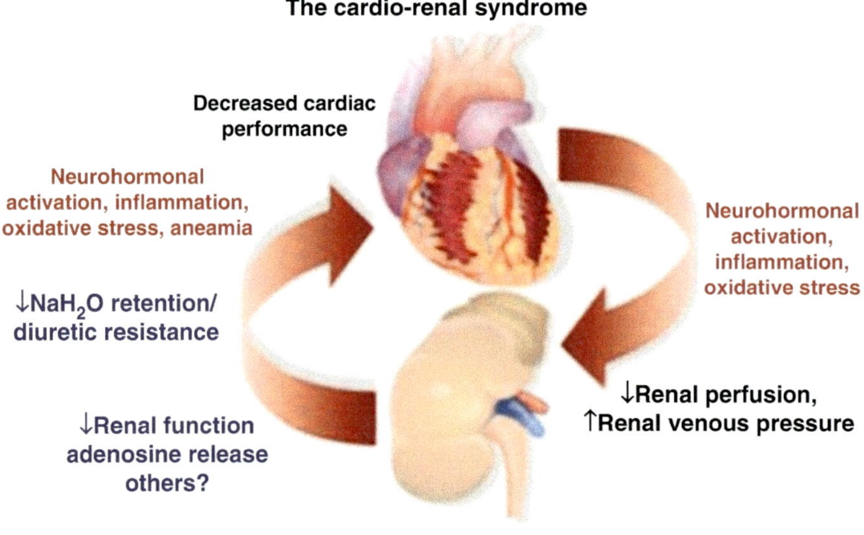

Fig. 10.3 Cardiorenal interactions in heart failure and kidney disease. Most of the mechanisms may be activated by each of the two conditions and are able to affect both cardiac and renal function. The mechanisms involved in the pathologic interactions between the heart and the kidney include hemodynamic abnormalities, neurohormonal activation, inflammation, and local intrarenal events (Reproduced with permission from Metra et al. [213])

10.5   Consequences of Congestion and Neurohormonal Activation in the Kidney and in Other Regional Circulatory System in the Abdomen

Many critically important changes occur in the kidney in the setting of cardiac dysfunction and neurohormonal activation (Fig. 10.3). When RBF decreases as a result of decreased cardiac output (CO), neurohormonally induced efferent arteriolar vasoconstriction, or increased central venous pressure (CVP), the kidney strives to maintain glomerular filtration rate (GFR) by increasing filtration fraction (FF) [43]. In normal conditions, FF is approximately 20–25 %, increases above this value in HF, and can rise above 50 % when congestion is complicated by increased intra-abdominal pressure. As explained below, increased FF in itself augments sodium reabsorption, an event which is magnified by increased SNA and RAAS activation. Different transporters mediate active transfer of sodium across the luminal side of proximal tubular cells. However, because the proximal tubules have a highly permeable epithelium, sodium can easily return to the lumen so that net sodium reabsorption is governed by passive Starling forces between the peritubular capillaries and renal interstitium. In congestive HF, because of an increased FF, the oncotic pressure in the peritubular capillaries (πPC) is higher, which stimulates sodium and water reabsorption into the vasculature. Because the kidney is an encapsulated organ, when congestion is present, the interstitial fluid hydrostatic pressure (PIF) and the peritubular capillaries hydrostatic pressure (PPC) are both increased, whereas the interstitial fluid oncotic pressure (πIF) drops because of increased lymph flow, which removes interstitial proteins. This also favors net sodium and water reabsorption into the vasculature [44–51]. Abnormally high-sodium reabsorption in the proximal tubule has profound consequences on the rest of the nephron. Under normal circumstances, the macula densa senses increased sodium chloride delivery because active chloride transport requires ATP, which is ultimately converted to adenosine. This substance, which is released from cells of the macula densa, has a paracrine vasoconstrictive effect on the afferent arteriole. This effect, known as tubuloglomerular feedback (TGF), protects the glomerulus from hyperfiltration injury. In congestive HF, due to increased sodium chloride reabsorption in the proximal tubule, chloride delivery to the macula densa is reduced and intracellular chloride levels are low. This stimulates NOS I and COX-2 activation and release of NO and PGE2. Both NO and PGE2 stimulate the granulosa cells of the afferent arteriole to secrete renin which activates angiotensin II, thus perpetuating a vicious cycle of neurohormonal activation and worsening congestion. It is also important to consider that loop diuretics, which are used in large numbers of ambulatory and in the majority of hospitalized HF patients, inhibit the Na+/K+/2Cl− co-transporter in the thick portion of the ascending loop of Henle, further reducing macula densa uptake of sodium chloride and escalating neurohormonal activation [43]. The distal convoluted tubules and collecting ducts reabsorb $\leq$10 % of the total amount of sodium filtered by the glomerulus. In contrast to the part of the nephron proximal to the macula densa, where net fractional sodium reabsorption is kept relatively constant under normal circumstances, distal fractional sodium reabsorption rates are highly variable depending on tubular flow rate, and levels of aldosterone and arginine vasopressin [52–54]. Therefore, it is the distal nephron which determines the urinary sodium concentration and osmolality. However, a prerequisite for the ability of the distal nephron to maintain a neutral sodium balance is adequate delivery of sodium. In congestive HF, because of increased fractional reabsorption in the proximal tubules and often decreased GFR in individual nephrons, tubular flow might be low in the distal part of the nephron despite significant systemic fluid excess. In addition, the increased levels of aldosterone and arginine vasopressin further stimulate reabsorption of the remaining tubular fluid. It is the decreased distal tubular flow which causes aldosterone breakthrough, which leads to secondary hyperaldosteronism despite therapy with adequate doses of RAAS inhibitors [55, 56]. Furthermore, prolonged exposure to loop diuretics produces adaptive hypertrophy of distal tubular cells, which increases local sodium reabsorption and aldosterone secretion. Indeed, experimental data shows that distal tubular cells adaptation to loop diuretics can be significantly attenuated by administration of aldosterone antagonists or thiazide diuretics [55, 57].

The escalating congestion resulting from the cardiorenal interactions outlined above has profound implications for all abdominal vascular systems, including the splanchnic, intestinal, hepatic, and splenic circulations [58]. In the splanchnic microcirculation, net filtration rate is determined by Starling forces, (PC -PIF) – (πC- πIF), which favor filtration throughout the entire length of the capillary bed. When capillary hydrostatic pressure increases as a result of congestion, filtration pressure is even higher [58]. Because the interstitium has low compliance, the excess filtrated fluid is drained directly into lymphatic capillaries, so that there is only a slight increase in interstitial fluid volume. Splanchnic lymphatic flow can increase as much as 20 times its normal value [59]. Because increased lymphatic flow removes interstitial proteins, the drop in interstitial oncotic pressure reduces filtration and the accumulation of fluid in the interstitium. Once lymphatic flow cannot increase further and interstitial compliance increases, interstitial fluid begins to accumulate [60]. When lymph flow can no longer adequately remove interstitial proteins, protein-rich edema accumulates to the point of compressing lymphatic vessels which further impairs lymph flow.

The intestinal microcirculation is characterized by a countercurrent system that enables extensive exchange of oxygen (O_2) between arterioles and venules. This O_2 "short circuit" creates a gradient with the lowest partial O_2 pressure at the villus tip [61–63]. During congestive HF, low perfusion, venous congestion, and sympathetically mediated arteriolar vasoconstriction in the splanchnic microcirculation stimulate O_2 exchange between arterioles and venules, exaggerating the O_2 gradient between the villus base and tip. This causes villus tip ischemia which is responsible for epithelial cells dysfunction and loss of intestinal barrier function. As a result, lipopolysaccharide or endotoxin, produced by gram-negative bacteria residing in the gut lumen, enters the systemic circulation and contributes to escalate the HF inflammatory milieu [61–63].

In the liver, hepatocytes continuously produce adenosine from the breakdown of ATP. Adenosine accumulates in the perisinusoidal space, which is drained by the lymphatic system. When portal blood flow is reduced because of α receptor–mediated vasoconstriction, lymph flow decreases and intrahepatic adenosine concentration increases. Adenosine then stimulates hepatic afferent nerves, which have synaptic connections with renal efferent sympathetic nerves. These events intensify renal vasoconstriction and sodium retention [58].

The splenic sinusoids are freely permeable to plasma proteins. As a result, their colloid osmotic pressure is the same as that of the surrounding lymphatic matrix. Therefore, fluid transport between the two spaces is dictated by differences in hydrostatic pressure. Transient congestion of the splanchnic venous system results in increased hydrostatic pressure inside the splenic sinusoids so that more fluid is transferred to the lymphatic matrix and buffered inside the lymphatic reservoirs of the spleen [64]. In congestive HF, increased cardiac filling pressures increase the production of atrial natriuretic peptide (ANP) which produces splenic arterial vasodilatation and venous vasoconstriction. These hemodynamic changes promote the shift of fluid into the perivascular third space of the spleen. Storage of large amounts of fluid in the spleen may lead to perceived central hypovolemia which further stimulates neurohormonal activity and perpetuates the vicious circle of congestion-driven SNA and RAAS enhancement. Moreover, when the splenic lymphatic circulation becomes overloaded, additional accumulation of interstitial edema occurs [58].

10.6 Autonomic Crosstalk in the Different Types of Cardiorenal Syndrome

According to a widely accepted definition, the cardiorenal syndrome is a pathophysiologic disorder of the heart and kidneys whereby acute or chronic dysfunction in one organ may induce acute or chronic dysfunction in the other organ. On the basis of this definition, five types of the cardiorenal syndrome have been identified and each has unique aspects of autonomic crosstalk between the heart and the kidney [65].

10.6.1 Cardiorenal Syndrome Type 1

This type of CRS is defined as abrupt worsening of cardiac function, such as it occurs with acute cardiogenic shock or ADHF, leading to acute kidney injury (AKI). Hemodynamic abnormalities play a crucial role in the pathogenesis of the CRS type 1 and trigger decreased renal arterial flow, renal oxygen consumption, and GFR and increased renal vascular resistance [66].

Different ADHF hemodynamic profiles have been identified on the basis of individual patients' adequacy of perfusion, assessed by measurement of CO, and extent of increase in cardiac filling pressures [67]. Since patients' clinical characteristics, treatment, and outcomes vary for different hemodynamic profiles, the pathophysiology of CRS type 1 may differ according to the hemodynamic milieu in which it occurs [67, 68]. The occurrence of AKI during ADHF is not restricted to an individual hemodynamic profile and may in fact be related to shifts in hemodynamic conditions when ADHF worsens or in response to treatment.

When CRS type 1 develops in patients with significant reductions in CO, with or without an increase in cardiac filling pressures, it is highly likely to be associated with a reduction in RBF. In ADHF, the relationship between CO, RBF, and intrarenal blood flow distribution remains unclear. However, it is plausible that activation of SNA and RAAS resulting from a significant reduction in intravascular volume will cause renal afferent (and, to a lesser extent, efferent) arteriolar vasoconstriction, leading to a decrease in RBF and renal perfusion pressure. If a low CO is associated with systemic arterial hypotension, renal perfusion pressure may decrease despite a relatively normal renal venous pressure, because renal autoregulation may be unable to compensate for the low blood pressure if the intravascular fluid volume is reduced. The finding of severely decreased RBF and GFR in the setting of reduced CO can therefore indicate that renal autoregulation is impaired [65].

An elevated CVP, which is readily transmitted to the renal vein, directly influences renal perfusion pressure [68–71]. In addition, because the kidney is an encapsulated organ, high renal venous pressure increases renal interstitial hydrostatic pressure. If this exceeds tubular hydrostatic pressure, the tubules collapse. Consequently, increasing intratubular pressure opposes filtration and therefore decreases GFR [65]. This mechanism is supported by experimental data showing a linear decrease in GFR upon increases in renal venous pressure, especially during volume expansion [72]. The response of renal autoregulation to increased renal venous pressure is unknown. However, it has been proposed that higher intrarenal levels of angiotensin II and SNA can indirectly influence arteriolar tone [72, 73].

It is more difficult to explain how the CRS type 1 occurs in ADHF patients with relatively preserved CO. If RBF is sufficiently reduced to be associated with a decreased GFR, it follows that in this situation, the drop in RBF is disproportionate to the decline in CO. This can occur with uni- or bilateral renal artery stenosis, which is estimated to occur in up to 40 % of patients with coexisting HF and CKD [74]. Other factors that may contribute to the development of the CRS type 1 in ADHF patients with preserved CO include (a) chronic use of RAAS inhibitors that impair the renal autoregulatory response to reductions in intravascular volume, (b) use of nonsteroidal anti-inflammatory drugs (NSAID) which may block TGF that would normally produce afferent arteriolar vasodilatation in response to a decreased intravascular fluid volume, and (c) preexisting arterial hypertension which may be associated with a reduction in functional nephrons [43, 65, 75].

It is also important to note that in patients with relatively preserved CO, the relative impact of increased CVP on renal perfusion pressure may not be as high as in patients with intravascular volume depletion. However, according to the mechanisms described earlier, an elevated CVP can still reduce GFR due to increased renal interstitial pressure and neurohormonal activation within the kidney and other regional circulations [67–71].

Biomarker evidence of neurohormonal activation includes the elevation in the levels of natriuretic peptides, mid-regional pro-adrenomedullin, and copeptin [75]. Indeed, ADHF patients with baseline elevation of natriuretic peptide levels and concomitant increase in cardiac filling pressures are at the highest risk for the development of the CRS type 1 [76].

10.6.2 Cardiorenal Syndrome Type 2

This type of CRS is characterized by chronic abnormalities in cardiac function leading to kidney injury or dysfunction. As such, the temporal relationship between the heart and kidney disease is an important aspect of the definition. While observational data clearly show that chronic heart and kidney disease commonly coexist, most studies lack information on whether cardiac dysfunction truly preceded renal abnormalities [77–80]. Thus, the mere coexistence of cardiovascular disease and CKD is not sufficient to make a diagnosis of true CRS type 2 which requires evidence that HF is the underlying cause of the onset and progression of CKD. One clear example is that of an acute myocardial infarction resulting in chronic LV dysfunction followed by the onset of renal function impairment or progression of pre-existing CKD. The predominant mechanisms leading from cardiac to renal dysfunction include neurohormonal activation, chronic renal hypoperfusion and venous congestion, inflammation, and oxidative stress. In addition, recurrent ADHF hospitalizations may contribute to the onset and progression of renal impairment [81] (Fig. 10.4). In patients with HF, the frequency of HF admissions has been

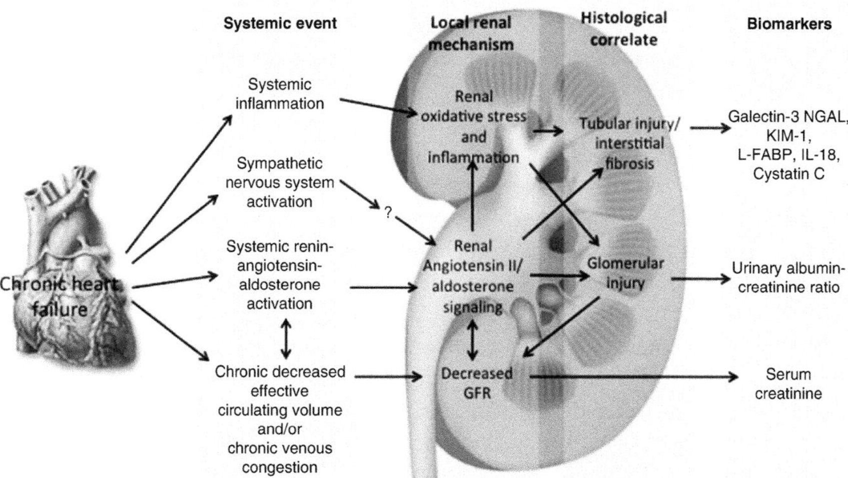

Fig. 10.4 Predominant pathophysiologic mechanisms of CRS2 in stable chronic HF. *NGAL* neutrophil gelatinase-associated lipocalin, *KIM-1* kidney injury molecule-1, *L-FABP* L-Fatty acid binding protein, *IL-18* interleukin-18, *GFR* glomerular filtration rate (Reproduced with permission from ADQI. Reproduced from Acute Dialysis Quality Initiative 10, under the terms of the Creative Commons Attribution License. Available at: www.ADQI.org. Accessed 2 July 2015)

shown to be independently associated with development of CKD most likely as a result of recurrent episodes of AKI caused both by the hemodynamic abnormalities and the treatment of ADHF [82]. In fact, animal models and epidemiologic studies have shown that repeated episodes of AKI lead to the development and progression of CKD [83].

As described earlier in the chapter, experimental models of chronic HF have shown that neurohormonally induced efferent arteriolar vasoconstriction in response to reduced glomerular plasma flow increases FF to preserve GFR. When these hemodynamic abnormalities persist for extended time periods (3–6 months in the rat model), glomerular pathologic changes ensue, as evidenced by albuminuria, podocyte injury, and focal glomerulosclerosis [43]. Eventually, when increased FF becomes inadequate to preserve filtration in individual glomeruli, GFR begins to decline. Importantly, many of these changes appear to be related to systemic and local renal increases in SNA and RAAS activation [43].

One of the principal roles of a normally functioning cardiorenal axis is the maintenance of extracellular fluid volume homeostasis. A complex system of volume and pressure sensors, afferent and efferent feedback loops, local and distant vasoactive substances, and neurohormonal systems with built-in redundancies serves to continuously monitor and adapt to changing extracellular fluid volume and blood pressure. When these systems are intact and function normally, they respond rapidly to constantly changing hemodynamics and volume status to ensure adequate tissue perfusion and oxygen delivery. The essential effector mechanisms are the SNA and RAAS. When significant cardiac dysfunction occurs, declining CO and consequent reduction in blood volume in the renal arterial circulation trigger activation of both SNA and RAAS [84]. It has long been recognized that the kidneys of patients with HF release substantial amounts of renin into the circulation [85], which, in turn, leads to increased A II production. By binding to AT1 receptor, A II has broad-reaching effects, including vasoconstriction-mediated increase in systemic vascular resistance, venous tone, and congestion. In addition, A II has potent central nervous system effects including increased thirst, SNA activation and non-osmotic release of vasopressin. In the kidney, A II increases the already high proximal tubular sodium reabsorption and, through preferential constriction of the efferent arteriole, glomerular FF. The latter, as described earlier, increases the oncotic pressure in PC, thus facilitating further return of sodium and water into the circulation [86].

Elevated CVP may have an especially important role in WRF in patient with HFpEF and hypertension. Indeed, in a canine model, renal venous hypertension, independent of changes in systemic arterial blood pressure, led not only to decreased renal blood flow and GFR but also to increased renin release [87, 88]. This provides further evidence that, in HF, renal abnormalities can be caused by neurohormonally induced venous hypertension and congestion in the absence of a decrease in effective circulating blood volume. In addition, the chronic activation of the SNS and RAAS may also contribute to the progression of preexisting CKD. Intrarenal levels of NE, A II, albuminuria, renal function, podocyte injury, and reactive oxygen species production were examined in an animal model of chronic volume overload, created by surgically induced aortic regurgitation in uninephrectomized rats [89]. Chronic volume overload led to predictable changes in the cardiac structure and function with associated increases in both intrarenal SNA and RAAS activity. Importantly, progressive kidney injury could be prevented by renal denervation and A II receptor blockade. Based on these findings, it is plausible that SNA and local A II activation stimulate NADPH oxidase–dependent reactive oxygen species generation in the kidney, which, in turn, causes podocyte injury and albuminuria [89].

Another effect of A II production is stimulation of release from the adrenal gland of aldosterone, which further augments sodium reabsorption in the distal nephron, aggravating pressure and volume overload. Aldosterone has also been implicated in progression of CKD and renal fibrosis [90]. Increased renal aldosterone levels promote oxidative stress. Through paracrine glycoprotein galectin-3 signaling, upregulation of the pro-fibrotic cytokine transforming growth factor-β (TGF-β) leads to increased fibronectin, which promotes renal fibrosis and glomerulosclerosis [91]. In Dahl salt-sensitive HF rats, the combination of ACE and aldosterone inhibition prevented histologic renal damage and lowered both creatinine and proteinuria to control levels. These findings suggest interplay of hypertension-induced and HF-associated renal injury with a related and mutually perpetuating pathophysiology. Inflammation is another non-hemodynamic mechanism contributing to the progression of CKD in the setting of HF [91].

The importance of SNA and RAAS activation in the HF clinical setting is underscored by the unquestionable benefits of RAAS antagonists and beta-blockers which are now the backbone of guidelines-directed medical therapy (GDMT) in HF patients. A detailed description of the studies bringing neurohormonal antagonists to the forefront of HF therapy is beyond the scope of this chapter. However, some aspects of these studies which are especially relevant to the CRS type 2 deserve mention. In the SOLVD study of enalapril in chronic HF, the net deterioration of eGFR from baseline to 14 days was slightly greater in the enalapril group compared to placebo. While early worsening of renal function was associated with increased mortality in the placebo group, it was free from adverse prognostic significance in the enalapril group [92]. Similarly, diabetic patients showed a decreased proteinuria with enalapril treatment [93]. An additional multivariable analysis suggested that despite a higher incidence of early worsening renal function in the enalapril group, there was no risk of longer term deterioration of eGFR compared with placebo [93–97]. Similar findings emerged from studies of aldosterone antagonists and beta-blockers [98]. Nevertheless, the role of neurohormonal antagonists in the prevention of the progression of CRS type 2 remains unclear.

It is important to note that a slight, expected, increase in creatinine, particularly in trials with inhibitors of RAAS, does not necessarily mean a progression of the CRS type 2.

Cardiac resynchronization therapy can improve hypoperfusion in HF as indicated by an increase in GFR by 2.7 ml/min in patients with GFR between 30 and 60 ml/min [99]. The use of LVADs has been shown to improve renal function early after device implantation. The reasons why this improvement appears to be transient have not been elucidated [100].

10.6.3 Cardiorenal Syndrome Type 3

The cardiorenal syndrome type 3, also called the acute renocardiac syndrome, is defined as an episode of AKI which precipitates and contributes to the development of acute cardiac injury and/or dysfunction [65]. There is limited data available describing the role of neurohormonal activation, specifically the SNS and RAAS in the pathophysiology of CRS type 3. However, activation of the SNS is a hallmark of both AKI and acute HF [65]. The enhancement of renal SNS activity and its consequent effect on NE spillover from nerve terminals during AKI [101] may impair myocardial function through several mechanisms, including direct effects of NE, disturbances in myocardial Ca2+ homeostasis, increase in myocardial oxygen demand which increases the risk of subendocardial ischemia, cardiomyocyte apoptosis mediated through β1-adrenergic receptor stimulation, stimulation of α1-adrenergic receptor–mediated cardiomyocyte hypertrophy, and direct RAAS activation [102]. Heightened adrenergic drive can stimulate β1-adrenergic receptors in the juxtaglomerular apparatus of the kidneys contributing to reduced renal blood flow and heightened rennin release and further RAAS activation. Maladaptive RAAS activation in AKI contributes to A II release, vasoconstriction, and further impairment of extracellular fluid homeostasis. In addition, A II contributes to vasoconstriction-mediated increase of systemic vascular resistance. It is also known that A II can directly modify myocardial structure and function, contribute to myocyte hypertrophy, and precipitate apoptosis in cardiomyocyte cultures [103–105]. Furthermore, A II is a potent stimulator of a number of cell signaling pathways including those involved in oxidative stress, inflammation, and the regulation of the extracellular matrix [105]. In a dog model of renal ischemia/reperfusion injury, increased RAAS activity was implicated in the observed reduction of coronary responsiveness to acetylcholine, adenosine, bradykinin, and L-arginine. In addition, renal ischemia/reperfusion injury was associated with increased myocardial oxygen consumption at rest. While a definitive role for the RAAS was conclusively shown, these findings imply that AKI may directly contribute to impaired coronary vasoreactivity and elevated myocardial oxygen consumption both of which can potentially increase the risk of myocardial ischemia and major cardiovascular events [105–110] (Fig. 10.5).

10.6.4 Cardiorenal Syndrome Type 4

This type of CRS occurs when CKD (e.g., chronic glomerular disease) contributes to decreased cardiac function, cardiac hypertrophy, and increased risk of adverse cardiovascular events.

The multiple and complex mechanisms which produce mutually detrimental interactions between the kidney and the heart in the CRS type IV are beyond the scope of this chapter and the discussion is limited to the potential roles of neurohormonal activation. However, it is important to note that the risks for cardiovascular complications in patients with eGFRs <30 ml/min/1.73 m^2 are up to tenfold higher than those with eGFRs >60 ml/min/1.73 m^2 [111]. This startling prevalence of cardiovascular complications exceeds the risk expected from typical risk factors, such as hypertension and

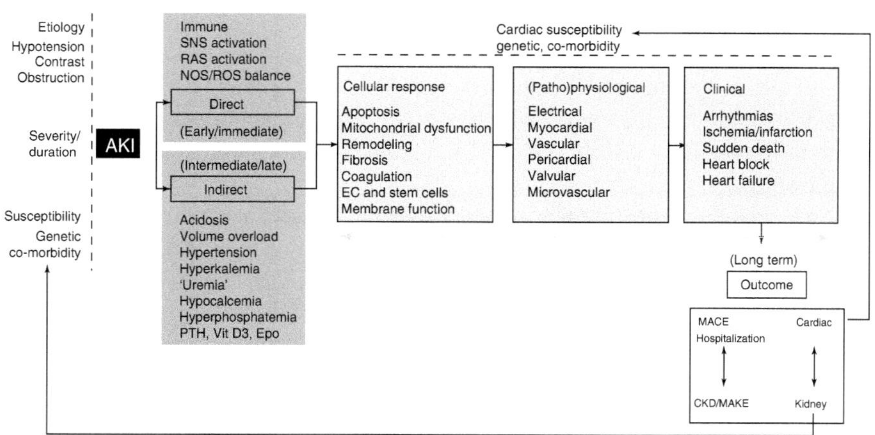

Fig. 10.5 Summary of the demographic contributors, clinical susceptibilities, and pathophysiologic mechanisms for development of CRS type 3. *AKI* acute kidney disease, *SNS* sympathetic nervous system, *RAS* renin angiotensin system, *NOS* nitric oxygen synthase, *PTH* parathyroid hormone, *Vit D3* vitamin D3, *Epo* erythropoietin, *EC* erythropoietic cells, *CKD* chronic kidney disease (Reproduced from Acute Dialysis Quality Initiative 10, under the terms of the Creative Commons Attribution License. Available at: www.ADQI.org. Accessed 2 July 2015)

hyperlipidemia, and suggests that the loss of renal function may directly contribute to the development of cardiovascular complications [111–115].

The renal response to impaired GFR can lead to activation of multiple compensatory pathways including upregulation of the RAAS and SNA as well as activation of the calcium-parathyroid axis. These physiologic responses can be due to underlying diseases such as hypertension or diabetes or can be a response to the functional decline of either the heart or the kidney. The loss of renal mass leads to the accumulation of total body sodium and water with the subsequent stimulation of A II and aldosterone production. The resulting hypertension coupled with direct effects of A II and aldosterone on cardiac myocytes accelerates left ventricular hypertrophy and cardiac fibrosis. Pathologic adaptations to increasing wall thickness contribute to a loss of capillary density, secondary myocardial fibrosis, and further compensatory hypertrophy [114]. Moreover, the progressive loss of nephron mass inherent to CKD leads to accumulation of salt and water which secondarily contributes to hypertension and pressure and volume overload. These same conditions contribute to LVH through upregulation of RAAS and subsequent release of pro-fibrotic factors such as galectin-3, TGF-β, and endogenous cardiac steroids [116]. In addition, prolonged periods of hemodynamic stress can induce cardiac remodeling which includes the increased expression of interstitial myofibroblasts, a cell type that is not present in normal myocardium and has high fibrogenic potential.

10.6.5 Cardiorenal Syndrome Type 5

This CRS occurs when an overwhelming insult leads to the simultaneous development of acute kidney injury (AKI) and acute cardiac dysfunction. The CRS type 5 encompasses a wide spectrum of disorders that acutely involve the heart and kidney, such as sepsis and drug toxicity where both the heart and the kidney are involved secondarily to the underlying process [65]. The CRS type 5 may develop in the presence or absence of previously impaired organ function. In contrast to the acute CRS type 5, its chronic counterpart, which occurs, for example in liver cirrhosis, has a more insidious onset and the kidney and cardiac dysfunction may develop slowly until overt decompensation occurs.

An essential feature of sepsis is the dissociation between the systemic circulation and the microcirculation in various organs [117]. Especially in the early phases of sepsis, profound microcirculatory changes can develop, despite apparently normal systemic hemodynamics [116–120]. Microcirculatory changes, such as lower blood flow velocities and heterogeneous perfusion patterns, strongly correlate with morbidity and mortality rates [118]. Sepsis can cause both left and right ventricular dilatation and dysfunction, which renders the heart less responsive to fluid resuscitation and catecholamine treatment [119]. Although cardiac dysfunction during sepsis can become severe enough to resemble cardiogenic shock, in the majority of cases, it can be reversed within 7–10 days [120, 121]. Moreover, as long as intravascular volume is maintained, tachycardia and reduced vascular tone may actually contribute to preserve or even increase CO in many patients. Myocardial blood flow or energy metabolism is not as important as previously thought in the development of depressed cardiac function during sepsis [122], which instead appears to be predominantly caused by myocardial depressant factors, including pro-inflammatory cytokines and components of the complement system [122–126].

In experimental models, it has been shown that, regardless of a normal or hyperdynamic systemic circulation, only animals that developed AKI during sepsis have increased renal vascular resistance. These findings are consistent with those of observational clinical studies [127]. Sepsis also affects central neuronal pathways including the SNA, the RAAS, and the hypothalamus-pituitary-adrenal axis, all of which affect cardiac and/or renal function, as repeatedly pointed out in this chapter. Importantly, the severity of sepsis-induced SNA dysfunction is strongly correlated with morbidity and mortality [128, 129]. The hallmark of increased SNA during sepsis is decreased HRV, which has been shown to be associated with the release of inflammatory mediators, such as IL-6, IL-10, and CRP [129, 130]. Data on kidney abnormalities due to sepsis-related autonomic dysfunction are largely preclinical. Interestingly, in a number of animal models, sepsis-induced changes in renal SNA do not appear directly affect renal blood flow [131]. The RAAS activation during sepsis has been deemed to reflect the body's attempt to restore and maintain an adequate blood pressure. Although counterintuitive, recent experimental and limited clinical data suggest that RAAS blockade might be beneficial, since RAAS activation has also been implicated in endothelial dysfunction, organ failure, and even mortality during severe sepsis [131–134]. Experimental studies have also shown that RAAS activation has detrimental effects on renal function during sepsis [135–138]. During experimental bacteremia, administration of ACE inhibitors improved creatinine clearance and urine output. Furthermore, during experimental endotoxemia, administration of a selective A II type 1 receptor antagonist improved renal blood flow and oxygenation.

Sepsis also causes complex alterations of hypothalamus-pituitary-adrenal signaling, which in some patients results in severe adrenal insufficiency [139]. This in turn triggers increased production of pro-inflammatory cytokines, free radicals, and prostaglandins as well as inhibition of chemotaxis and expression of adhesion molecules. Indeed, short-term administration of moderate-dose glucocorticoids has been shown to reduce the need for vasopressors and length of stay in the intensive care unit [139–141].

Although no definitive data are available on the cardiorenal crosstalk which occurs during sepsis, some specific pathophysiologic mechanisms appear plausible: a reduced cardiac output can reduce renal perfusion, further aggravating sepsis-induced kidney injury; fluid overload due to AKI can lead to overt HF in an already dilated and hypocontractile heart; finally, AKI-induced metabolic acidosis can impair contractility and increases heart rate, worsening myocardial stress [127–139]. Beside the hemodynamic effects of the failing heart on the renal circulation, there are also cardiac changes due to impaired fluid clearance by the kidney. Furthermore, sound experimental evidence shows that AKI itself leads to distant organ function [142]. In a murine model, AKI was associated to decreased cardiac contractility and apoptosis, which was attenuated by treatment with an anti-TNF drug [143]. Cardiac hypertrophy and an increase in cardiac macrophages have also been demonstrated in the setting of sepsis-related AKI [142, 144]. This has particularly profound effects on the brain, which extend to systemic neuroendocrine responses during sepsis [145, 146]. Maintaining hemodynamic stability and maintaining tissue perfusion are key components for preventing CRS type 5 in the hyperacute phase of sepsis. Although fluid resuscitation is essential in early sepsis, continued administration of high fluid volumes can contribute to circulatory congestion and its deleterious consequences, including the development of CRS type 5 [147–150].

The management of cardiac dysfunction in the hyperacute and acute phases of sepsis requires a careful balance between fluid administration to maintain adequate filling pressures and the use of vasoactive drugs to improve cardiac contractility. Although vasopressors can help to restore blood pressure, their indiscriminate use can decrease CO by increasing afterload, especially if hypovolemia is present. Norepinephrine is the preferred vasoconstrictor (α-adrenergic effects with some inotropic effects via its moderate β-adrenergic effects). This drug, which increases systemic blood pressure but decreases renal perfusion in normal conditions, can increase renal perfusion during sepsis [151]. The use of phosphodiesterase inhibitors should be based on careful consideration of their inotropic effects versus their vasodilatatory actions. Although it is a strong vasoconstrictor, vasopressin should be used cautiously as it may have detrimental effects on cardiac output and splanchnic perfusion [152]. Vasopressin paradoxically increases urine output and possibly creatinine clearance in patients with septic shock [151–155]. However, it remains unclear what the target systemic and intrarenal blood pressures should be to optimize renal function [152]. There is no role for dopamine to improve renal hemodynamics and function [156], and there have been limited studies with fenoldopam [157].

The role of the calcium-sensitizer levosimendan in the prevention of the CRS type 5 during sepsis is unknown [158].

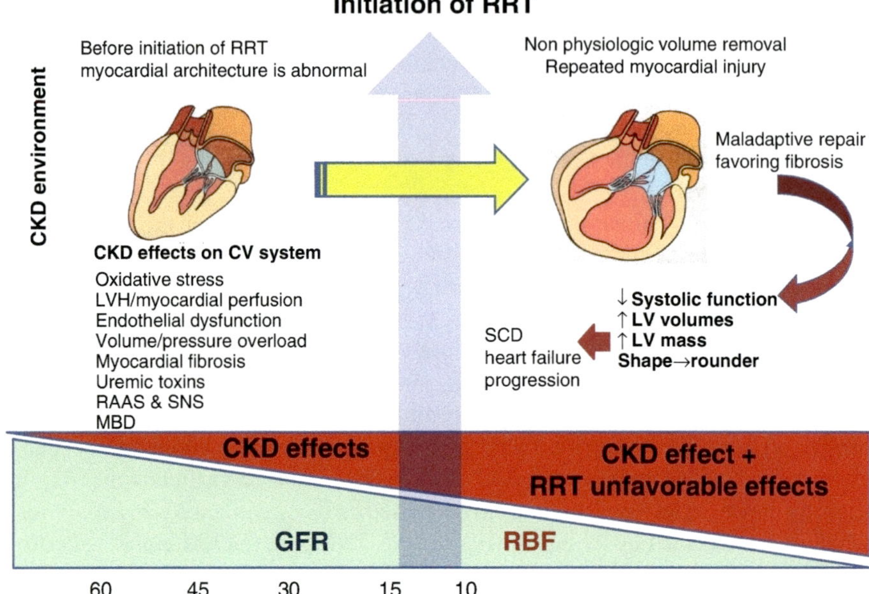

Fig. 10.6 Declining glomerular filtration rate (*GFR*) is associated with multiple stressors upon the cardiovascular (*CV*) system including volume/pressure overload, oxidative stress, and activation of the renin angiotensin system (*RAAS*) and neurohumoral pathways. Prior to the initiation of renal replacement therapy, the heart undergoes maladaptive responses including reduced diastolic compliance, left ventricular hypertrophy (*LVH*), reduction in myocardial capillary density, and uremia-induced myocardial fibrosis. Following the initiation of renal replacement therapy, "nonphysiologic" fluid removal worsens myocardial ischemia leading to progressive heart failure and sudden cardiac death. *CKD* chronic kidney disease, *SNS* sympathetic nervous system, *MBD* metabolic and bone disorder, *RRT* renal replacement therapy, *RBF* renal blood flow, *LV* left ventricle, *SCD* sudden cardiac death

Currently, there are no specific drug-based interventions for renal dysfunction in sepsis. General supportive measures include avoidance of nephrotoxic agents, maintenance of an adequate perfusion pressure, and intervention with dialysis. Diuretics have limited roles in the CRS type 5 [155, 158]. Instead, continuous renal replacement therapy should be considered and implemented early, but further studies are needed to validate this concept (Fig. 10.6).

10.7 Non-pharmacological Modulation of the Autonomic Cardiorenal Crosstalk in Heart Failure

10.7.1 Renal Denervation

The pathophysiologic mechanisms involved in the autonomic cardiorenal crosstalk raise the question whether renal denervation may produce benefit in HF patients [6]. The discussion which follows will not include studies conducted in resistant hypertension and is rather focused on the available data on the effects of renal denervation in

HF [159]. The renal denervation procedure consists of the delivery of low-energy radiofrequency lesions within the renal arteries using electrode catheters positioned just proximal to the origin of the second-order renal artery branch. The technical aspects and potential adverse events of the procedure have been extensively described elsewhere. The ablation of the sympathetic afferent and efferent nerves to the renal arteries should produce a significant reduction in SNA. In HF patients, attenuation of SNA should augment natriuresis, decrease cardiac filling pressures, and potentially improve overall cardiac function [6, 160–162]. Limited data exists on use of renal denervation in HF patients. The principal aim of the Renal Denervation in Patients With Advanced Heart Failure (REACH) pilot study was to examine the safety of renal denervation in a normotensive population with chronic HF [163]. Despite receiving GDMT, the seven study subjects had no hypotension or syncopal episodes while their renal function remained stable over a 6-month period. This very small pilot study also showed a trend toward an improvement in symptoms and exercise capacity [163]. Among 51 NYHA class III and IV HF patients randomized to renal nerves ablation plus optimal medical therapy vs. optimal medical therapy alone, the renal denervation arm had a trend toward reduced HF hospitalizations and improvement in LVEF over a follow-up period of 12 months [164]. These preliminary results are encouraging, but they must be substantiated by larger randomized studies with a longer follow-up. The Renal Denervation in Patients With Advanced Heart Failure (REACH) study (NCT01538992), which was to be a prospective, double-blinded, randomized study on the safety and effectiveness of renal denervation in 100 patients with chronic systolic HF, has been withdrawn prior to enrollment [165]. The Renal Denervation in Patients With Chronic Heart Failure & Renal Impairment Clinical Trial (Symplicity HF) (NCT01392196) is listed on the website clinicaltrials.gov as "active but not recruiting" at the time of this writing [166]. Despite these disappointing events, recent evidence suggesting that renal denervation may reduce left ventricular hypertrophy independent of a drop in blood pressure has raised interest in exploring its role in HF with preserved EF [167]. Pilot studies have also shown that renal denervation may have beneficial effects on glucose metabolism, heart rate, and atrial and ventricular arrhythmias [168–173]. All these comorbidities are characterized by an increased sympathetic tone which is known to adversely affect outcomes in HF patients.

Extreme caution should be used in extrapolating the effects of renal denervation in hypertension studies to those that can occur in an HF population. The long-term impact of renal artery damage is unknown, particularly in HF patients with an already declining renal function. Solid data on the individual variability in renal innervation patterns and in the contribution of the SNA to HF progression are lacking. The pathophysiological implications of renal denervation should be subjected to additional rigorous investigation before this approach can be added to the armamentarium of HF therapies.

10.7.2 Vagal Nerve Stimulation

The vagal nerve originates in the medulla and innervates essentially all the organs in the neck, thorax, and abdomen. The cervical vagal nerve contains both unmyelinated and myelinated nerve fibers. Afferents from the gastrointestinal tract, heart, and lungs outnumber the parasympathetic efferents to the visceral organs. The left vagal nerve gives rise to cardiac efferents that regulate cardiac contractility and the AV node, while efferent fibers in the right vagal nerve act on the sinoatrial node to regulate heart rate [174, 175]. Notably, the mammalian vagal nerve fibers are divided into type A, B, and C. The type of fibers recruited influences the clinical impact of therapies aimed at their modulation. It has been known for more than three decades that there is a strong association between depressed vagal reflexes (as assessed by BRS) and risk of ventricular arrhythmias in the early postinfarction period [176, 177]. Almost two decades ago, the Autonomic Tone and Reflexes After Myocardial Infarction (ATRAMI) study showed that markers of autonomic activity (BRS and HRV) were useful in the risk stratification of patients after a myocardial infarction [178]. Specifically, a depressed BRS in patients with reduced cardiac function identified patients at high risk for HF and arrhythmic mortality [178]. Vagal nerve stimulation (VNS), already used for the treatment of epilepsy and medically refractory depression, is now under investigation also as a treatment for HF [179–183]. The benefit of VNS is due to its central and peripheral antiadrenergic effects and to its anti-apoptotic and anti-inflammatory actions [184]. The role of VNS in HF is supported by the evidence that reduced vagal activity in ADHF is associated with greater hemodynamic abnormalities and increased mortality [182–184]. The improved long-term survival observed in a rodent model of HF induced by myocardial infarction is attributed to the fact that vagal stimulation prevents ischemia-induced loss of connexin 43 thereby improving electrical instability [185]. Additional experimental evidence has shown that VNS improves structural remodeling and EF and reduces a number of inflammatory markers such as TNF-α and interleukin-6 [186].

The apparatus for vagal nerve stimulation is an implantable system that delivers electrical impulses via an asymmetric bipolar multi-contact cuff electrode around the vagal nerve in cervical area. The stimulation electrode is tunneled to the infraclavicular region and attached to the pulse generator. The system used in the CardioFit study (BioControl Medical Ltd, Yehudi, Israel) consists of an asymmetric bipolar multi-contact cuff electrode specifically designed to preferentially activate the vagal efferent fibers in the right cervical vagal nerve. The stimulation lead is designed to recruit efferent vagal B-fibers, with minimal activation of A-fibers, which could have central adverse effects [187]. A right ventricular sensing electrode is placed to prevent excessive bradycardia from VNS. The implantation procedure requires a multidisciplinary team which includes a surgeon and a cardiac electrophysiologist. The stimulation intensities needed to stimulate the appropriate nerve fibers are variable. Stimulation amplitude is gradually up-titrated to achieve targets of approximately 5.5 mA and a heart rate reduction of 5–10 beats, in the absence of adverse effects [188]. The CardioFit trial was an open-label multicenter pilot study in 32 patients with NYHA class II–IV and LVEF <35 %. There were significant improvements in NYHA class ($p<0.001$) and reduction in LV systolic volumes ($p=0.02$) which were sustained at 1 year. However, 26 serious adverse events occurred in 13/32 patients (40.6 %), including three deaths and two clearly device-related AEs (postoperative pulmonary edema and need of surgical revision). Expected nonserious device-related AEs (stimulation-related neck pain, cough, impaired swallowing, dysphonia, nausea, and indigestion) occurred early but were reduced and eventually resolved after stimulation intensity adjustment [188]. The ongoing INcrease Of VAgal TonE in congestive heart failure (INOVATE-HF) trial is a randomized, multicenter (USA and European sites), open-label phase III trial which aims to enroll 650 patients (NYHA class III, LVEF $\leq$40 %, LV end-diastolic dimension 50–80 mm) in a 3:2 randomization scheme to active VNS therapy versus standard of care without implant [189]. The primary efficacy end point of this trial is a composite of all-cause mortality or HF hospitalization. Another multicenter randomized, double-blind, phase II trial, Neural Cardiac Therapy for Heart Failure Study (NECTAR-HF, NCT01385176), is examining the clinical efficacy of direct right VNS in 250 HF patients [190].

The full therapeutic potential of VNS may be due to multiple effects, including heart rate reduction, SNA attenuation, RAAS inhibition, restoration of BRS, suppression of pro-inflammatory cytokines, and decrease in gap junction remodeling [191]. The main challenges to widespread application of VNS include patient selection and identification of the most appropriate pacing protocol. It is possible that patients demonstrating higher baseline SNA may have the best response to SNA, whereas those with ischemic HF and a high scar burden may derive less benefit from neuromodulation therapies. Although intravascular VNS may be possible through stimulation of the coronary sinus ostium and/or superior vena cava to slow down heart rate and prolong AV conduction, many technical challenges remain with respect to selective recruitment of the appropriate vagal fibers, pain perception, and stimulation protocols [192].

Overall, the early data shows that VNS is feasible, safe, and effective in HF patients. However, the encouraging results of pilot studies must be confirmed in larger multicenter randomized studies.

10.7.3   Carotid Baroreceptor Stimulation

Carotid baroreflexes play a critical role in blood pressure regulation through modulation of SNA [193–195]. The carotid baroreceptors are mechanoreceptors located in the carotid sinus and aortic arch, which are stretch sensitive to distension of the vessel wall. Afferent signals from these high-pressure baroreceptors reach the nucleus tractus solitarius in the dorsal medulla of the brainstem and are processed in the ventrolateral medulla, from which the signals controlling the SNA are transmitted to the rest of the body [196]. Activation of high-pressure baroreceptors reduces SNA and enhances the vagal tone [197, 198]. Although carotid sinus stimulation was used to treat angina and hypertension more than 50 years ago, its application was abandoned due to technical limitations and the introduction of effective pharmacological therapies. Renewed interest in the use of BRS as a therapy for HF has been stimulated by evidence that baroreceptor desensitization plays a critical role in the onset and progression of the cardiorenal syndrome despite use of GDMT. In addition, technological advances have improved the clinical application of BRS [199]. In dogs with pacing-induced HF, BRS was associated with lower plasma NE levels and improved survival [200]. Reduction in SNA by BRS can also decrease the effects of A II on myocardial hypertrophy, endothelial dysfunction, and increased vascular resistance and extracellular fluid volume, all of which mediate progression of HF [200–202]. Increased baroreceptor activity can be achieved with either bilateral or unilateral carotid sinus stimulation. The most investigated apparatus for BRS is Rheos system (CVRx, Inc., Minneapolis, MN, USA) which has three components: an implantable pulse generator, carotid sinus leads, and the programmer. The pulse generator is implanted in the infraclavicular region and is connected to two electrode leads that are connected to the perivascular tissue of the two carotid sinuses. The procedure requires an experienced team consisting of a vascular surgeon, electrophysiologist, anesthesiologist, and HF specialist. The second generation of the system (Barostim neo, CVRx, Inc., Minneapolis, MN, USA) consists of a pulse generator and only one carotid sinus electrode. This system consists of a reduced-size electrode which delivers less power and has the potential for a simpler implant and fewer adverse effects. There are few ongoing studies of BRS in patients with both HfrEF and HFpEF. The CVRx® Rheos® Diastolic Heart Failure Trial, a prospective, randomized, double-blind trial examining the safety/efficacy of BRS in 60 subjects has recently been completed and publication of the results is anticipated [203]. The Rheos HOPE4HF Trial is an ongoing open-label randomized study examining the impact of bilateral baroreflex stimulation in 540 patients with diastolic HF (LVEF >40 %). The Barostim neo System in the Treatment of Heart Failure, Barostim HOPE4HF [Hope for Heart Failure], Study (NCT01720160) enrolled patients with NYHA class III HF and LVEF ≤35 % on GDMT at 45 centers in the USA, Canada, and Europe. Subjects were randomly assigned to receive ongoing GDMT alone or ongoing GDMT plus baroreceptor activation therapy (BAT) (treatment group) for 6 months. The primary safety end point was system- and procedure-related major adverse neurological and cardiovascular events. The primary efficacy end points were changes in NYHA functional class, quality-of-life score, and 6-min hall walk distance. One hundred forty-six patients were randomized, 70 to control and 76 to treatment. The major adverse neurological and cardiovascular event-free rate was 97.2 %. Patients assigned to BAT, compared with control group patients, experienced improvements in the distance walked in 6 min (60.0 m vs. 1.5 m; $p=0.004$), quality-of-life score (−17.0 points vs. 2.1 points; $p<0.001$), and NYHA class ($p=0.002$). The BAT significantly reduced NT-proBNP ($p=0.02$) and was associated with a trend toward fewer days hospitalized for HF ($p=0.08$) [204].

Alternative strategies to examine the stimulation of carotid sinus nerves via endovascular stimulation with a catheter in the internal jugular vein are also being investigated (ACES II study, Acute Carotid Sinus Endovascular Stimulation Study) [205]. Some newer systems are also evaluating the placement of endovascular stents with external sources of energy to stimulate the carotid baroreceptors.

10.7.4 Spinal Cord Stimulation

Spinal cord stimulation (SCS) is a therapy approved by the FDA for the treatment of chronic pain and medically refractory angina. This therapy involves the placement of a stimulation electrode in the epidural space tunneled to a pulse generator in the paraspinal lumbar region. The distal poles of the electrode are placed in the region of the fourth and fifth thoracic vertebrae. Spinal cord stimulation is applied at 90 % of the motor threshold at a frequency of 50 Hz with a pulse width of 200 ms width for 2 h, three times a day. Several studies have shown that SCS may have a cardioprotective effect, largely mediated through a vagal-dependent mechanism, which reduces heart rate and blood pressure. The SCS at thoracic vertebra T1 may increase the sinus cycle length and prolong intracardiac conduction, and both effects appear to be vagally mediated [206].

Preclinical work using a canine postinfarction HF model has also demonstrated that SCS administered during coronary artery balloon occlusion may reduce infarct size and suppress ventricular arrhythmias [206–208]. The most robust evidence that SCS may have a role in the treatment of HF is the preclinical work undertaken in a canine model of chronic HF resulting from a myocardial infarction induced by embolization of the left anterior descending coronary artery. Animals were then randomized to receive SCS, medical therapy, or a combination of SCS and medical therapy over a 10-week period. Spinal cord stimulation was performed at T4, at 90 % the motor threshold, three times a day for 2 h each. The groups receiving SCS or medical therapy had a significantly greater decline in BNP and NE levels, combined with a marked reduction in the number of spontaneous ventricular arrhythmias. The greatest increase in LVEF occurred in animals treated with SCS. Another study in a pig model yielded similar results. It also appears that VT suppression and improvement in cardiac function are specific to a particular spinal segment and stimulation threshold. Significant and similar effects may be obtained with stimulation at 90 % of the motor threshold at the T1 or T4 level [207, 208].

On the basis of this preclinical work, there are a number of studies assessing the efficacy and safety of this modality in systolic HF patients. The SCS HEART (Spinal cord stimulation for Heart Failure, NCT01362725) study, a non-randomized, open-label safety study of 20 patients with NYHA class III or IV and LVEF between 20 and 35 % on GDMT is listed as "active but not recruiting" [209]. A similar status is listed for the DEFEAT-HF study (Determining the Feasibility of spinal cord neuromodulation for the treatment of chronic HF, NCT01112579) [210]. Another small, open-label, single-arm, safety and efficacy study (Trial of autonomic neuromodulation for treatment of chronic HF, TAME-HF, NCT01820130) has been withdrawn prior to enrollment [211]. The reasons for the fate of these trials are unknown.

10.7.5 Developing Therapies

The cardiac plexus lies within the adventitia of the great vessels between the ascending aorta and pulmonary artery. This plexus receives innervation from postganglionic sympathetic and preganglionic parasympathetic cardiac autonomic nerves. According to recent data in a canine model, endovascular cardiac plexus stimulation increases LV contractility without increasing heart rate [212]. Transcutaneous or endovascular approaches to stimulate the vagal nerve are being developed. Ongoing research is aimed at identifying novel sensor approaches to measure autonomic activity.

Conclusion

The autonomic nervous system modulates the function of both heart and kidney to maintain intravascular volume homeostasis. Excessive sympathetic activation in HF initiates and maintains mutually detrimental interactions between the heart and the kidney which play key role in the progression of both HF and kidney disease. Innovative non-pharmacological interventions that can favorably alter the cardiac and renal autonomic tone are currently being investigated. Renal denervation, which disrupts the renal nerves from the renal artery, may restore neurohormonal balance to facilitate favorable myocardial remodeling and improve congestion. Vagal nerve and carotid baroreceptor stimulation have been shown in separate pilot studies to improve functional status and cardiac function. In experimental work, spinal cord stimulation has been shown to be beneficial in HF. Multiple clinical trials are currently evaluating the safety and efficacy of these therapeutic strategies in the treatment of HF. While these modalities show promise, additional investigation is sorely needed before they can be widely used in the treatment of the cardiorenal syndrome.

References

1. May CN, Frithiof R, Hood SG, McAllen RM, McKinley MJ, Ramchandra R. Specific control of sympathetic nerve activity to the mammalian heart and kidney. Exp Physiol. 2009;95:34–40.
2. Morrison SF. Differential control of sympathetic outflow. Am J Physiol Regul Integr Comp Physiol. 2001;281:R683–98.
3. Watson AM, Mogulkoc R, McAllen RM, May CN. Stimulation of cardiac sympathetic nerve activity by central angiotensinergic mechanisms in conscious sheep. Am J Physiol Regul Integr Comp Physiol. 2004;286:R1051–6.
4. Frithiof R, Ramchandra R, Hood SG, May CN, Rundgren M. The hypothalamic paraventricular nucleus mediates sodium induced changes in cardiovascular and renal function in conscious sheep. Am J Physiol Regul Integr Comp Physiol. 2009;397:R185–93.
5. Ramchandra R, Hood SG, Watson AM, May CN. Responses of cardiac sympathetic nerve activity to changes in circulating volume differ in normal and heart failure sheep. Am J Physiol Regul Integr Comp Physiol. 2008;295:R719–26.
6. Sobotka PA, Krum H, Böhm M, Francis DP, Schlaich MP. The role of renal denervation in the treatment of heart failure. Curr Cardiol Rep. 2012;14:285–92.
7. Parati G, Esler M. The human sympathetic nervous system: its relevance in hypertension and heart failure. Eur Heart J. 2012;33:1058–66.
8. Macefield V, Wallin BG, Vallbo AB. The discharge behaviour of single vasoconstrictor motoneurones in human muscle nerves. J Physiol (Lond). 1994;481:799–809.
9. Lambert E, Straznicky N, Schlaich MP, et al. Differing patterns of sympathoexcitation in normal weight and obesity-related hypertension. Hypertension. 2007;50:862–8.
10. Lambert G. The assessment of human sympathetic nervous system activity from measurements of norepinephrine turnover. Hypertension. 1988;11:3–20.
11. Friberg P, Meredith I, Jennings G, Lambert G, Fazio V, Esler M. Evidence of increased renal noradrenaline spillover rate during sodium restriction in man. Hypertension. 1990;16:121–30.
12. Hasking G, Esler M, Jennings G, Burton D, Johns J, Korner P. Norepinephrine spillover to plasma in congestive heart failure: evidence of increased overall and cardiorenal sympathetic nervous activity. Circulation. 1986;73:615–21.

13. Parati G, Saul JP, Di Rienzo M, Mancia G. Spectral analysis of blood pressure and heart rate variability in evaluating cardiovascular regulation. A critical appraisal. Hypertension. 1995;25:1276–86.
14. Saul JP, Berger RD, Albrecht P, Stein SP, Chen MH, Cohen RJ. Transfer function analysis of the circulation: unique insights into cardiovascular regulation. Am J Physiol Heart Circ Physiol. 1991;261:H1231–45.
15. Van de Borne P, Rahnama M, Mezzetti S, et al. Contrasting effects of phentolamine and nitroprusside on neural and cardiovascular variability. Am J Physiol Heart Circ Physiol. 2001;281:H559–65.
16. Parati G, Mancia G, Di Rienzo M, Castiglioni P, Taylor JA, Studinger P. Point: counterpoint cardiovascular variability is/is not an index of autonomic control of circulation. J Appl Physiol. 2006;101:676–82.
17. Parati G, Di Rienzo M, Mancia G. How to measure baroreflex sensitivity: from the cardiovascular laboratory to daily life. J Hypertens. 2000;18:7–19.
18. Parati G, di Rienzo M, Bertinieri G, et al. Evaluation of the baroreceptor-heart rate reflex by 24-hour intra-arterial blood pressure monitoring in humans. Hypertension. 1988;12:214–22.
19. Pagani M, Somers V, Furlan R, et al. Changes in autonomic regulation induced by physical training in mild hypertension. Hypertension. 1988;12:600–10.
20. Robbe HW, Mulder LJ, Ruddel H, et al. Assessment of baroreceptor reflex sensitivity by means of spectral analysis. Hypertension. 1987;10:538–43.
21. Grassi M, Esler M. How to assess sympathetic activity in humans. J Hypertens. 1999;17:719–34.
22. Tripsodiakis F, Karayannis G, Giamouzis G, Skoularigis J, Louridas G, Butler J. The sympathetic nervous system in heart failure: physiology, pathophysiology and clinical implications. J Am Coll Cardiol. 2009;54:1747–62.
23. Verberne HJ, Brewster LM, Somsen GA, van Eck-Smit BL. Prognostic value of myocardial 123I-metaiodobenzylguanidine (MIBG) parameters in patients with heart failure: a systematic review. Eur Heart J. 2008;29:1147–59.
24. Tamaki S, Yamada T, Okuyama Y, et al. Cardiac iodine-123 metaiodobenzylguanidine imaging predicts sudden cardiac death independently of left ventricular ejection fraction in patients with chronic heart failure and left ventricular systolic dysfunction: results from a comparative study with signal-averaged electrocardiogram, heart rate variability, and QT dispersion. J Am Coll Cardiol. 2009;53:426–35.
25. Jacobson AF, Lombard J, Banerjee G, Camici PG. 123I-mIBG scintigraphy to predict risk for adverse cardiac outcomes in heart failure patients: design of two prospective multicenter international trials. J Nucl Cardiol. 2009;16:113–21.
26. DiBona GF, Kopp UC. Neural control of renal function. Physiol Rev. 1997;77:75–97.
27. DiBona GF. Neural control of the kidney: past, present, and future. Hypertension. 2003;41:621–4.
28. Bell-Reuss E, Trevino DL, Gottschalk CW. Effect of renal sympathetic nerve stimulation on proximal water and sodium reabsorption. J Clin Invest. 1976;57:1104–7.
29. Zanchetti AS. Neural regulation of renin release: experimental evidence and clinical implications in arterial hypertension. Circulation. 1977;56:691–8.
30. Kirchheim H, Ehmke H, Persson P. Sympathetic modulation of renal hemodynamics, renin release and sodium excretion. Klin Wochenschr. 1989;67:858–64.
31. Shlipak MG, Massie BM. The clinical challenge of cardiorenal syndrome. Circulation. 2004;110:1514–7.
32. Katholi RE, Hageman GR, Whitlow PL, et al. Hemodynamic and afferent renal nerve responses to intrarenal adenosine in the dog. Hypertension. 1983;5:I149–54.
33. Campese VM, Kogosov E. Renal afferent denervation prevents hypertension in rats with chronic renal failure. Hypertension. 1995;25:878–82.
34. Hausberg M, Kosch M, Harmelink P, et al. Sympathetic nerve activity in end-stage renal disease. Circulation. 2002;106:1974–9.
35. Schlaich M, Krum H, Walton T, Lambert G, Sobotka P, Esler M. A novel catheter based approach to denervate the human kidney reduces blood pressure and muscle sympathetic

nerve activity in a patient with end stage renal disease and hypertension. J Hypertens. 2009;27 Suppl 4:s437.

36. Zucker IH. Novel mechanisms of sympathetic regulation in chronic heart failure. Hypertension. 2006;48:1005–11.
37. Levine TB, Francis GS, Goldsmith SR, et al. Activity of the sympathetic nervous system and renin-angiotensin system assessed by plasma hormone levels and their relation to hemodynamic abnormalities in congestive heart failure. Am J Cardiol. 1982;49:1659–66.
38. Cohn JN, Levine TB, Olivari MT, et al. Plasma norepinephrine as a guide to prognosis in patients with chronic congestive heart failure. N Engl J Med. 1984;311:819–23.
39. Goldsmith SR, Sobotka PA, Bart BA. The sympathorenal axis in hypertension and heart failure. J Card Fail. 2010;16:369–73.
40. Cohn JN, Pfeffer MA, Rouleau J, et al. Adverse mortality effect of central sympathetic inhibition with sustained release moxonidine in patients with heart failure (MOXCON). Eur J Heart Fail. 2003;5:659–67.
41. Nozawa T, Igawa A, Fujii N, et al. Effects of long-term renal sympathetic denervation on heart failure after myocardial infarction in rats. Heart Vessels. 2002;16:51–6.
42. Francis GS, Siegel RM, Goldsmith SR, et al. Acute vasoconstrictor response to intravenous furosemide in patients with chronic congestive heart failure. Activation of the neurohumoral axis. Ann Intern Med. 1985;103:1–6.
43. Verbrugge FH, Dupont M, Steels P, et al. The kidney in congestive heart failure: are natriuresis, sodium, and diuretics really the good, the bad and the ugly? Eur J Heart Fail. 2014;16:133–42.
44. Gibson DG, Marshall JC, Lockey E. Assessment of proximal tubular sodium reabsorption during water diuresis in patients with heart disease. Br Heart J. 1970;32:399–405.
45. Lewy JE, Windhager EE. Peritubular control of proximal tubular fluid reabsorption in the rat kidney. Am J Physiol. 1968;214:943–54.
46. Grandchamp A, Boulpaep EL. Pressure control of sodium reabsorption and intercellular backflux across proximal kidney tubule. J Clin Invest. 1974;54:69–82.
47. Gottschalk CW, Mylle M. Micropuncture study of pressures in proximal tubules and peritubular capillaries of the rat kidney and their relation to ureteral and renal venous pressures. Am J Physiol. 1956;185:430–9.
48. Burnett Jr JC, Knox FG. Renal interstitial pressure and sodium excretion during renal vein constriction. Am J Physiol. 1980;238:F279–82.
49. Haddy FJ, Scott J, Fleishman M, Emanuel D. Effect of change in renal venous pressure upon renal vascular resistance, urine and lymph flow rates. Am J Physiol. 1958;195:97–110.
50. Lebrie SJ, Mayerson HS. Influence of elevated venous pressure on flow and composition of renal lymph. Am J Physiol. 1960;198:1037–40.
51. Ott CE, Haas JA, Cuche JL, Knox FG. Effect of increased peritubule protein concentration on proximal tubule reabsorption in the presence and absence of extracellular volume expansion. J Clin Invest. 1975;55:612–20.
52. Lote CJ, Snape BM. Collecting duct flow rate as a determinant of equilibration between urine and renal papilla in the rat in the presence of a maximal antidiuretic hormone concentration. J Physiol. 1977;270:533–44.
53. Allen GG, Barratt LJ. Effect of aldosterone on the transepithelial potential difference of the rat distal tubule. Kidney Int. 1981;19:678–86.
54. Woodhall PB, Tisher CC. Response of the distal tubule and cortical collecting duct to vasopressin in the rat. J Clin Invest. 1973;52:3095–108.
55. Schrier RW. Aldosterone 'escape' vs 'breakthrough'. Nat Rev Nephrol. 2010;6:61.
56. Tang WH, Vagelos RH, Yee YG, Benedict CR, Willson K, Liss CL, Fowler MB. Neurohormonal and clinical responses to high- versus low-dose enalapril therapy in chronic heart failure. J Am Coll Cardiol. 2002;39:70–8.
57. Kim GH. Long-term adaptation of renal ion transporters to chronic diuretic treatment. Am J Nephrol. 2004;24:595–605.
58. Verbrugge FH, Dupont M, Steels P, et al. Abdominal contributions to cardiorenal dysfunction in congestive heart failure. J Am Coll Cardiol. 2013;62:485–95.

59. Aukland K, Reed RK. Interstitial-lymphatic mechanisms in the control of extracellular fluid volume. Physiol Rev. 1993;73:1–78.
60. Guyton AC. Interstitial fluid pressure. II. Pressure-volume curves of interstitial space. Circ Res. 1965;16:452–60.
61. Sandek A, Rauchhaus M, Anker SD, von Haehling S. The emerging role of the gut in chronic heart failure. Curr Opin Clin Nutr Metab Care. 2008;11:632–9.
62. Ding J, Magnotti LJ, Huang Q, Xu DZ, Condon MR, Deitch EA. Hypoxia combined with Escherichia coli produces irreversible gut mucosal injury characterized by increased intestinal cytokine production and DNA degradation. Shock. 2001;16:189–95.
63. Magnusson M, Magnusson KE, Denneberg T. Impaired gut barrier in experimental chronic uremic rats. Miner Electrolyte Metab. 1992;18:288–92.
64. Sultanian R, Deng Y, Kaufman S. Atrial natriuretic factor increases splenic microvascular pressure and fluid extravasation in the rat. J Physiol. 2001;533:273–80.
65. Ronco C, Haapio M, House A, Anavekar N, Bellomo R. Cardiorenal syndrome. J Am Coll Cardiol. 2008;52:1527–39.
66. Hanada S, Takewa Y, Mizuno T, Tsukiyan T, Taenaka Y, Tatsumi E. Effect of the technique for assisting renal blood circulation on ischemic kidney in acute cardiorenal syndrome. J Artif Organs. 2012;15:140–5.
67. Stevenson LW, Perloff JK. The limited reliability of physical signs for estimating hemodynamics in chronic heart failure. JAMA. 1989;261:884–8.
68. Nohria A, Tsang SW, Fang JC, Lewis EF, Jarcho JA, Mudge GH, Stevenson LW. Clinical assessment identifies hemodynamic profiles that predict outcomes in patients admitted with heart failure. J Am Coll Cardiol. 2003;41:1797–804.
69. Mullens W, Abrahams Z, Francis GS, Sokos G, Taylor DO, Starling RC, Young JB, Tang WH. Importance of venous congestion for worsening of renal function in advanced decompensated heart failure. J Am Coll Cardiol. 2009;53:589–96.
70. Damman K, van Deursen VM, Navis G, Voors AA, van Veldhuisen DJ, Hillege HL. Increased central venous pressure is associated with impaired renal function and mortality in a broad spectrum of patients with cardiovascular disease. J Am Coll Cardiol. 2009;53:582–8.
71. Nohria A, Hasselblad V, Stebbins A, et al. Cardiorenal interactions: insights from the ESCAPE trial. J Am Coll Cardiol. 2008;51:1268–74.
72. Uthoff H, Breidthardt T, Klima T, et al. Central venous pressure and impaired renal function in patients with acute heart failure. Eur J Heart Fail. 2011;13:432–9.
73. Fiksen-Olsen MJ, Strick DM, Hawley H, Romero JC. Renal effects of angiotensin II inhibition during increases in renal venous pressure. Hypertension. 1992;19:II137–41.
74. De Silva R, Loh H, Rigby AS, et al. Epidemiology, associated factors, and prognostic outcomes of renal artery stenosis in chronic heart failure assessed by magnetic resonance angiography. Am J Cardiol. 2007;100:273–9.
75. Maisel A, Xue Y, Shah K, Mueller C, et al. Increased 90-day mortality in patients with acute heart failure with elevated copeptin: secondary results from the Biomarkers in Acute Heart Failure (BACH) study. Circ Heart Fail. 2011;4:613–20.
76. Shah RV, Truong QA, Gaggin HK, Pfannkuche J, Hartmann O, Januzzi Jr JL. Mid-regional pro-atrial natriuretic peptide and pro-adrenomedullin testing for the diagnostic and prognostic evaluation of patients with acute dyspnoea. Eur Heart J. 2012;33:2197–205.
77. Maisel AS, Katz N, Hillege HL, Shaw A, et al. Acute Dialysis Quality Initiative Consensus Group: biomarkers in kidney and heart disease. Nephrol Dial Transplant. 2011;26:62–74.
78. Heywood JT, Fonarow GC, Costanzo MR, Mathur VS, Wigneswaran JR, Wynne J. High prevalence of renal dysfunction and its impact on outcome in 118,465 patients hospitalized with acute decompensated heart failure: a report from the ADHERE database. J Card Fail. 2007;13:422–30.
79. Hebert K, Dias A, Delgado MC, et al. Epidemiology and survival of the five stages of chronic kidney disease in a systolic heart failure population. Eur J Heart Fail. 2010;12:861–5.
80. Cruz DN, Bagshaw SM. Heart-kidney interaction: epidemiology of cardiorenal syndromes. Int J Nephrol. 2010;2011:351291. doi:10.4061/2011/351291.

81. Bagshaw SM, Cruz DN, Aspromonte N, et al. Epidemiology of cardio-renal syndromes: workgroup statements from the 7th ADQI Consensus Conference. Nephrol Dial Transplant. 2010;25:1406–16.
82. Setoguchi S, Stevenson LW, Schneeweiss S. Repeated hospitalizations predict mortality in the community population with heart failure. Am Heart J. 2007;154:260–6.
83. Tanaka K, Ito M, Kodama M, et al. Longitudinal change in renal function in patients with idiopathic dilated cardiomyopathy without renal insufficiency at initial diagnosis. Circ J. 2007;71:1927–31.
84. Chawla LS, Kimmel PL. Acute kidney injury and chronic kidney disease: an integrated clinical syndrome. Kidney Int. 2012;82:516–24.
85. Bongartz LG, Cramer MJ, Doevendans PA, Joles JA, Braam B. The severe cardiorenal syndrome: 'Guyton revisited'. Eur Heart J. 2005;26:11–7.
86. Merrill AJ, Morrison JL, Branno ES. Concentration of renin in renal venous blood in patients with chronic heart failure. Am J Med. 1946;1:468.
87. Ichikawa I, Pfeffer JM, Pfeffer MA, Hostetter TH, Brenner BM. Role of angiotensin II in the altered renal function of congestive heart failure. Circ Res. 1984;55:669–75.
88. Kishimoto T, Maekawa M, Abe Y, Yamamoto K. Intrarenal distribution of blood flow and renin release during renal venous pressure elevation. Kidney Int. 1973;4:259–66.
89. Rafiq K, Noma T, Fujisawa Y, et al. Renal sympathetic denervation suppresses de novo podocyte injury and albuminuria in rats with aortic regurgitation. Circulation. 2012;125:1402–13.
90. Remuzzi G, Cattaneo D, Perico N. The aggravating mechanisms of aldosterone on kidney fibrosis. J Am Soc Nephrol. 2008;19:1459–62.
91. Onozato ML, Tojo A, Kobayashi N, Goto A, Matsuoka H, Fujita T. Dual blockade of aldosterone and angiotensin II additively suppresses TGF-β and NADPH oxidase in the hypertensive kidney. Nephrol Dial Transplant. 2007;22:1314–22.
92. Testani JM, Kimmel SE, Dries DL, Coca SG. Prognostic importance of early worsening renal function after initiation of angiotensin-converting enzyme inhibitor therapy in patients with cardiac dysfunction. Circ Heart Fail. 2011;4:685–91.
93. Capes SE, Gerstein HC, Negassa A, Yusuf S. Enalapril prevents clinical proteinuria in diabetic patients with low ejection fraction. Diabetes Care. 2000;23:377–80.
94. Bansal N, Tighiouart H, Weiner D, Griffith J, Vlagopoulos P, Salem D, Levin A, Sarnak MJ. Anemia as a risk factor for kidney function decline in individuals with heart failure. Am J Cardiol. 2007;99:1137–42.
95. Ljungman S, Kjekshus J, Swedberg K. Renal function in severe congestive heart failure during treatment with enalapril – the Cooperative North Scandinavian Enalapril Survival Study (CONSENSUS) Trial. Am J Cardiol. 1992;70:479–87.
96. Hillege HL, van Gilst WH, van Veldhuisen DJ, Navis G, Grobbee DE, de Graeff PA, de Zeeuw D. Accelerated decline and prognostic impact of renal function after myocardial infarction and the benefits of ACE inhibition: the CATS randomized trial. Eur Heart J. 2003;24:412–20.
97. Anand IS, Bishu K, Rector TS, Ishani A, Kuskowski MA, Cohn JN. Proteinuria, chronic kidney disease, and the effect of an angiotensin receptor blocker in addition to an angiotensin-converting enzyme inhibitor in patients with moderate to severe heart failure. Circulation. 2009;120:1577–84.
98. Jackson CE, Solomon SD, Gerstein HC, et al. Albuminuria in chronic heart failure: prevalence and prognostic importance. Lancet. 2009;374:543–50.
99. Boerrigter G, Costello-Boerrigter LC, Abraham WT, et al. Cardiac resynchronization therapy improves renal function in human heart failure with reduced glomerular filtration rate. J Card Fail. 2008;14:539–46.
100. Sandner SE, Zimpfer D, Zrunek P, et al. Renal function and outcome after continuous flow left ventricular assist device implantation. Ann Thorac Surg. 2009;87:1072–8.
101. Kobuchi S, Tanaka R, Shintani T, et al. Mechanisms underlying the renoprotective effect of GABA against ischemia/reperfusion-induced renal injury in rats. J Pharmacol Exp Ther. 2011;338:767–74.

102. Li C, Zhang D, Han S, et al. Synthesis, electronic properties, and applications of indium oxide nanowires. Ann N Y Acad Sci. 2003;1006:104–21.
103. Singh K, Xiao L, Remondino A, Sawyer DB, Colucci WS. Adrenergic regulation of cardiac myocyte apoptosis. J Cell Physiol. 2001;189:257–65.
104. Kim S, Iwao H. Molecular and cellular mechanisms of angiotensin II-mediated cardiovascular and renal diseases. Pharmacol Rev. 2000;52:11–34.
105. Kajstura J, Cigola E, Malhotra A, et al. Angiotensin II induces apoptosis of adult ventricular myocytes in vitro. J Mol Cell Cardiol. 1997;29:859–70.
106. Kawano H, Do YS, Kawano Y, et al. Angiotensin II has multiple profibrotic effects in human cardiac fibroblasts. Circulation. 2000;101:1130–7.
107. Yap SC, Lee HT. Acute kidney injury and extrarenal organ dysfunction: new concepts and experimental evidence. Anesthesiology. 2012;116:1139–48.
108. Kingma Jr JG, Vincent C, Rouleau JR, Kingma I. Influence of acute renal failure on coronary vasoregulation in dogs. J Am Soc Nephrol. 2006;17:1316–24.
109. Desai KV, Laine GA, Stewart RH, et al. Mechanics of the left ventricular myocardial interstitium: effects of acute and chronic myocardial edema. Am J Physiol Heart Circ Physiol. 2008;294:H2428–34.
110. Nath KA, Grande JP, Croatt AJ, et al. Transgenic sickle mice are markedly sensitive to renal ischemia-reperfusion injury. Am J Pathol. 2005;166:963–72.
111. Go AS, Chertow GM, Dongjie Fan D, McCulloch CE, Hsu CY. Chronic kidney disease and the risks of death, cardiovascular events, and hospitalization. N Engl J Med. 2004;351:1296–305.
112. Beattie JN, Soman SS, Sandberg KR, Yee J, Borzak S, Garg M. Determinants of mortality after myocardial infarction in patients with advanced renal dysfunction. Am J Kidney Dis. 2001;37:1191–200.
113. Anavekar NS, McMurray JJ, Velazquez EJ, Solomon SD, Kober L, Rouleau JL. Relation between renal dysfunction and cardiovascular outcomes after myocardial infarction. N Engl J Med. 2004;351:1285–95.
114. Rostand SG, Kirk KA, Rutsky EA. Dialysis-associated ischemic heart disease: insights from coronary angiography. Kidney Int. 1984;25:653–9.
115. Parfey PS, Harnett JD, Foley RN. Heart failure and ischemic heart disease in chronic uremia. Curr Opin Nephrol Hypertens. 1995;4:105–10.
116. Bogrov AY, Shapiro JI. Endogenous digitalis: pathophysiologic roles and therapeutic applications. Nat Clin Pract Nephrol. 2008;4:378–92.
117. Lundy DJ, Trzeciak S. Microcirculatory dysfunction in sepsis. Crit Care Clin. 2009;25:721–31.
118. Trzeciak S, et al. Early microcirculatory perfusion derangements in patients with severe sepsis and septic shock: relationship to hemodynamics, oxygen transport, and survival. Ann Emerg Med. 2007;49:88–98.
119. Sakr Y, et al. Persistent microcirculatory alterations are associated with organ failure and death in patients with septic shock. Crit Care Med. 2004;32:1825–31.
120. Lambermont B, et al. Effects of endotoxic shock on right ventricular systolic function and mechanical efficiency. Cardiovasc Res. 2003;59:412–8.
121. Jardin F, et al. Sepsis-related cardiogenic shock. Crit Care Med. 1990;18:1055–60.
122. Parker MM, et al. Profound but reversible myocardial depression in patients with septic shock. Ann Intern Med. 1984;100:483–90.
123. Dhainaut JF, Huyghebaert MF, Monsallieret JF, et al. Coronary hemodynamics and myocardial metabolism of lactate, free fatty acids, glucose, and ketones in patients with septic shock. Circulation. 1987;75:533–41.
124. Niederbichler AD, Hoesel LM, Westfallet MV, et al. An essential role for complement C5a in the pathogenesis of septic cardiac dysfunction. J Exp Med. 2006;203:53–61.
125. Kumar A, Thota V, Dee L, et al. Tumor necrosis factor-α and interleukin-1β are responsible for in vitro myocardial cell depression induced by human septic shock serum. J Exp Med. 1996;183:949–58.

126. Torre-Amione G, Kapadia S, Benedict C, et al. Proinflammatory cytokine levels in patients with depressed left ventricular ejection fraction: a report from the Studies of Left Ventricular Dysfunction (SOLVD). J Am Coll Cardiol. 1996;27:1201–6.
127. Lerolle N, Guérot E, Faisyet C, et al. Renal failure in septic shock: predictive value of Doppler-based renal arterial resistive index. Intensive Care Med. 2006;32:1553–9.
128. Murugan R, Karajala-Subramanyam V, Lee M, et al. Acute kidney injury in non-severe pneumonia is associated with an increased immune response and lower survival. Kidney Int. 2010;77:527–35.
129. Papaioannou VE, Dragoumanis C, Theodorouet V, et al. Relation of heart rate variability to serum levels of C-reactive protein, interleukin-6 and -10 in patients with sepsis and septic shock. J Crit Care. 2009;24:625.e1–e7.
130. Schmidt H, Hoyer DH, Hennen R, et al. Autonomic dysfunction predicts both 1- and 2-month mortality in middle-aged patients with multiple organ dysfunction syndrome. Crit Care Med. 2008;36:967–70.
131. Ramchandra R, Wan L, Hood SG, et al. Septic shock induces distinct changes in sympathetic nerve activity to the heart and kidney in conscious sheep. Am J Physiol Regul Integr Comp Physiol. 2009;297:R1247–53.
132. Meijvis SC, et al. Prognostic value of serum angiotensin-converting enzyme activity for outcome of community-acquired pneumonia. Clin Chem Lab Med. 2011;49:1525–32.
133. Nakada TA, Russell JA, Boyd JH, et al. Association of angiotensin II type 1 receptor-associated protein gene polymorphism with increased mortality in septic shock. Crit Care Med. 2011;39:1641–8.
134. Doerschug KC, Delsing AS, Schmidt GA, Ashare A. Renin-angiotensin system activation correlates with microvascular dysfunction in a prospective cohort study of clinical sepsis. Crit Care. 2010;14:R24.
135. Shen L, Mo H, Cai L, et al. Losartan prevents sepsis-induced acute lung injury and decreases activation of nuclear factor-κB and mitogen-activated protein kinases. Shock. 2009;31:500–6.
136. Hagiwara S, Iwasaka H, Matumoto S, et al. Effects of an angiotensin-converting enzyme inhibitor on the inflammatory response in in vivo and in vitro models. Crit Care Med. 2009;37:626–33.
137. Nitescu N, Grimberg E, Guron G. Low-dose candesartan improves renal blood flow and kidney oxygen tension in rats with endotoxin-induced acute kidney dysfunction. Shock. 2008;30:166–72.
138. Mortensen EM, Restrepo MI, Copeland LA, et al. Impact of previous statin and angiotensin II receptor blocker use on mortality in patients hospitalized with sepsis. Pharmacotherapy. 2007;27:1619–26.
139. Soni A, Pepper GM, Wyrwinski PM, et al. Adrenal insufficiency occurring during septic shock: incidence, outcome, and relationship to peripheral cytokine levels. Am J Med. 1995;98:266–71.
140. Annane D, Bellissant E, Bollaert PE, et al. Corticosteroids in the treatment of severe sepsis and septic shock in adults: a systematic review. JAMA. 2009;301:2362–75.
141. Sligl WI, Milner Jr DA, Sundar S, et al. Safety and efficacy of corticosteroids for the treatment of septic shock: a systematic review and meta-analysis. Clin Infect Dis. 2009;49:93–101.
142. Kelly KJ. Distant effects of experimental renal ischemia/reperfusion injury. J Am Soc Nephrol. 2003;14:1549–58.
143. Grams ME, Rabb H. The distant organ effects of acute kidney injury. Kidney Int. 2012;81:942–8.
144. Burchill L, Velkoska E, Dean RG, Lew RA, Smith AI, Levidiotis V, Burrell LM. Acute kidney injury in the rat causes cardiac remodelling and increases angiotensin-converting enzyme 2 expression. Exp Physiol. 2008;93:622–30.
145. Liu M, Liang Y, Chigurupati S, et al. Acute kidney injury leads to inflammation and functional changes in the brain. J Am Soc Nephrol. 2008;19:1360–70.

146. Tokuyama H, Kelly DJ, Zhang Y, Gow RM, Gilbert RE. Macrophage infiltration and cellular proliferation in the non-ischemic kidney and heart following prolonged unilateral renal ischemia. Nephron Physiol. 2007;106:54–62.
147. Liu KD, Taylor TB, Ancukiewicz M, et al. Acute kidney injury in patients with acute lung injury: impact of fluid accumulation on classification of acute kidney injury and associated outcomes. Crit Care Med. 2011;39:2665–71.
148. Macedo E, Bouchard J, Soroko SH, et al. Fluid accumulation, recognition and staging of acute kidney injury in critically-ill patients. Crit Care. 2010;14:R82.
149. Bellomo R, Prowle JR, Echeverri JE, et al. Fluid management in septic acute kidney injury and cardiorenal syndromes. Contrib Nephrol. 2010;165:206–18. Basel Karger.
150. Boyd JH, Forbes J, Nakada T, et al. Fluid resuscitation in septic shock: a positive fluid balance and elevated central venous pressure are associated with increased mortality. Crit Care Med. 2011;39:259–65.
151. Redfors B, Bragadottir G, Sellgren J, Swärd K, Ricksten SE, et al. Effects of norepinephrine on renal perfusion, filtration and oxygenation in vasodilatory shock and acute kidney injury. Intensive Care Med. 2011;37:60–7.
152. Guzman JA, Rosado AE, Kruse JA. Vasopressin vs. norepinephrine in endotoxic shock: systemic, renal, and splanchnic hemodynamic and oxygen transport effects. J Appl Physiol. 2003;95:803–9.
153. Gordon AC, Russell JA, Walley KR, et al. The effects of vasopressin on acute kidney injury in septic shock. Intensive Care Med. 2010;36:83–91.
154. Deruddre S, Cheisson G, Mazoit GC, Vicaut E, Benhamou D, Duranteau J, et al. Renal arterial resistance in septic shock: effects of increasing mean arterial pressure with norepinephrine on the renal resistive index assessed with Doppler ultrasonography. Intensive Care Med. 2007;33:1557–62.
155. Bellomo R, Wan L, May C. Vasoactive drugs and acute kidney injury. Crit Care Med. 2008;36(suppl):S179–86.
156. Schmoelz M, Schelling G, Dunker M, Irlbeck M, et al. Comparison of systemic and renal effects of dopexamine and dopamine in norepinephrine-treated septic shock. J Cardiothorac Vasc Anesth. 2006;20:173–8.
157. Cobas M, Paparcuri G, De La Pena M, Cudemus G, Barquist E, Varon A, et al. Fenoldopam in critically ill patients with early renal dysfunction. A crossover study. Cardiovasc Ther. 2011;29:280–4.
158. Nigwekar SU, Waikar SS. Diuretics in acute kidney injury. Semin Nephrol. 2011;31:523–34.
159. Singh JP, Kandala J, Camm AJ. Non-pharmacological modulation of the autonomic tone to treat heart failure. Eur Heart J. 2014;35:77–85.
160. Symplicity HTN-1 Investigators. Catheter-based renal sympathetic denervation for resistant hypertension: durability of blood pressure reduction out to 24 months. Hypertension. 2011;57:911–7.
161. Schlaich MP, Sobotka PA, Krum H, Lambert E, Esler MD. Renal sympathetic-nerve ablation for uncontrolled hypertension. N Engl J Med. 2009;361:932–4.
162. Mahfoud F, Ukena C, Schmieder RE, et al. Ambulatory blood pressure changes after renal sympathetic denervation in patients with resistant hypertension. Circulation. 2013;128:132–40.
163. Davies JE, Manisty CH, Petraco R, et al. First-in-man safety evaluation of renal denervation for chronic systolic heart failure: primary outcome from REACH-Pilot study. Int J Cardiol. 2013;1(62):189–92.
164. Ozaki Y. European Society of Cardiology (ESC) Congress Report from Munich 2012. Circ J. 2012;76:2530–5.
165. Renal Artery Denervation in Chronic Heart Failure Study (REACH). Available at: https://clinicaltrials.gov/ct2/results?term=NCT01538992. Accessed 30 June 2015.
166. Renal denervation in patients with advanced heart failure (SIMPLICITY HF). Available at: https://clinicaltrials.gov/ct2/results?term=NCT01392196. Accessed 30 June 2015.

167. Brandt MC, Mahfoud F, Reda S, Schirmer SH, Erdmann E, Bohm M, Hoppe UC. Renal sympathetic denervation reduces left ventricular hypertrophy and improves cardiac function in patients with resistant hypertension. J Am Coll Cardiol. 2012;59:901–9.

168. Zile MR, Little WC. Effects of autonomic modulation: more than just blood pressure. J Am Coll Cardiol. 2012;59:910–2.

169. Mahfoud F, Schlaich M, Kindermann I, et al. Effect of renal sympathetic denervation on glucose metabolism in patients with resistant hypertension: a pilot study. Circulation. 2011;123:1940–6.

170. Linz D, Mahfoud F, Schotten U, Ukena C, Neuberger HR, Wirth K, Bohm M. Renal sympathetic denervation suppresses postapneic blood pressure rises and atrial fibrillation in a model for sleep apnea. Hypertension. 2012;60:172–8.

171. Pokushalov E, Romanov A, Corbucci G, et al. A randomized comparison of pulmonary vein isolation with versus without concomitant renal artery denervation in patients with refractory symptomatic atrial fibrillation and resistant hypertension. J Am Coll Cardiol. 2012;60:1163–70.

172. Ukena C, Bauer A, Mahfoud F, et al. Renal sympathetic denervation for treatment of electrical storm: first-in-man experience. Clin Res Cardiol. 2012;101:63–7.

173. Ukena C, Mahfoud F, Spies A, et al. Effects of renal sympathetic denervation on heart rate and atrioventricular conduction in patients with resistant hypertension. Int J Cardiol. 2012;167:2846–51.

174. Van Stee EW. Autonomic innervation of the heart. Environ Health Perspect. 1978;26:151–8.

175. Armour JA. Cardiac neuronal hierarchy in health and disease. Am J Physiol Regul Integr Comp Physiol. 2004;287:R262–71.

176. Vanoli E, De Ferrari GM, Stramba-Badiale M, et al. Vagal stimulation and prevention of sudden death in conscious dogs with a healed myocardial infarction. Circ Res. 1991;68:1471–81.

177. Billman GE, Schwartz PJ, Stone HL. Baroreceptor reflex control of heart rate: a predictor of sudden cardiac death. Circulation. 1982;66:874–80.

178. La Rovere MT, Bigger Jr JT, Marcus FI, Mortara A, Schwartz PJ. Baroreflex sensitivity and heart-rate variability in prediction of total cardiac mortality after myocardial infarction. ATRAMI (Autonomic Tone and Reflexes After Myocardial Infarction) Investigators. Lancet. 1998;351:478–84.

179. Heck C, Helmers SL, DeGiorgio CM. Vagus nerve stimulation therapy, epilepsy, and device parameters: scientific basis and recommendations for use. Neurology. 2002;59(6 Suppl 4):S31–7.

180. Rush AJ, Marangell LB, Sackeim HA, et al. Vagus nerve stimulation for treatment- resistant depression: a randomized, controlled acute phase trial. Biol Psychiatry. 2005;58:347–54.

181. Schwartz PJ, De Ferrari GM, Sanzo A, et al. Long term vagal stimulation in patients with advanced heart failure: first experience in man. Eur J Heart Fail. 2008;10:884–91.

182. Milby AH, Halpern CH, Baltuch GH. Vagus nerve stimulation for epilepsy and depression. Neurotherapeutics. 2008;5:75–85.

183. Li M, Zheng C, Sato T, Kawada T, Sugimachi M, Sunagawa K. Vagal nerve stimulation markedly improves long-term survival after chronic heart failure in rats. Circulation. 2004;109:120–4.

184. Olshansky B, Sabbah HN, Hauptman PJ, Colucci WS. Parasympathetic nervous system and heart failure: pathophysiology and potential implications for therapy. Circulation. 2008;118:863–71.

185. Ando M, Katare RG, Kakinuma Y, et al. Efferent vagal nerve stimulation protects heart against ischemia-induced arrhythmias by preserving connexin43 protein. Circulation. 2005;112:164–70.

186. Zhang Y, Popovic ZB, Bibevski S, et al. Chronic vagus nerve stimulation improves autonomic control and attenuates systemic inflammation and heart failure progression in a canine high-rate pacing model. Circ Heart Fail. 2009;2:692–9.

187. Anholt TA, Ayal S, Goldberg JA. Recruitment and blocking properties of the CardioFit stimulation lead. J Neural Eng. 2011;8:034004.
188. De Ferrari GM, Crijns HJ, Borggrefe M, et al. Chronic vagus nerve stimulation: a new and promising therapeutic approach for chronic heart failure. Eur Heart J. 2011;32:847–55.
189. Hauptman PJ, Schwartz PJ, Gold MR, et al. Rationale and study design of the increase of vagal tone in heart failure study: INOVATE-HF. Am Heart J. 2012;163:954–62.
190. Neural cardiac therapy for heart failure study (NECTAR-HF). https://clinicaltrials.gov/ct2/show/NCT01385176. Accessed 30 June 2015.
191. Sabbah HN, Ilsar I, Zaretsky A, Rastogi S, Wang M, Gupta RC. Vagus nerve stimulation in experimental heart failure. Heart Fail Rev. 2011;16:171–8.
192. Bianchi S, Rossi P, Della Scala A, et al. Atrioventricular (AV) node vagal stimulation by transvenous permanent lead implantation to modulate AV node function: safety and feasibility in humans. Heart Rhythm. 2009;6:1282–6.
193. McCubbin JW, Green JH, Page IH. Baroreceptor function in chronic renal hypertension. Circ Res. 1956;4:205–10.
194. Chapleau MW, Hajduczok G, Abboud FM. Mechanisms of resetting of arterial baroreceptors: an overview. Am J Med Sci. 1988;295:327–34.
195. Thrasher TN. Unloading arterial baroreceptors causes neurogenic hypertension. Am J Physiol Regul Integr Comp Physiol. 2002;282:R1044–53.
196. Biaggioni I, Whetsell WO, Jobe J, Nadeau JH. Baroreflex failure in a patient with central nervous system lesions involving the nucleus tractus solitarii. Hypertension. 1994;23:491–5.
197. Robertson D, Hollister AS, Biaggioni I, et al. The diagnosis and treatment of baroreflex failure. N Engl J Med. 1993;329:1449–55.
198. Heusser K, Tank J, Engeli S, et al. Carotid baroreceptor stimulation, sympathetic activity, baroreflex function, and blood pressure in hypertensive patients. Hypertension. 2010;55:619–26.
199. Creager MA. Baroreceptor reflex function in congestive heart failure. Am J Cardiol. 1992;69:10G–5; discussion 15G–16G.
200. Zucker IH, Hackley JF, Cornish KG, et al. Chronic baroreceptor activation enhances survival in dogs with pacing-induced heart failure. Hypertension. 2007;50:904–10.
201. Higashi T, Kobayashi N, Hara K, Shirataki H, Matsuoka H. Effects of angiotensin II type 1 receptor antagonist on nitric oxide synthase expression and myocardial remodeling in Goldblatt hypertensive rats. J Cardiovasc Pharmacol. 2000;35:564–71.
202. Nishida Y, Ding J, Zhou MS, Chen QH, Murakami H, Wu XZ, Kosaka H. Role of nitric oxide in vascular hyper-responsiveness to norepinephrine in hypertensive Dahl rats. J Hypertens. 1998;16:1611–8.
203. CVRx I. Health outcomes prospective evaluation for heart failure with EF ≥40%. In: CVRx I. Rheos HOPE4HF Study. https://clinicaltrials.gov/ct2/show/NCT00957073. Accessed 30 June 2015.
204. Abraham WT, Zile MR, Weaver FA, et al. Baroreflex activation therapy for the treatment of heart failure with a reduced ejection fraction. JACC Heart Fail. 2015;3:487–96.
205. Management MCRD. Acute carotid sinus endovascular stimulation II study. Available at http://www.clinicaltrials.gov/ct2/show/NCT01458483. Accessed 30 June 2015.
206. Olgin JE, Takahashi T, Wilson E, Vereckei A, Steinberg H, Zipes DP. Effects of thoracic spinal cord stimulation on cardiac autonomic regulation of the sinus and atrioventricular nodes. J Cardiovasc Electrophysiol. 2002;13:475–81.
207. Lopshire JC, Zhou X, Dusa C, et al. Spinal cord stimulation improves ventricular function and reduces ventricular arrhythmias in a ca nine postinfarction heart failure model. Circulation. 2009;120:286–94.
208. Isa ZF, Zhou X, Unholy MR, Rosenberger J, Bhatia D, Groh WJ, Miller JM, Zipes DP. Thoracic spinal cord stimulation reduces the risk of ischemic ventricular arrhythmias in a postinfarction heart failure canine model. Circulation. 2005;111:3217–20.

209. Medical SJ. Spinal cord stimulation for heart failure as a restorative treatment. Available at http://www.clinicaltrials.gov/ct2/show/NCT01362725. Accessed 30 June 2015.
210. Management MCRD. Determining the feasibility of spinal cord neuromodulation for the treatment of chronic heart failure. Available at http://www.clinicaltrials.gov/ct2/show/NCT01112579. Accessed 30 June 2015.
211. Medical SJ. Trial of autonomic neuroModulation for trEatment of chronic heart failure. Available at http://www.clinicaltrials.gov/ct2/show/NCT01820130. Accessed 30 June 2015.
212. Kobayashi M, Sakurai S, Takaseya T, et al. Effects of percutaneous stimulation of both sympathetic and parasympathetic cardiac autonomic nerves on cardiac function in dogs. Innovations (Phila). 2012;7:282–9.
213. Metra M, Cotter G, Gheorghiade M, Dei Cas L, Voors AA. The role of the kidney in heart failure. Eur Heart J. 2012;33:2135–43.

Vagal Stimulation in Heart Failure: An Anti-inflammatory Intervention?

11

Gaetano M. De Ferrari, Peter J. Schwartz, Alice Ravera, Veronica Dusi, and Laura Calvillo

11.1 Background Leading to Vagal Stimulation in Heart Failure

Heart failure (HF) is accompanied by an autonomic imbalance usually characterised by both increased sympathetic activity and withdrawal of vagal activity. Sympathetic activation in the setting of decreased systolic function includes appropriate reflex compensatory responses to impaired systolic function as well as excitatory stimuli inducing adrenergic responses in excess of homeostatic requirements [1, 2]. Therefore, even though cardiac adrenergic drive initially supports the performance of the failing heart, long-term activation of the sympathetic nervous system is deleterious and, accordingly, beta-adrenergic blocker treatment is beneficial [3].

G.M. De Ferrari (✉)
Department of Cardiology, Fondazione IRCCS Policlinico San Matteo,
Viale Golgi, 19, Pavia 27100, Italy

Department of Molecular Medicine, University of Pavia, Pavia, Italy

Cardiovascular Clinical Research Center, Fondazione IRCCS Policlinico San Matteo,
Pavia, Italy
e-mail: g.deferrari@smatteo.pv.it

P.J. Schwartz
IRCCS Istituto Auxologico Italiano, Center for Cardiac Arrhythmias of Genetic Origin,
Milan, Italy

A. Ravera • V. Dusi
Department of Cardiology, Fondazione IRCCS Policlinico San Matteo,
Viale Golgi, 19, Pavia 27100, Italy

Department of Molecular Medicine, University of Pavia, Pavia, Italy

L. Calvillo
Laboratory of Cardiovascular Genetics, IRCCS Istituto Auxologico Italiano, Milan, Italy

© Springer International Publishing Switzerland 2016
E. Gronda et al. (eds.), *Heart Failure Management: The Neural Pathways*,
DOI 10.1007/978-3-319-24993-3_11

The possibility that markers of vagal activity such as heart rate variability and baroreflex sensitivity (BRS) could be of prognostic value was first suggested in a post-myocardial infarction conscious canine model [4, 5] and subsequently confirmed in several studies in patients with a recent myocardial infarction (MI) [6–9].

Arterial baroreflex-mediated heart rate responses to drug-induced blood pressure changes are significantly blunted in patients with HF [10, 11]. It is recognised that the arterial baroreceptor reflex vagal control of heart rate is impaired relatively early in HF, at variance with the preserved baroreflex regulation of muscle sympathetic nerve activity, albeit from a higher baseline value [2]. The impairment in the cardiopulmonary baroreflex-mediated inhibition of sympathetic discharge markedly contributes to the increase in sympathetic activity observed in patients with HF [2, 12, 13]. Additionally, patients with HF show a defect in the transmission of nerve impulses at the level of the parasympathetic ganglion, leading to a reduced efferent vagal activity directed to the heart [14].

The baroreflex heart rate response to blood pressure increase was assessed in a group of almost 300 HF patients by Mortara et al. [15]. Baroreflex sensitivity was significantly correlated with left ventricular (LV) ejection fraction, cardiac index and pulmonary artery wedge pressure. During follow-up, patients in the lower quartile of BRS had an almost threefold increase in the composite end point of cardiac death, nonfatal cardiac arrest and status 1 priority transplantation. At multivariable analysis, BRS was an independent predictor of death after adjustment for noninvasive known risk factors but not when haemodynamic indexes were also considered. However, in patients with severe mitral regurgitation, BRS remained a strong prognostic marker independent of haemodynamic function.

The predictive role of blunted vagal baroreflexes was subsequently confirmed and shown to be independent from anti-adrenergic treatment with beta-blockers [16]. In a group of almost 400 HF patients with heart rate variability measured from an implanted cardiac resynchronisation device, markers of reduced vagal activity were associated with increased mortality and further vagal withdrawal was found to precede acute decompensation [17].

11.2 Experimental Studies on Vagal Stimulation

11.2.1 Arrhythmia Models

In 1859, Einbrodt published the results of investigations assessing the effects of vagal stimulation on several cardiovascular parameters [18]. He observed that during vagal stimulation, dogs were less likely to die while delivering current to the ventricle, a fascinating demonstration of the increase in ventricular fibrillation (VF) threshold caused by vagal stimulation reported more than 100 years later [19, 20].

After the observation by Scherlag et al. [21] in 1970 suggesting a potential anti-arrhythmic effect of vagal stimulation following myocardial ischaemia, Kent et al. [22] and Myers et al. [23] found that vagal stimulation reduced the risk of VF in anesthetised dogs with anterior myocardial ischaemia. In the latter study, the protective effect was not influenced by preventing the heart rate decrease and only mildly reduced by decentralising the nerve thus abolishing afferent activation. Different conclusions were reached by Yoon et al. [19, 24] who suggested that the favourable effects on VF were heart rate dependent during acute myocardial ischaemia and due to an anti-adrenergic action in the absence of myocardial ischaemia.

We studied the influence of the autonomic nervous system in a conscious canine animal model for sudden death in which atropine favoured the occurrence of VF [25] and BRS predicted the risk of VF [5]. In this model, we performed a study in which two groups of dogs susceptible to VF underwent a further exercise and ischaemia test either with no additional intervention (control group) or with right vagal stimulation started a few seconds after the beginning of coronary occlusion [26]. VF occurred in 23 of 25 (92 %) control animals, but only in 3 of 26 (11.5 %) vagally stimulated dogs. In the vagal stimulation test, heart rate (HR) during ischaemia was, on the average, 85 beats/min lower than in the control test (170 ± 36 vs. 255 ± 33 beats/min). When heart rate was kept, by atrial pacing, at the level attained in the control tests, 5 of the 9 animals (55 %) remained protected from VF. In this same model, pharmacological muscarinic activation was less effective in the prevention of VF compared to propranolol but caused a significantly lower reduction in left ventricular dP/dt max [27].

In an acute murine model of 30-min left coronary artery occlusion [28], vagal stimulation confirmed a striking antiarrhythmic effect and prevented more than 50 % of the loss of connexin43 induced by ischaemia in the control group.

11.2.2 Ischaemia-Reperfusion Models

It was shown in the 1970s that myocardial reperfusion after ischaemia may cause malignant arrhythmias [29]. We found that vagal stimulation strikingly decreased reperfusion arrhythmias, an effect that was partially heart rate dependent [30]. The effect of vagal activation on ischaemia/reperfusion injury will be discussed later in this chapter.

11.2.3 Heart Failure Models

In the last decade the effects of chronic electrical right-sided vagal nerve stimulation (VNS) have been assessed in three different and well-established animal models of congestive heart failure (CHF).

The first of these studies was carried out by the Japanese group of Kenji Sunagawa and the results were published in 2004 [31]. Two weeks after a large (more than 40 % of the left ventricular wall) anterior myocardial infarction leading to HF, surviving rats were randomised to vagal and sham-stimulated groups. Right vagus nerve was stimulated intermittently – 10 s every minute – using an implantable radio-controlled stimulator (Fig. 11.1). The 6-week duration of VNS was mainly

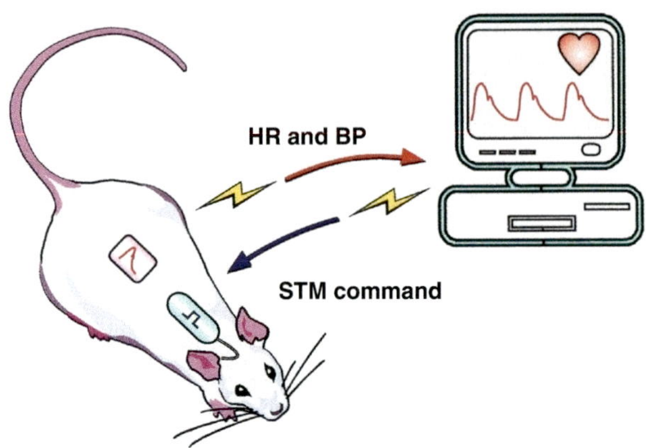

Fig. 11.1 Neural interface approach to stimulate the vagal nerve. While monitoring heart rate through an implantable transmitter, a remote control system adjusted the intensity of electrical pulses of an implantable miniature radio-controlled electrical stimulator (Reproduced with permission from Li et al. [31])

determined by generator's life and the intensity was adjusted to reduce heart rate (HR) by 20–30 bpm from a starting value of 360 bpm. After 140 days, treated rats had significantly lower plasmatic levels of both norepinephrine and BNP compared with the sham-operated rats, despite no significant difference in infarct size (as expected since the relatively long time elapsed between coronary ligation and the beginning of VNS). These long-term neurohormonal effects were associated with improvement in left ventricular (LV) haemodynamics and with a strong impact on 20-week survival (86 % vs. 50 %). Interestingly, the long-term mortality rate of untreated CHF rats after left coronary ligation was similar to what already observed in 1985 in a pioneer work by Pfeffer et al. [32]. On the other hand, the protective effect of VNS appeared to be greater than those of captopril described by Pfeffer, since approximately 40 % of the captopril-treated CHF rats died at 140 days, while VNS reduced the mortality rate to less than 20 %.

Shortly after, the group of Hani Sabbah evaluated the effects of cervical VNS in a canine model of intracoronary microembolisation-induced HF [33]. First (2005), they demonstrated that LV volumes and function significantly improved after 3 months of monotherapy with VNS compared with sham-operated animals. The VNS system used (CardioFit, BioControl) had a feedback HR control set to reduce basal HR by approximately 10 %. They also assessed mRNA and protein expression of TNF-α, IL-6, NOS isoforms and connexin-43 (Cx43) in LV tissue. Long-term therapy with VNS significantly decreased both TNF-α and IL-6, tended to normalise the expression of NOS isoforms in the failing LV myocardium and was associated with a major increase in the expression of Cx43. This is a protein-forming gap junctions which is reduced or redistributed from intercalated discs to lateral cell borders in HF [34], increasing susceptibility to arrhythmia in failing hearts [35]. Finally, histology of the right vagus nerve showed normal fascicles and cellular structure when compared to the left vagus. Subsequently (2007), the same group demonstrated that a 3-month combination therapy of VNS and beta-blockade (metoprolol) improved LV haemodynamics beyond what seen with beta-blockade alone (+9.8±0.6 % vs. +5.5±1.2 %). More recently [36], they performed a crossover study using a different VNS system (Boston Scientific Corporation) specifically set with a low stimulation intensity, not affecting HR. Twenty-six canines were enrolled in VNS monotherapy vs control or a crossover study, with crossover occurring at 3 months. Not only in the 6-month stimulated group but also in the crossover study VNS resulted in a significant benefit in LV parameters. Moreover, VNS led to improvement of the plasmatic and tissual biomarkers assessed, including NT-proBNP, pro-ANP and multiple inflammatory molecules (TNF-α, IL-6, BCL-2, caspase-3, Cx43 and the 3 isoforms of NO synthase).

Finally, Zhang et al. [37] studied the effects of chronic VNS in a different canine model of HF, namely, high-rate ventricular pacing. All dogs underwent 8 weeks of high-rate ventricular pacing with concomitant VNS (at an intensity reducing sinus heart rate ≈20 bpm) in the active group and no stimulation in the sham control group. Also, in this study, the treated group showed meaningful benefits in LV haemodynamics, plasmatic levels of inflammatory biomarkers (CRP) and neurohormones (norepinephrine and angiotensin II) despite the fact that HR was not allowed to change due to ventricular pacing. Furthermore, heart rate variability and baroreflex sensitivity, two important markers of autonomic dysfunction in HF, were both significantly improved in VNS dogs.

11.3   Mechanism of Action of Vagal Stimulation

Several mechanisms may contribute to the beneficial effects of vagal stimulation.

Heart rate may decrease acutely during stimulation, albeit minimally if the intensity of stimulation is low and chronically if the autonomic balance is shifted to a less-marked sympathetic dominance. An anti-sympathetic effect is exerted at several levels: centrally because of afferent vagal stimulation and peripherally at both pre- and postsynaptic levels.

Vagal stimulation produces anti-apoptotic effects, facilitates release of NO and has been demonstrated to exert anti-inflammatory effects. The overall mechanisms of action of vagal stimulation are discussed in recent reviews [1, 38–40].

This paper will focus on what we believe is the most intriguing mechanism, namely, the anti-inflammatory effect.

11.4   Inflammation in Heart Failure

Following the original observation by Levine et al. in 1990 of an enhanced inflammatory response associated with HF [41], numerous studies provided evidence of the relationship between inflammation and the severity of HF, its progression and outcome. Notably, inflammatory mediators have been proposed as markers of HF presence, severity or prognosis [42].

There are currently two main recognised inflammatory mechanisms involved in HF: the release of pro-inflammatory cytokines and soluble factors by immune cells, and the dysregulation of nitric oxide synthase in the heart.

The main cytokines up-regulated in HF are the TNF superfamily; the IL-1 family, including IL-1β, IL-18 and IL-6; and a wide range of factors such as s-ICAM-1 or HMGB1 [43]. These mediators have been recognised as pivotal contributors to the development of the main features of HF by a wide range of studies, conducted either in experimental models or in man. These studies showed that high cytokine levels correlate with impaired systolic function and low ejection fraction in experimental models of HF [44–46]. Moreover, pro-inflammatory cytokines negatively influence left ventricular remodelling by activating different biochemical mediators, promoting cardiomyocyte hypertrophy [47] and apoptosis [48], as well as extracellular matrix degradation [49], with the net effect of causing left ventricular dilation [49]. Beside these effects, pro-inflammatory cytokines also cause endothelial dysfunction [50] and abnormalities in the cellular metabolism, as well as the systemic syndrome known as *cardiac cachexia*, typical of end-stage HF [51]. However, these cytokines do not exert solely deleterious effects, since some of their actions appear to be cardioprotective. For instance, the presence of TNF and IL-6 contributes to limit apoptosis and promote cardiac repair after myocardial ischaemia [52].

The second important inflammatory mechanism associated with HF is the dysregulation of the signalling molecule NO (nitric oxide). NO is synthesised in the heart by three different isoforms of NO synthase (NOS): neuronal NOS (NOS1), endothelial NOS (NOS3) and inducible NOS (NOS2). NOS1 and NOS3 are constitutively expressed in the normal heart, whereas NOS2 is produced in response to TNF and IL-6 in conditions such as in heart failure. NOS1 and NOS3 produce physiological amounts of NO that protect the myocardium from adrenergic stimuli and wall stress, preventing arrhythmias and remodelling. Conversely, NOS2 produces excessive amounts of NO that result in myocardial dysfunction and decreased response to catecholamines [53–55]. Heart failure is characterised by an excess of NO and the coexistence of reactive oxygen species (ROS) and NO. This occurs because of alterations in NOS isoforms produced by the inflammatory process. Namely, NOS2 is up-regulated by TNF, whereas NOS1 is downregulated. This particular pattern produces an increase of myocardial concentrations of NO, playing a role in the transition from adaptive to maladaptive remodelling [43].

11.5 Anti-cytokine Therapies

The growing knowledge of the role of inflammation in heart failure led to studies aimed at reducing this inflammatory response and its consequences. Drugs antagonising cytokines were investigated starting with TNF due to its central role in the inflammatory process associated with heart failure. Indeed, TNF levels are strongly associated with heart failure and its severity [56, 57]. Also, encouraging results were found in *in vitro* tests [58] and preclinical studies [59] with the anti-TNF agent etanercept. However, the results of the clinical studies with either etanercept [60] or the anti-TNF antibody infliximab [61] were very discouraging since these agents were ineffective and even worsened HF in some cases.

Although targeting inflammation still remains a promising strategy to positively influence the natural history of HF, the failure of anti-cytokine-based trials suggests that the complexity of the cytokine network requires a less simplistic approach. Interfering with a single cytokine such as TNF may eliminate its negative effects but without preserving the potentially beneficial ones. Indeed, there is growing evidence that cytokines classically considered pro-inflammatory exert also anti-inflammatory effects. A better strategy could be the modulation, rather than the suppression, of cytokine production since a balanced immune response is necessary to respond to injury and restore health, in agreement with the *cytokine theory of diseases* [62].

11.6 The Cholinergic Anti-inflammatory Pathway

At the beginning of this century, the revolutionary hypothesis emerged that the immune activation could be modulated by the nervous system through parasympathetic activity. Tracey proposed that the autonomic nervous system could influence inflammation, in a way similar to its influences on the inner splanchno-thoracic organs, through unconscious reflex pathways that maintain the fine homeostasis of the immune system [63]. This so-called inflammatory reflex can sense inflammation through vagal afferents and responds with an increase of vagal efferent activity. This *cholinergic anti-inflammatory pathway* can inhibit further release of pro-inflammatory mediators through the action of acetylcholine on macrophages and other immune cells.

The existence of this pathway was first suggested in 2000 by Borovikova et al. [64] who showed that electrical stimulation of the vagal nerve in endotoxemic mice inhibits the macrophagic release of TNF and other pro-inflammatory cytokines, without affecting the production of anti-inflammatory cytokines, as IL-10, thus preventing the development of shock. Few years later, Pavlov and colleagues demonstrated that intrathecal administration of muscarinic agonists in endotoxemic rats increases vagal outflow, provoking a rise of instantaneous heart rate variability (HRV) and a drop of pro-inflammatory cytokine levels [65]. Further evidence of the activity of the *cholinergic anti-inflammatory pathway* was found not only in sepsis but also in experimental models of various diseases such as haemorrhagic shock [66], rheumatoid arthritis [67], pancreatitis [68] and ischaemia and reperfusion of the lung [69] and heart [70, 71].

11.7 Physiology of the Cholinergic Anti-inflammatory Pathway

As every visceral reflex, the *cholinergic anti-inflammatory pathway* is made up by an afferent arc providing input to a central integrative point and an efferent arc acting on the target cells to modify their activity (Fig. 11.2). The afferent arc is constituted of vagal sensitive neurons that fire in response to the presence of IL-1, TNF

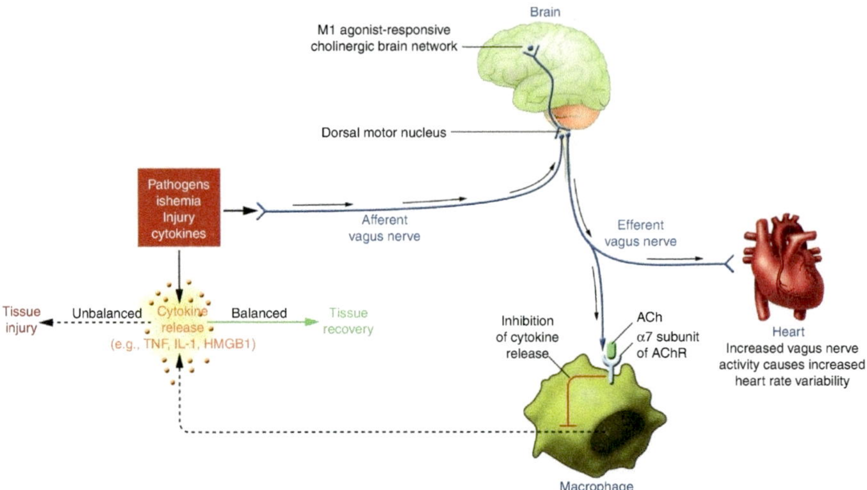

Fig. 11.2 Cholinergic anti-inflammatory pathway balances cytokine production. Several forms of injury lead to inflammatory response with cytokines release. If this reaction is excessive, these mediators can cause disease. The cholinergic anti-inflammatory pathway inhibits cytokine production through the key receptor alpha7-nicotinic AChR expressed on macrophages, polymorphonuclear cells, endothelium and other cells. Vagal fibres also exert favourable autonomic modulation at cardiac level (Reproduced with permission from Tracey [72])

and other inflammatory cytokines, detected by glomic cells situated in most organs and tissues. These sensitive neurons project to the hypothalamus and the brainstem, in the nucleus of the solitary tract. In the brainstem, a neural network processes the information and regulates the outflow from vagal nuclei such as the nucleus ambiguous and the dorsal motor nucleus where the efferent vagal neurons are located. These vagal fibres release acetylcholine in the inner organs and in the spleen, the major repository of pro-inflammatory monocytes and macrophages. Acetylcholine binds the α7 subunity of the nicotinic receptor, situated on the surface of macrophages, endothelial cells and B and T cells. The activation of the receptor generates inhibition of the production of pro-inflammatory cytokines, as TNF, IL-1, IL-6 and IL-8, without influencing the production of anti-inflammatory cytokines, such as IL-10. Efferents to the adrenal gland favour the production of corticosteroids, providing an additional anti-inflammatory mechanism [72, 73].

11.8 Cholinergic Anti-inflammatory Pathway as Therapeutic Target

The *cholinergic anti-inflammatory pathway* may provide the possibility to prevent the deleterious effects of an excessive inflammatory and immune response without suppressing it completely.

In a rat model of ischaemia and reperfusion injury (widely accepted as an inflammatory process) obtained by suprarenal aortic clamping, Bernik et al. showed that vagal stimulation attenuated TNF levels in liver, serum and heart and reduced hypotension and shock [74]. In a mouse model of laparotomy and intestinal manipulation, de Jonge et al. showed that the anti-inflammatory action of alpha-7nAChR activation in peritoneal macrophages was associated with activation of the Jak2/Stat3 signalling pathway, resulting in inhibition of the synthesis of pro-inflammatory cytokines [75]. Interestingly, the same Jak/Stat pathway was found to be implicated in the early phase of ischaemic preconditioning: cardioprotection provided by preconditioning was blocked by AG490 which inhibited Jak2/Stat3 phosphorylation [76, 77]. Furthermore, Dawn et al. showed that both IL-6 and TNF-α are involved in the development of ischaemic preconditioning; specifically, TNF seems to act via the activation of NF-kB and AP1 transcription factors [78, 79]. These findings appear in agreement with the concept that remote conditioning is likely to confer its protective effects through efferent vagal activity [80]. A key mechanism leading to reperfusion injury is the prolonged opening of a nonspecific pore in the inner mitochondrial membrane (permeability transition pore, PTP) leading to ATP depletion, activation of death messengers such as caspases and ultimately to cell death [81]. In a murine model of ischaemia/reperfusion associated with fixed rate pacing [82], vagal stimulation improved LV systolic and diastolic pressures, prevented downregulation of the anti-apoptotic protein Bcl-2 and suppressed caspase-3 activation. These favourable effects were abolished by a PTP opener, atractyloside. These findings are in agreement with the recent demonstration that the cholinergic nicotinic anti-inflammatory pathway is the main mechanism of protection in case of remote vascular injury after cardiac ischemia and reperfusion. Indeed vagal stimulation not only improved cardiac function but also up-regulated M3AChR and alpha7nAChR and ameliorated vascular function and degradation of endothelial structure in mesenteric arteries [83].

Additionally, it was recently reported that vagal nerve stimulation decreases the inflammatory response to haemorrhage and improves coagulation in a model of haemorrhagic shock [84]. Also, Schulte et al. showed that vagal activity may play a major role in maintaining haemodynamic stability and cardiac immune homeostasis during septic shock in a model of systemic inflammation [85].

Overall, this new scenario led investigators to evaluate the potential of a pharmacological approach to enhance vagal activity thereby activating the cholinergic anti-inflammatory pathway without using electrical devices. A promising agent appears GTS-21, a selective alpha7-nicotinic acetylcholine receptor agonist. In a murine model of endotoxemia and severe sepsis, GTS-21 inhibited TNF, HMGB-1 and NF-kB and improved survival [86]. Recently, Kox et al. reported an anti-inflammatory effect of this agent on the innate immune response during experimental human endotoxemia [87]. Oral administration of GTS-21 was found to be safe in human volunteers and, although no significant differences in inflammatory markers were found between subjects in the active and placebo arm, within the GTS-21-treated group, higher plasma concentrations correlated with lower levels of TNF-α,

IL-6 and IL-1RA after intravenous injection of 2 ng/kg Escherichia coli-derived lipopolysaccharides.

Several years ago GTS-21 was found to be able to attenuate the impairment of spatial cognitive deficit and the progressive neuronal degeneration induced by permanent occlusion of the bilateral common carotid arteries in rats [88], thus suggesting that this compound may be beneficial for the treatment of neurodegenerative diseases following chronic cerebral hypoperfusion. Also, pretreatment with a cholinergic agonist, nicotine or GTS-21 significantly attenuated both renal dysfunction and tubular necrosis induced by experimental renal ischaemia in rats [89].

11.9 Cholinergic Anti-inflammatory Pathway and Inflammation in Heart Failure

Given the fact that vagal nerve stimulation showed a remarkable ability to modulate innate immune responses in various inflammatory diseases, it would appear logical to assess the potential of vagal stimulation to normalise the inflammatory status associated with heart failure.

The main theoretical advantage in stimulating vagus nerve instead of inhibiting inflammation by pharmacological intervention is that the cholinergic pathway is an already existing physiological anti-inflammatory mechanism which may be simply reinforced or fine-tuned. This is particularly attractive after the failure of pharmacological interventions targeting the inflammatory responses in heart failure [60].

Very relevant appears the recent study by Ismahil and colleagues [90] highlighting the role of monocytes/macrophages and dendritic cells in chronic heart failure. In a murine experimental model of heart failure, pro-inflammatory macrophages and monocytes were found to be increased both in the heart and in blood but decreased in the spleen which, undergoes marked remodelling in HF. The authors demonstrated that the spleen is essential for the progression of remodelling and inflammation in HF since splenectomy reversed inflammation and remodelling in mice with HF, whereas splenocytes from mice with HF to injected in recipient healthy mice homed in the heart and eventually caused the typical symptoms of HF.

11.10 Clinical Studies with Vagal Stimulation

Clinically, chronic vagal stimulation (VS) has been used for the management of drug-refractory epilepsy [91] and, more recently, depression [92].

Three clinical studies of VS in patients with systolic HF have been reported so far. Table 11.1 summarises the main baseline characteristics of the patients enrolled. The CardioFit pilot study – an extension of the first-in-man single-centre feasibility study [93] – used the CardioFit 5000 device (BioControl Medical, Yehud, Israel), a system including, in addition to a right vagal nerve electrode, a right ventricular sensing lead allowing VS to be synchronised to the QRS complex and withheld in case of low heart rate. This open-label phase II study [94] enrolled 32 patients in total (94 % men; mean

Table 11.1 Patients' characteristics at baseline in the three published VS clinical studies

Parameter	CardioFit	ANTHEM-HF	NECTAR-HF
Patients number	32	60	96 (87 paired data)
Age (years)	56 ± 11	51 ± 12	59 ± 11
NYHA class II/III/IV	15/15/2	34/26/0	14/73/0
Ischaemic HF (%)	62	75	67
Patients taking BB (%)	97 %	100 %	94 %
Patients taking ACE-i or ARB (%)	97 %	85 %	ACE-i 78 %, ARB 25 %
Patients taking MRA (%)	97 %	75 %	70
LVEF baseline (%)	23 ± 8	32 ± 7	30 ± 6
LVESV baseline (ml)	185 ± 63	108 ± 40	155 ± 58
ICD/CRT-D/no device	19/0/13	0/0/60	73/9/13

ACE-i angiotensin-converting enzyme inhibitor, *ARB* angiotensin receptor blocker, *BB* beta-blocker, *CRT* cardiac resynchronisation therapy, *HF* heart failure, *LVEF* left ventricular ejection fraction, *LVESV* left ventricular end-systolic volume, *MRA* mineralocorticoid receptor antagonist

age 56 ± 11 years) with a history of chronic NYHA class II–IV HF and an LVEF of 23 ± 8 %. All patients were receiving optimal medical therapy (OMT) and 19 patients had an implantable cardioverter-defibrillator (ICD). Vagal stimulation intensity was mostly limited by patient's symptoms and was uptitrated to 4.1 ± 1.2 mA (with 1–2 pulses per cardiac cycle). The heart rate was minimally affected acutely during stimulation but decreased significantly during the study from 82 ± 13 to 76 ± 13 b/min. After a follow-up of 6 months, 59 % of patients improved by at least one NYHA class and both the distance on the 6-min walk test and the Minnesota Living with Heart Failure Questionnaire quality-of-life score improved significantly. Blinded echocardiography revealed a non-significant decrease in LV end-diastolic volume index, a significant reduction in LV end-systolic volume index and a significant increase in LVEF (from 22 ± 7 % to 29 ± 8 %). Follow-up in a group of patients at 1 and 2 years showed persistence of the increase in LVEF.

A VS system with no RV sensing lead was used in the Autonomic Regulation Therapy via Left or Right Cervical Vagus Nerve Stimulation in Patients with Chronic Heart Failure (ANTHEM-HF) study [95], an open-label phase II trial that enrolled 60 patients with NYHA class II and III HF, LVEF <40 % and QRS <150 ms. Patients were randomised to either left or right cervical VS uptitrating the amplitude over a 10-week period and reaching an average value of 2.0 ± 0.6 mA; then, they were followed for 6 months. Procedure and device-related complications appeared low. In the pooled right + left VS analysis, LVEF increased by 4.5 % ($p < 0.05$), whereas the co-primary efficacy end point, LV end-systolic volume, decreased non-significantly by 4.1 ml. A non-significant trend towards greater improvement with right VS was observed. There was a significant improvement in the Minnesota Living with Heart Failure score and 77 % of patients improved by at least one NYHA.

The Neural Cardiac Therapy for Heart Failure (NECTAR-HF) study was a phase II study which enrolled 96 patients with NYHA class II and III HF, an LVEF <35 %, a QRS <130 ms and LV end-diastolic diameter >55 mm. At variance with the previous study, all patients received a right-sided device implant and were randomised 2:1 to active treatment or sham treatment (with the device on only during the titration visits) for the first 6 months; thereafter, all patients received active treatment. The device used in NECTAR-HF was similar to that used in ANTHEM, also lacking an RV lead [96]. The stimulation intensity was 1.3 ± 0.8 mA. There were no major safety concerns; an assessment of blinding performed at 6 months revealed that 70 % of the patients assigned to active treatment correctly guessed their randomisation group. There was no effect on primary efficacy end point, which was the change in LV end-systolic diameter at 6-month follow-up [97]. Several secondary end points, including LV end-diastolic dimension, LV end-systolic volume, LVEF, peak V02, and N-terminal pro-hormone brain natriuretic peptide, were also not different between groups. On the other hand, statistically significant improvements were found in the active therapy group in quality of life for the Minnesota Living with Heart Failure Questionnaire ($p < 0.049$) and the New York Heart Association class ($p < 0.032$).

Overall, the three studies yielded different results. Although several factors may account for this discrepancy, two possibilities deserve to be mentioned. First, only one trial was controlled and (albeit partially) blinded and it was the one with neutral findings (NECTAR-HF). Second, the amplitude reached by vagal stimulation was very different in the three studies. Lower frequencies of stimulation allow greater amplitudes to be reached with tolerable side effects. Accordingly, the stimulation intensity varied in the three studies: it was 1.3 ± 08 mA in NECTAR-HF (range 0.3–3.5), stimulating at 20 Hz; 2.0 ± 0.6 mA in ANTHEM (maximum amplitude allowed 3 mA), stimulating at 10 Hz; and 4.2 ± 1.2 mA (range 1.1–5.5) in the CardioFit pilot trial, stimulating at 1–2 Hz. Higher amplitudes allow a greater recruitment of nerve fibres. Experimental studies in conscious dogs have shown that amplitudes such as those used in the NECTAR-HF study, albeit providing an improvement in LV function [36], recruit only a minority of the fibres in the cervical vagal trunk [98]. Thus, it is likely that the lower amplitude of VS in NECTAR-HF and ANTHEM recruited an insufficient number of vagal fibres and that this could have played a major role in the different results.

Hopefully, the picture will be more clear when the results of the ongoing Increase of Vagal Tone in Heart Failure (INOVATE-HF) study [99] will be available (likely in 2017). This is an international, multicentre randomised clinical trial assessing safety and efficacy of the CardioFit™ vagal stimulation system in patients with symptomatic HF who are on optimal medical treatment [99]. INOVATE-HF is randomising 650 patients with NYHA class III symptoms, an LVEF ≤ 40 % and LV end-diastolic dimensions 50–80 mm in a 3:2 ratio to either active treatment (implanted) or continuation of medical therapy (not implanted). The primary end point of the study is the composite of all-cause mortality or unplanned HF hospitalisation equivalent, using a time to first event analysis.

Conclusions

Vagal nerve stimulation is a promising new approach for patients with chronic heart failure whose clinical usefulness needs to be assessed in large randomised clinical trials. Activation of the cholinergic anti-inflammatory pathway is likely to play an important role in the favourable effects of vagal stimulation.

Conflict of Interest Disclosures GMDF is a consultant for Boston Scientific; PJS for BioControl Medical Ltd.

References

1. Floras JS. Sympathetic nervous system activation in human heart failure: clinical implications of an updated model. J Am Coll Cardiol. 2009;54:375–85.
2. Brack KE, Winter J, Ng GA. Mechanisms underlying the autonomic modulation of ventricular fibrillation initiation-tentative prophylactic properties of vagus nerve stimulation on malignant arrhythmias in heart failure. Heart Fail Rev. 2013;18:389–408.
3. Hunt SA, Abraham WT, Chin MH, Feldman AM, Francis GS, Ganiats TG, Jessup M, Konstam MA, Mancini DM, Michl K, Oates JA, Rahko PS, Silver MA, Stevenson LW, Yancy CW. 2009 focused update incorporated into the ACC/AHA 2005 guidelines for the diagnosis and management of heart failure in adults: a report of the American College of Cardiology Foundation/American Heart Association Task Force on Practice Guidelines. Circulation. 2009;119:e391–479.
4. Billman GE, Schwartz PJ, Stone HL. Baroreceptor reflex control of heart rate: a predictor of sudden cardiac death. Circulation. 1982;66:874–80.
5. Schwartz PJ, Vanoli E, Stramba Badiale M, De Ferrari G, Billman GE, Foreman RD. Autonomic mechanisms and sudden death. New insights from analysis of baroreceptor reflexes in conscious dogs with and without a myocardial infarction. Circulation. 1988;78:969–79.
6. Kleiger RE, Miller JP, Bigger Jr JT, Moss AJ, The Multicenter Post Infarction Research Group. Decreased heart rate variability and its association with increased mortality after acute myocardial infarction. Am J Cardiol. 1987;59:256–62.
7. La Rovere MT, Bigger JT, Marcus F, Mortara A, Schwartz PJ. ATRAMI (Autonomic Tone and Reflexes After Myocardial Infarction), Baroreflex sensitivity and heart-rate variability in prediction of total cardiac mortality after myocardial infarction. Lancet. 1998;351:478–84.
8. Schmidt G, Malik M, Barthel P, Schneider R, Ulm K, Rolnitzky L, Camm AJ, Bigger Jr JT, Schomig A. Heart-rate turbulence after ventricular premature beats as a predictor of mortality after acute myocardial infarction. Lancet. 1999;353:1390–6.
9. De Ferrari GM, Sanzo A, Bertoletti A, Specchia G, Vanoli E, Schwartz PJ. Baroreflex sensitivity predicts long-term cardiovascular mortality after myocardial infarction even in patients with preserved left ventricular function. J Am Coll Cardiol. 2007;50:2285–90.
10. Eckberg DL, Drabinsky M, Braunwald E. Defective cardiac parasympathetic control in patients with heart disease. N Engl J Med. 1971;285:877–83.
11. Ferguson DW, Berg WJ, Roach PJ, Oren RM, Mark AL. Effects of heart failure on baroreflex control of sympathetic neural activity. Am J Cardiol. 1992;69:523–31.
12. Dibner Dunlap ME, Smith ML, Kinugawa T, Thames MD. Enalapatrilat augments arterial and cardiopulmonary baroreflex control of sympathetic nerve activity in patients with heart failure. J Am Coll Cardiol. 1996;27:358–64.
13. Dibner Dunlap ME. Arterial or cardiopulmonary baroreflex control of sympathetic nerve activity in heart failure? Am J Cardiol. 1992;70:1640–2.
14. Bibevski S, Dunlap ME. Evidence for impaired vagus nerve activity in heart failure. Heart Fail Rev. 2011;16:129–35.
15. Mortara A, La Rovere MT, Pinna GD, Prpa A, Maestri R, Febo O, Pozzoli M, Opasich C, Tavazzi L. Arterial baroreflex modulation of heart rate in chronic heart failure: clinical and hemodynamic correlates and prognostic implications. Circulation. 1997;96:3450–8.

16. La Rovere MT, Pinna GD, Maestri R, Robbi E, Caporotondi A, Guazzotti G, Sleight P, Febo O. Prognostic implications of baroreflex sensitivity in heart failure patients in the beta-blocking era. J Am Coll Cardiol. 2009;53:193–9.

17. Adamson PB, Smith AL, Abraham WT, Kleckner KJ, Stadler RW, Shih A, Rhodes MM, InSync III Model 8042 and Attain OTW Lead Model 4193 Clinical Trial Investigators. Continuous autonomic assessment in patients with symptomatic heart failure: prognostic value of heart rate variability measured by an implanted cardiac resynchronization device. Circulation. 2004;110:2389–94.

18. Einbrodt E. Ueber Herzreizung und ihr Verhaeltnis zum Blutdruck. Akademie der Wissenschaften (Vienna). Sitzungsberichte. 1859;38:345.

19. Yoon MS, Han J, Tse WW, Rogers R. Effects of vagal stimulation, atropine, and propranolol on fibrillation threshold of normal and ischemic ventricles. Am Heart J. 1977;93:60–5.

20. Kolman BS, Verrier RL, Lown B. The effect of vagus nerve stimulation upon vulnerability of the canine ventricle: role of the sympathetic-parasympathetic interactions. Circulation. 1975;52:578–85.

21. Scherlag BJ, Helfant RH, Haft JI, Damato AN. Electrophysiology underlying ventricular arrhythmias due to coronary ligation. Am J Physiol. 1970;219:1665–71.

22. Kent KM, Smith ER, Redwood DR, Epstein SE. Electrical stability of acutely ischemic myocardium: influences of heart rate and vagal stimulation. Circulation. 1973;47:291–8.

23. Myers RW, Pearlman AS, Hyman RM, Goldstein RA, Kent KM, Goldstein RE, Epstein SE. Beneficial effects of vagal stimulation and bradycardia during experimental acute myocardial ischemia. Circulation. 1974;49:943–7.

24. Yoon MS, Fondacaro JD, Han J. Effects of vagal stimulation and atropine on ventricular arrhythmias during acute coronary occlusion. J Electrocardiol. 1978;11:27–31.

25. De Ferrari GM, Vanoli E, Stramba-Badiale M, Hull Jr SS, Foreman RD, Schwartz PJ. Vagal reflexes and survival during acute myocardial ischemia in conscious dogs with a healed myocardial infarction. Am J Physiol. 1991;261:H63–9.

26. Vanoli E, De Ferrari GM, Stramba-Badiale M, Hull Jr SS, Foreman RD, Schwartz PJ. Vagal stimulation and prevention of sudden death in conscious dogs with a healed myocardial infarction. Circ Res. 1991;68:1471–81.

27. De Ferrari GM, Salvati P, Grossoni M, Ukmar G, Vaga L, Patrono C, Schwartz PJ. Pharmacologic modulation of the autonomic nervous system in the prevention of sudden cardiac death. A study with propranolol, methacholine and oxotremorine in conscious dogs with a healed myocardial infarction. J Am Coll Cardiol. 1993;22:283–90.

28. Ando M, Katare RG, Kakinuma Y, Zhang D, Yamasaki F, Muramoto K, Sato T. Efferent vagal nerve stimulation protects heart against ischemia-induced arrhythmias by preserving connexin43 protein. Circulation. 2005;112:164–70.

29. Murdock DK, Loeb JM, Euler DE, Randall WC. Electrophysiology of coronary reperfusion. A mechanism for reperfusion arrhythmias. Circulation. 1980;61:175–82.

30. Zuanetti G, De Ferrari GM, Priori SG, Schwartz PJ. Protective effect of vagal stimulation on reperfusion arrhythmias in cats. Circ Res. 1987;61:429–35.

31. Li M, Zheng C, Sato T, Kawada T, Sugimachi M, Sunagawa K. Vagal nerve stimulation markedly improves long-term survival after chronic heart failure in rats. Circulation. 2004;109:120–4.

32. Pfeffer MA, Pfeffer JM, Steinberg C, Finn P. Survival after an experimental myocardial infarction: beneficial effects of long-term therapy with captopril. Circulation. 1985;72:406–12.

33. Sabbah HN, Ilsar I, Zaretsky A, Rastogi S, Wang M, Gupta RC. Vagus nerve stimulation in experimental heart failure. Heart Fail Rev. 2011;16:171–8.

34. Jongsma HJ, Wilders R. Gap junctions in cardiovascular disease. Circ Res. 2000;86:1193–7.

35. Severs NJ, Bruce AF, Dupont E, Rothery S. Remodelling of gap junctions and connexin expression in diseased myocardium. Cardiovasc Res. 2008;80:9–19.

36. Hamann JJ, Ruble SB, Stolen C, Wang M, Gupta RC, Rastogi S, Sabbah HN. Vagus nerve stimulation improves left ventricular function in a canine model of chronic heart failure. Eur J Heart Fail. 2013;15:1319–26.

37. Zhang Y, Popovic ZB, Bibevski S, Fakhry I, Sica DA, Van Wagoner DR, Mazgalev TN. Chronic vagus nerve stimulation improves autonomic control and attenuates systemic inflammation and heart failure progression in a canine high-rate pacing model. Circ Heart Fail. 2009;2: 692–9.
38. Olshansky B, Sabbah HN, Hauptman PJ, Colucci WS. Parasympathetic nervous system and heart failure: pathophysiology and potential implications for therapy. Circulation. 2008;118:863–71.
39. De Ferrari GM, Schwartz PJ. Vagus nerve stimulation: from pre-clinical to clinical application: challenges and future directions. Heart Fail Rev. 2011;16:195–203.
40. De Ferrari GM. Vagal stimulation in heart failure. J Cardiovasc Transl Res. 2014;7:310–20.
41. Levine B, Kalman J, Mayer L, Fillit HM, Packer M. Elevated circulating levels of tumor necrosis factor in severe chronic heart failure. N Engl J Med. 1990;323:236–41.
42. Hartupee J, Mann DL. Positioning of inflammatory biomarkers in the heart failure landscape. J Cardiovasc Transl Res. 2013;6:485–92.
43. Li W, Olshansky B. Inflammatory cytokines and nitric oxide in heart failure and potential modulation by vagus nerve stimulation. Heart Fail Rev. 2011;16:137–45.
44. Pagani FD, Baker LS, Hsi C, Knox M, Fink MP, Visner MS. Left ventricular systolic and diastolic dysfunction after infusion of tumor necrosis factor-alpha in conscious dogs. J Clin Invest. 1992;90:389–98.
45. Hosenpud JD, Campbell SM, Mendelson DJ. Interleukin-1-induced myocardial depression in an isolated beating heart preparation. J Heart Transplant. 1989;8:460–4.
46. Kinugawa K, Takahashi T, Kohmoto O, Yao A, Aoyagi T, Momomura S, Hirata Y, Serizawa T. Nitric oxide-mediated effects of interleukin-6 on [Ca2+]i and cell contraction in cultured chick ventricular myocytes. Circ Res. 1994;75:285–95.
47. Yokoyama T, Nakano M, Bednarczyk JL, McIntyre BW, Entman M, Mann DL. Tumor necrosis factor-alpha provokes a hypertrophic growth response in adult cardiac myocytes. Circulation. 1997;95:1247–52.
48. Krown KA, Page MT, Nguyen C, Zechner D, Gutierrez V, Comstock KL, Glembotski CC, Quintana PJ, Sabbadini RA. Tumor necrosis factor alpha-induced apoptosis in cardiac myocytes. Involvement of the sphingolipid signaling cascade in cardiac cell death. J Clin Invest. 1996;98:2854–65.
49. Weber KT. Cardiac interstitium in health and disease: the fibrillar collagen network. J Am Coll Cardiol. 1989;13:1637–52.
50. Anker SD, Volterrani M, Egerer KR, Felton CV, Kox WJ, Poole-Wilson PA, Coats AJ. Tumour necrosis factor alpha as a predictor of impaired peak leg blood flow in patients with chronic heart failure. QJM. 1998;91:199–203.
51. Anker SD, Ponikowski PP, Clark AL, Leyva F, Rauchhaus M, Kemp M, Teixeira MM, Hellewell PG, Hooper J, Poole-Wilson PA, Coats AJ. Cytokines and neurohormones relating to body composition alterations in the wasting syndrome of chronic heart failure. Eur Heart J. 1999;20:683–93.
52. Frangogiannis NG, Smith CW, Entman ML. The inflammatory response in myocardial infarction. Cardiovasc Res. 2002;53:31–47.
53. Sawyer DB, Colucci WS. Nitric oxide in the failing myocardium. Cardiol Clin. 1998;16:657–64, viii.
54. Sharma R, Coats AJ, Anker SD. The role of inflammatory mediators in chronic heart failure: cytokines, nitric oxide, and endothelin-1. Int J Cardiol. 2000;72:175–86.
55. Umar S, van der Laarse A. Nitric oxide and nitric oxide synthase isoforms in the normal, hypertrophic, and failing heart. Mol Cell Biochem. 2010;333:191–201.
56. Baumgarten G, Knuefermann P, Mann DL. Cytokines as emerging targets in the treatment of heart failure. Trends Cardiovasc Med. 2000;10:216–23.
57. Seta Y, Shan K, Bozkurt B, Oral H, Mann DL. Basic mechanisms in heart failure: the cytokine hypothesis. J Card Fail. 1996;2:243–9.
58. Kapadia S, Torre-Amione G, Yokoyama T, Mann DL. Soluble TNF binding proteins modulate the negative inotropic properties of TNF-alpha in vitro. Am J Physiol. 1995;268:H517–25.

59. Bozkurt B, Kribbs SB, Clubb Jr FJ, Michael LH, Didenko VV, Hornsby PJ, Seta Y, Oral H, Spinale FG, Mann DL. Pathophysiologically relevant concentrations of tumor necrosis factor-alpha promote progressive left ventricular dysfunction and remodeling in rats. Circulation. 1998;97:1382–91.

60. Mann DL, McMurray JJ, Packer M, Swedberg K, Borer JS, Colucci WS, Djian J, Drexler H, Feldman A, Kober L, Krum H, Liu P, Nieminen M, Tavazzi L, van Veldhuisen DJ, Waldenstrom A, Warren M, Westheim A, Zannad F, Fleming T. Targeted anticytokine therapy in patients with chronic heart failure: results of the Randomized Etanercept Worldwide Evaluation (RENEWAL). Circulation. 2004;109:1594–602.

61. Chung ES, Packer M, Lo KH, Fasanmade AA, Willerson JT, Anti-TNF Therapy Against Congestive Heart Failure Investigators. Randomized, double-blind, placebo-controlled, pilot trial of infliximab, a chimeric monoclonal antibody to tumor necrosis factor-alpha, in patients with moderate-to-severe heart failure: results of the anti-TNF Therapy Against Congestive Heart Failure (ATTACH) trial. Circulation. 2003;107:3133–40.

62. Czura CJ, Tracey KJ. Autonomic neural regulation of immunity. J Intern Med. 2005;257:156–66.

63. Tracey KJ. The inflammatory reflex. Nature. 2002;420:853–9.

64. Borovikova LV, Ivanova S, Zhang M, Yang H, Botchkina GI, Watkins LR, Wang H, Abumrad N, Eaton JW, Tracey KJ. Vagus nerve stimulation attenuates the systemic inflammatory response to endotoxin. Nature. 2000;405:458–62.

65. Pavlov VA, Ochani M, Gallowitsch-Puerta M, Ochani K, Huston JM, Czura CJ, Al-Abed Y, Tracey KJ. Central muscarinic cholinergic regulation of the systemic inflammatory response during endotoxemia. Proc Natl Acad Sci U S A. 2006;103:5219–23.

66. Guarini S, Cainazzo MM, Giuliani D, Mioni C, Altavilla D, Marini H, Bigiani A, Ghiaroni V, Passaniti M, Leone S, Bazzani C, Caputi AP, Squadrito F, Bertolini A. Adrenocorticotropin reverses hemorrhagic shock in anesthetized rats through the rapid activation of a vagal anti-inflammatory pathway. Cardiovasc Res. 2004;63:357–65.

67. Saeed RW, Varma S, Peng-Nemeroff T, Sherry B, Balakhaneh D, Huston J, Tracey KJ, Al-Abed Y, Metz CN. Cholinergic stimulation blocks endothelial cell activation and leukocyte recruitment during inflammation. J Exp Med. 2005;201:1113–23.

68. van Westerloo DJ, Giebelen IA, Florquin S, Daalhuisen J, Bruno MJ, de Vos AF, Tracey KJ, van der Poll T. The cholinergic anti-inflammatory pathway regulates the host response during septic peritonitis. J Infect Dis. 2005;191:2138–48.

69. Webster JI, Tonelli L, Sternberg EM. Neuroendocrine regulation of immunity. Annu Rev Immunol. 2002;20:125–63.

70. Mioni C, Bazzani C, Giuliani D, Altavilla D, Leone S, Ferrari A, Minutoli L, Bitto A, Marini H, Zaffe D, Botticelli AR, Iannone A, Tomasi A, Bigiani A, Bertolini A, Squadrito F, Guarini S. Activation of an efferent cholinergic pathway produces strong protection against myocardial ischemia/reperfusion injury in rats. Crit Care Med. 2005;33:2621–8.

71. Calvillo L, Vanoli E, Andreoli E, Besana A, Omodeo E, Gnecchi M, Zerbi P, Vago G, Busca G, Schwartz PJ. Vagal stimulation, through its nicotinic action, limits infarct size and the inflammatory response to myocardial ischemia and reperfusion. J Cardiovasc Pharmacol. 2011;58:500–7.

72. Tracey KJ. Physiology and immunology of the cholinergic antiinflammatory pathway. J Clin Invest. 2007;117:289–96.

73. Tracey KJ. Reflex control of immunity. Nat Rev Immunol. 2009;9:418–28.

74. Bernik TR, Friedman SG, Ochani M, DiRaimo R, Susarla S, Czura CJ, Tracey KJ. Cholinergic antiinflammatory pathway inhibition of tumor necrosis factor during ischemia reperfusion. J Vasc Surg. 2002;36:1231–6.

75. de Jonge WJ, van der Zanden EP, The FO, Bijlsma MF, van Westerloo DJ, Bennink RJ, Berthoud HR, Uematsu S, Akira S, van den Wijngaard RM, Boeckxstaens GE. Stimulation of the vagus nerve attenuates macrophage activation by activating the Jak2-STAT3 signaling pathway. Nat Immunol. 2005;6(8):844–51.

76. Booz GW, Day JN, Baker KM. Interplay between the cardiac renin angiotensin system and JAK-STAT signaling: role in cardiac hypertrophy, ischemia/reperfusion dysfunction, and heart failure. J Mol Cell Cardiol. 2002;34:1443–53.

77. Hattori R, Maulik N, Otani H, Zhu L, Cordis G, Engelman RM, Siddiqui MA, Das DK. Role of STAT3 in ischemic preconditioning. J Mol Cell Cardiol. 2001;33:1929–36.
78. Dawn B, Xuan YT, Guo Y, Rezazadeh A, Stein AB, Hunt G, Wu WJ, Tan W, Bolli R. IL-6 plays an obligatory role in late preconditioning via JAK-STAT signaling and upregulation of iNOS and COX-2. Cardiovasc Res. 2004;64:61–71.
79. Dawn B, Guo Y, Rezazadeh A, Wang OL, Stein AB, Hunt G, Varma J, Xuan YT, Wu WJ, Tan W, Zhu X, Bolli R. Tumor necrosis factor-alpha does not modulate ischemia/reperfusion injury in naïve myocardium but is essential for the development of late preconditioning. J Mol Cell Cardiol. 2004;37:51–61.
80. Donato M, Buchholz B, Rodríguez M, Pérez V, Inserte J, García-Dorado D, Gelpi RJ. Role of the parasympathetic nervous system in cardioprotection by remote hindlimb ischaemic preconditioning. Exp Physiol. 2013;98:425–34.
81. Shanmuganathan S, Hausenloy DJ, Duchen MR, Yellon DM. Mitochondrial permeability transition pore as a target for cardioprotection in the human heart. Am J Physiol Heart Circ Physiol. 2005;289:H237–42.
82. Katare RG, Ando M, Kakinuma Y, Arikawa M, Handa T, Yamasaki F, Sato T. Vagal nerve stimulation prevents reperfusion injury through inhibition of opening of mitochondrial permeability transition pore independent of the bradycardiac effect. J Thorac Cardiovasc Surg. 2009;137:223–31.
83. Zhao M, He X, Bi XY, Yu XJ, Gil Wier W, Zang WJ. Vagal stimulation triggers peripheral vascular protection through the cholinergic anti-inflammatory pathway in a rat model of myocardial ischemia/reperfusion. Basic Res Cardiol. 2013;108:345.
84. Rezende-Neto JB, Alves RL, Carvalho Jr M, Almeida T, Trant C, Kushmerick C, Andrade M, Rizoli SB, Cunha-Melo J. Vagus nerve stimulation improves coagulopathy in hemorrhagic shock: a thromboelastometric animal model study. J Trauma Manag Outcomes. 2014;8:15.
85. Schulte A, Lichtenstern C, Henrich M, Weigand MA, Uhle F. Loss of vagal tone aggravates systemic inflammation and cardiac impairment in endotoxemic rats. J Surg Res. 2014;188:480–8.
86. Pavlov VA, Ochani M, Yang LH, Gallowitsch-Puerta M, Ochani K, Lin X, Levi J, Parrish WR, Rosas-Ballina M, Czura CJ, Larosa GJ, Miller EJ, Tracey KJ, Al-Abed Y. Selective alpha7-nicotinic acetylcholine receptor agonist GTS-21 improves survival in murine endotoxemia and severe sepsis. Crit Care Med. 2007;35:1139–44.
87. Kox M, Pompe JC, Gordinou de Gouberville MC, van der Hoeven JG, Hoedemaekers CW, Pickkers P. Effects of the α7 nicotinic acetylcholine receptor agonist GTS-21 on the innate immune response in humans. Shock. 2011;36:5–11.
88. Nanri M, Miyake H, Murakami Y, Matsumoto K, Watanabe H. GTS-21, a nicotinic agonist, attenuates multiple infarctions and cognitive deficit caused by permanent occlusion of bilateral common carotid arteries in rats. Jpn J Pharmacol. 1998;78:463–9.
89. Yeboah MM, Xue X, Duan B, Ochani M, Tracey KJ, Susin M, Metz CN. Cholinergic agonists attenuate renal ischemia-reperfusion injury in rats. Kidney Int. 2008;74:62–9.
90. Ismahil MA, Hamid T, Bansal SS, Patel B, Kingery JR, Prabhu SD. Remodeling of the mononuclear phagocyte network underlies chronic inflammation and disease progression in heart failure: critical importance of the cardiosplenic axis. Circ Res. 2014;114:266–82.
91. Uthman BM, Reichl AM, Dean JC, Eisenschenk S, Gilmore R, Reid S, Roper SN, Wilder BJ. Effectiveness of vagus nerve stimulation in epilepsy patients, a 12-year observation. Neurology. 2004;63:1124–6.
92. Shuchman M. Approving the vagus-nerve stimulator for depression. N Engl J Med. 2007;356:1604–7.
93. Schwartz PJ, De Ferrari GM, Sanzo A, Landolina M, Rordorf R, Raineri C, Campana C, Revera M, Ajmone-Marsan N, Tavazzi L, Odero A. Long term vagal stimulation in patients with advanced heart failure. First experience in man. Eur J Heart Fail. 2008;10:884–91.
94. De Ferrari GM, Crijns HJGM, Borggrefe M, Milasinovic G, Smid J, Zabel M, Gavazzi A, Sanzo A, Dennert R, Kuschyk J, Raspopovic S, Klein H, Swedberg K, Schwartz PJ, for the CardioFit Multicenter Trial Investigators. Chronic vagus nerve stimulation: a new and promising therapeutic approach for chronic heart failure. Eur Heart J. 2011;32:847–55.

95. Premchand RK, Sharma K, Mittal S, Monteiro R, Dixit S, Libbus I, DiCarlo LA, Ardell JL, Rector TS, Amurthur B, KenKnight BH, Anand IS. Autonomic regulation therapy via left or right cervical vagus nerve stimulation in patients with chronic heart failure: results of the ANTHEM-HF Trial. J Card Fail. 2014;20(11):808–16. doi:10.1016/j.cardfail.2014.08.009.

96. De Ferrari GM, Tuinenburg AE, Ruble S, Brugada J, Klein H, Butter C, Wright DJ, Schubert B, Solomon S, Meyer S, Stein K, Ramuzat A, Zannad F. Rationale and study design of the NEuroCardiac TherApy foR Heart Failure Study: NECTAR-HF. Eur J Heart Fail. 2014;16:692–9.

97. Zannad F, De Ferrari GM, Tuinenburg AE, Wright D, Brugada J, Butter C, Klein H, Stolen C, Meyer S, Stein KM, Ramuzat A, Schubert B, Daum D, Neuzil P, Botman C, Caste MA, D'Onofrio A, Solomon SD, Wold N, Ruble SB. Chronic vagal stimulation for the treatment of low ejection fraction heart failure: results of the neural cardiac therapy for heart failure (NECTAR-HF) randomized controlled trial. Eur Heart J. 2015;36(7):425–33. doi:10.1093/eurheartj/ehu345.

98. Castoro MA, Yoo PB, Hincapie JG, Hamann JJ, Ruble SB, Wolf PD, Grill WM. Excitation properties of the right cervical vagus nerve in adult dogs. Exp Neurol. 2011;227:62–8.

99. Hauptman PJ, Schwartz PJ, Gold MR, Borggrefe M, Van Veldhuisen DJ, Starling RC, Mann DL. Rationale and study design of the increase of vagal tone in heart failure study: INOVATE-HF. Am Heart J. 2012;163:954–62.

Baroreflex Activation Therapy in Heart Failure

Guido Grassi and Eric G. Lovett

12.1 Background

As described throughout this monograph, renewed interest in therapies for heart failure (HF) which target the autonomic nervous system is driven by the fact that HF is characterized by autonomic imbalance and that patient outcomes continue to be poor despite significant advances in medical and device therapies. Not only does this lead to excess morbidity and mortality for patients, but it also incurs substantial costs to the healthcare system due to hospitalization associated with events of worsening HF, sudden cardiac death (SCD), and other cardiovascular events such as myocardial infarction and stroke. While the occurrence of these events is slightly higher for HF with reduced ejection fraction (HFrEF) as compared to HF with preserved ejection fraction (HFpEF), in both cases cardiovascular events are responsible for the majority of deaths [15]. Although unfortunate, this is not surprising in the case of HFpEF, which has no specifically indicated therapies. What is rather disheartening is that despite aggressive use of state-of-the-art medical therapies and cardiac rhythm management devices, SCD and circulatory failure remain, in equal proportion, the leading modes of death in HFrEF [48]. Circulatory failure is the predominant mode of death in HFpEF, although SCD accounts for approximately 7 % of deaths [15]. Clearly, there is ample justification for pursuit of new therapies

G. Grassi (✉)
Cardiovascular Department, IRCCS MultiMedica,
Via Milanese 300, Sesto San Giovanni (Milano), Lombardia 20 141, Italy

Clinica Medica, Dipartimento di Scienze della Salute, Università Milano-Bicocca,
Via Milanese 300, Sesto San Giovanni (Milano), Lombardia 20 141, Italy
e-mail: guido.grassi@unimib.it

E.G. Lovett
Research, CVRx, Inc,
9201 West Broadway Avenue, Suite 650, Minneapolis, MN 55445, USA
e-mail: elovett@cvrx.com

© Springer International Publishing Switzerland 2016
E. Gronda et al. (eds.), *Heart Failure Management: The Neural Pathways*,
DOI 10.1007/978-3-319-24993-3_12

when HFpEF patients have no additional options, and the last resorts of HFrEF patients are ventricular assist devices and allografts. New therapies must be developed to fill this gap, and autonomically mediated treatments represent an attractive and underutilized approach. Experience has shown, however, that such therapies must be targeted with care to maintain an ability to preserve dynamic homeostasis and to avoid untoward effects. An ideal autonomic therapy would fulfill these criteria and address the pathophysiology of HF at a level relevant for both HFrEF and HFpEF.

12.2 The Baroreflex: A Primary Regulator of Cardiovascular Function

Under normal conditions, circulatory function is tightly regulated to match organ perfusion to oxygen demand. This is accomplished through a host of mechanisms including local autoregulation [10]. At the level of integrative physiology, perfusion is coordinated by systemically active reflexes including the transient chemoreflex and diving reflex [1]. Due to its tonically active nature, the most important among these systemic reflexes is the baroreflex [52]. Teleologically, the apparent purpose of the baroreflex is to distribute blood flow among the major circulatory beds according to regional needs. This is accomplished by sensing perfusion with mechanoreceptors distributed throughout the circulatory system, including within the heart, veins, and arteries, and accordingly modulating regional vascular smooth muscle tone. Afferents from these receptors converge centrally in the nucleus of the solitary tract, where the signals are integrated and, through adjacent centers, coordinated signals are generated for efferent autonomic nerves leading to the arteries, veins, heart, and other organs (Fig. 12.1) [22, 52]. Although experimental evidence suggests these mechanoreceptors sense distention [6], they are generally referred to as baroreceptors because when they are stimulated in normal physiology, the most consistent and obvious effect is a change in systemic BP, usually accompanied by a concomitant change in heart rate. The amount of influence exerted by the various baroreceptor loci differs from region to region, with the carotid baroreceptors having the greatest impact on efferent regulation [33].

The buffering action of the baroreflex on the circulation is measured by baroreflex sensitivity (BRS), defined as the change in duration of the cardiac cycle per unit change in BP. In the case of important cardiovascular pathophysiologies such as HF and hypertension, BRS is depressed; thus, the baroreflex is less active than normal in regulating cardiovascular performance [28, 29]. While this is an interesting observation from the standpoint of mechanism, it is also of clinical consequence: depressed BRS has been linked to adverse outcomes in HF [39, 46]. Presumably, the link is mediated by the increased sympathetic and decreased parasympathetic nerve traffic which accompany reduced BRS. The cardiovascular implications of these changes include elevated heart rate and cardiac automaticity, increased arterial resistance and stiffness, decreased natriuresis, and reduced splanchnic blood flow

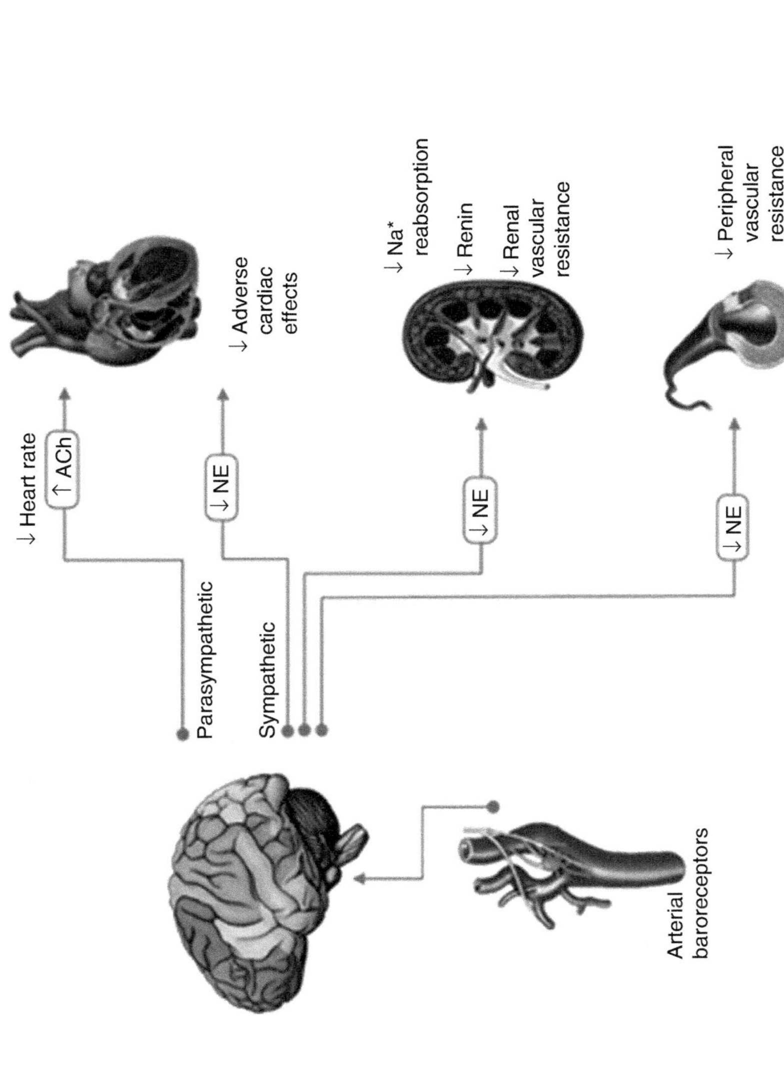

Fig. 12.1 Effects on cardiovascular and renal function due to reduced sympathetic and increased parasympathetic drive resulting from baroreflex activation. After Floras [22]

leading to increased blood volume and pressures in the pulmonary circuit and increased myocardial oxygen demand. Clinically, these effects translate to an environment conducive to arrhythmogenesis and worsening HF culminating in decompensation and circulatory failure. Importantly, reduced BRS appears to be driven at the receptor level rather than centrally [44], suggesting the premise that interventions which potentiate afferent carotid sinus nerve activity may improve BRS and associated outcomes.

Concordantly, direct assessment of efferent traffic has confirmed that therapies which counteract the effects of reduced BRS improve outcome in HFrEF. Muscle sympathetic nerve activity (MSNA), measured by microelectrodes percutaneously introduced into the peroneal nerve, provides a direct assessment of efferent traffic which parallels the activity of cardiac, renal, and other sympathetic nerves. MSNA is chronically decreased by treatments which indirectly affect sympathetic activity such as angiotensin-converting enzyme inhibitors, statins, and cardiac resynchronization therapy [27, 29, 30]. Beta-blocker therapy, which also improves outcome in HF but does not necessarily reduce sympathetic activity [7], interferes with efferent sympathetic activity by blocking receptors for norepinephrine while not antagonizing sympathetic cotransmitters including neuropeptide Y and adenosine triphosphate. In contrast, a therapy which produces indiscriminate sympatholysis worsens outcome in HF: the central alpha-agonist moxonidine produced excess mortality compared to placebo in the MOXCON trial [16, 21].

Given the link between reduced BRS, increased sympathetic tone, and adverse outcome in HF, it is logical to consider exogenous means of activating the baroreflex as a therapy. Although it was not conceived as such, medicinal use of digitalis is the most long-standing and widely used therapy. Digitalis acts, at least in part, by sensitizing baroreceptors so that BRS is increased [20]. Results from the DIG trial have shown that digitalis improves outcome in both HFrEF and HFpEF [2, 3]. Unfortunately, digitalis is difficult to apply practically due to its narrow therapeutic window and toxic effects from overdose [47], problems that can be exacerbated by diuretic therapy and renal dysfunction which are both common in HF.

Nonpharmacologic means have also been used to activate the baroreflex in HF. The technique of carotid massage has been known for centuries and remains in wide use today as a means of diagnosing and acutely treating conduction abnormalities and supraventricular arrhythmias. In a case series reported in the 1950s, it was also incorporated into a protocol for the treatment of acute decompensated HF. Patients improved when subjected to massage-induced baroreflex activation, with symptoms including hypertension, elevated heart rate, pulmonary edema, and dyspnea quickly resolving [4].

With the advent of active implantable device technology, a system was developed to transiently activate the baroreflex through direct stimulation of the carotid sinus nerve. The device was used in patients with refractory angina and symptom-limited functional capacity. Acute activation of the device in clinical trials was demonstrated to increase functional capacity [13] and reduce cardiac filling pressures [19]. Technological limitations and the development of bypass grafting precluded widespread use of the system, but the potential benefits had been demonstrated.

12.3   Baroreflex Activation Therapy (BAT)

Technological improvements in electronics and battery technology, coupled with continued poor outcome of HF patients, motivated the development of a new approach to chronically activate the baroreflex. The Barostim™ *neo*™ system (Fig. 12.2) consists of an implanted pulse generator with a form factor similar to a contemporary implanted defibrillator coupled to a carotid sinus lead. Implant of the electrode directly on the carotid sinus provides for chronic activation of the baroreflex without the need to surgically isolate the carotid sinus nerve. Improved device technology allows the system to continuously excite carotid baroreceptors for 3–4 years using a single battery. The system is implanted unilaterally, typically on the right side. The lead is affixed directly to the carotid sinus with sutures and subcutaneously tunneled to the pectoral region where the pulse generator is implanted. Right-sided implant is motivated by the fact that patients frequently have cardiac rhythm management devices preferentially placed on the left side and by clinical experience demonstrating that full therapeutic efficacy may be obtained with

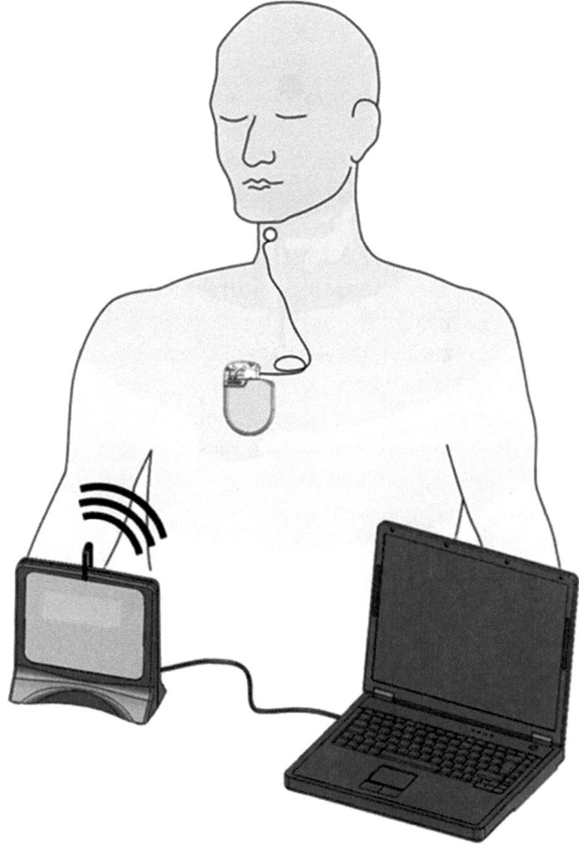

Fig. 12.2 Schematic depiction of the implantable baroreflex activation therapy system. A pulse generator similar in size to an implanted defibrillator delivers electrical stimulation via a lead implanted on the arterial surface in the vicinity of the carotid sinus. The system is controlled by a laptop computer running custom software. Information is exchanged between the computer and pulse generator through a radiofrequency communication link

unilateral, right-sided implant [18]. System implant time averages approximately 90 min for new implanters and is often less than 60 min among experienced implanters. The system safety profile is comparable to a pacemaker [36].

The implanted system is controlled by a programmer consisting of a laptop computer, custom software, and an antenna module. Programming and device status information is transmitted wirelessly via a radiofrequency link with a range of several meters. Therapy intensity is typically up-titrated over the course of the first 3 months using a standardized procedure and is then adapted as necessary according to patient needs. Programmable parameters include pulse amplitude, pulse width and pulse frequency, as well as duty cycle and the possibility of applying different therapy regimens based on time of day to accommodate diurnal rhythms.

12.4 Basic Science Supporting the Use of BAT in HF

An extensive literature exists on the physiologic effects of the baroreflex. It is too vast to be adequately described here, but an overview relevant to BAT in HF has been produced by Georgakopoulos and colleagues [26]. This review will focus on studies of the baroreflex conducted specifically with BAT.

12.4.1 Animal Studies

Acute studies of BAT in animal models have demonstrated sustained salutary effects on cardiac pump efficiency, arteries, veins, and myocardial automaticity. BAT intervention in normal canines significantly increases stroke volume and reduces heart rate while preserving cardiac output [23]. This is achieved by reducing systemic vascular resistance and arterial stiffness. Despite accompanying acute reductions in BP, average renal blood flow is unchanged while flow pulsatility increases [51]. The reduced myocardial oxygen demand, increased cardiac reserve, and maintained perfusion would be expected to improve functional capacity and protect against arrhythmogenic effects of myocardial ischemia in HF. Decreased pressure transmission with maintained perfusion through the renal artery may guard against increases in renin and help preserve renal function, thereby lessening the chances of developing cardiorenal syndrome.

In addition to arterial effects, venous capacitance is modulated by BAT. Acute BAT induces sustained transfer of blood volume from the arterial to the venous circulation in normal dogs [14]. At equal reductions in BP, BAT produces a comparable capacitance change but a more modest increase in arterial conductance as compared to sodium nitroprusside. BAT also reduces heart rate while nitroprusside increases it. Volume transfer in HF results in reduced cardiac filling pressures, thereby improving ejection as well as filling. Submaximal change in arterial conductance and reduced heart rate suggest that BAT provides greater reserve to adapt to physiologic need.

BAT also exerts electrophysiologic effects on the myocardium. In studies of normal dogs subjected to ischemia and infarction, BAT increased effective refractory period and action potential duration while reducing incidence of ventricular arrhythmia [42, 43]. In addition, BAT reduced cardiac sympathetic nerve traffic and the heart rate variability (HRV) low-frequency to high-frequency power ratio (LF/HF), indicating suppression of sympathetic nerve activity associated with ischemia and infarction.

The foregoing results are encouraging but raise an important question: if the baroreflex is constantly activated by BAT, has the ability of the cardiovascular system to adapt to physiologic need been compromised (i.e., is it possible that BAT lowers BRS)? Both acute and chronic studies indicate that the answer is no. In acute studies of rats, Avolio and colleagues demonstrated that reflex responses to bolus infusions of phenylephrine and sodium nitroprusside were not impaired by BAT [38]. Rather, the reduced BP driven by BAT acted as a new set point around which the reflex responses were superimposed. Calculations revealed that BAT actually increased BRS. Similarly, Iliescu reported that chronic BAT administered to obese hypertensive canines chronically increased BRS [37]. Thus, the acute hemodynamic improvements of BAT, coupled with improved adaptability of the cardiovascular system, would be expected to improve chronic HF.

Consistent with these expectations, chronic studies of BAT in two canine models of chronic HF demonstrated significant benefit. In a rapid pacing model, BAT doubled the duration of survival while reducing filling pressures and plasma norepinephrine [54]. In a microembolization HFrEF model, BAT increased ejection fraction, reduced cardiac fibrosis, and normalized myocyte intracellular factors associated with beta receptor signaling, a characteristic derangement in human HF [49]. A second study of the microembolization model demonstrated a protective effect of BAT against induction of ventricular arrhythmia lasting at least 6 months that was reversed 6 weeks after BAT withdrawal [50].

In summary, preclinical evaluations of BAT illustrate important mechanistic pathways through which BAT can benefit HF, including greater cardiac pump efficiency, reduced systemic vascular resistance, increased venous capacitance, as well as protection against myocardial ischemia, ventricular arrhythmia, and declining renal function. The effects are mediated through tonic reductions in sympathetic activity and increases in parasympathetic activity. Most importantly, BAT improves survival.

12.4.2 Human Studies

Mechanisms of BAT have also been explored in the clinical environment. Investigator-initiated substudies of feasibility and commercial hypertension patients have afforded opportunities to confirm that mechanisms observed in animal studies translate to patients. A study of HRV from serial Holter recordings found BAT chronically increased LF/HF ratio and decreased LF power, indicating reduced sympathetic activity and increased parasympathetic activity [51]. Moreover, the study found that BAT increased turbulence onset associated with premature ventricular contractions, implying that BAT increased BRS [40]. These findings were further validated by acute measurement of MSNA, which demonstrated a direct on-off relationship between initiation of BAT and reduction of efferent sympathetic traffic [34]. Pulse wave analysis of concomitantly acquired continuous BP exhibited improved ventricular-vascular coupling with reduction of wasted left ventricular external work and improved myocardial perfusion with an increase in subendocardial viability ratio [35].

Chronic hemodynamic improvements have also been observed clinically with BAT. From serial echocardiography and BP measurement, BAT was shown to reduce myocardial wall stress [24] and arterial elastance [25], indicating reduced filling pressures associated with diminished load. Importantly, cardiac contractility was not affected. Direct measurement of cardiac hemodynamics was also conducted in one patient [51]. Consistent with animal studies, BAT substantially increased stroke volume and reduced heart rate while maintaining cardiac output. Systemic vascular resistance and arterial stiffness diminished. Afterload was reduced and diastolic filling improved as assessed by peak filling rate despite reduced left atrial pressure, suggesting restoration of the ability of the left ventricle to enhance early filling. Taken as a whole, the clinical studies of mechanism strongly suggest that benefits of BAT observed in animals translate directly to the clinical environment.

12.4.3 BAT and Blood Pressure in HF

While results from basic science provide encouragement that BAT can benefit HF patients, it is appropriate to reflect on the implications of validating mechanisms of action in hypertensive patients. Hemodynamic and neural changes were accompanied by reductions in BP. For patients with HFpEF, this is generally not a concern, as many are hypertensive and contractile function is unimpaired. However, HFrEF patients are typically normotensive to hypotensive and with diminished cardiac contractility. Moreover, low BP has been associated with adverse outcomes in these patients [5].

In this context, it is important to consider the primary means by which BAT reduces BP, namely, through reduced arterial resistance and stiffness. The greater the contractile function of the heart, the more BP is diminished per unit reduction in arterial resistance [11]. Therefore, it is expected that BAT will reduce BP substantially in hypertensive patients but should have only modest effects in HFrEF patients. In some patients, contractile function may be so compromised that no change in BP is detectable at all. Because BAT does not affect cardiac contractility, acute changes will be dictated solely by reduced arterial smooth muscle tone. On a chronic basis, it is possible that BAT may even increase BP, for as the heart is chronically unloaded, pump function may recover. This could be further enhanced through reduced left atrial pressure as well as increased BRS and exercise tolerance.

12.5 Clinical Trials of BAT in HF

With thoroughly demonstrated mechanisms of action and successful proof-of-concept animal studies, the rationale for clinical application of BAT in HF is clear. If clinical results verify that BAT mechanisms of action are operative in HF, one would reasonably expect BAT to improve outcome for the reasons cited above.

12.5.1 First-in-Man Experience with BAT in HFrEF

An open-label, single-center feasibility study of BAT in HFrEF was undertaken to confirm the translation of basic science results to the clinical environment [31]. Patients were required to have NYHA class III HF, EF $\leq$ 40 %, 6-min hall walk distance (6MHWd) between 150 and 450 m while receiving optimal, stable medical therapy. Eleven patients were enrolled in the study and followed for 6 months. MSNA, clinical variables, and echocardiograms were collected at baseline, 3 months, and 6 months. MSNA was also recorded at 1 month. Results demonstrated a progressive decline in MSNA consistent with BAT up-titration, reaching a 30 % reduction at 6 months (Fig. 12.3). Concurrent with reduced MSNA were clinically significant improvements in BRS, NYHA class, 6-min walk distance, LVEF, and quality of life as assessed with the Minnesota Living with HF Questionnaire (QOL). BP and renal function were unchanged from baseline. It was also observed that the cumulative number of HF hospitalization days was dramatically reduced in the 6 months following activation as compared to the 6 months prior to enrollment

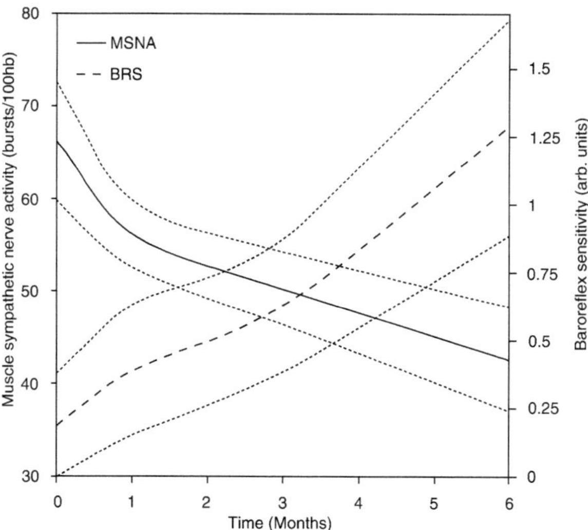

Fig. 12.3 Decreasing MSNA and increasing BRS trends observed in a study of 11 HFrEF patients receiving chronic BAT [31], as illustrated with exponential regression model fits paired with 95 % confidence intervals

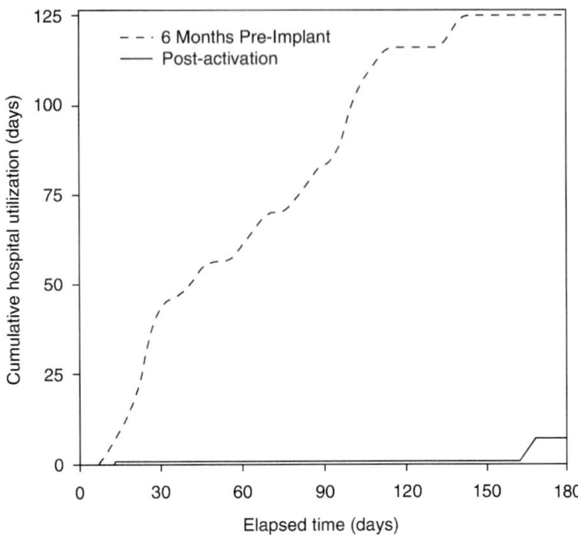

Fig. 12.4 Substantial reduction in hospital days accrued for worsening HFrEF in the 6 months before implant versus the 6 months following activation in the 11 patient cohort [31]

(Fig. 12.4). It has been recently reported that the clinical benefits can be observed at the long-term follow up of 21 months [32]. The long-term chronic BAT-dependent reductions in sympathetic activity is accompanied, in HFrEF, by an improvement in general clinical presentation, quality of life and functional capacity thus inducing an improvement in outcome.

12.5.2 The Global Barostim HF Randomized Trial in HFrEF

With proof-of-concept accomplished, a trial has been initiated to confirm therapeutic benefit can be translated to a large number of centers throughout the developed world. Eligibility criteria are similar to the open-label trial with EF limited to 35 % or less. Unlike the earlier study, which enrolled no patients receiving resynchronization therapy (CRT), the present trial allows enrollment of patients who have been receiving CRT for at least 6 months. Patients with atrial fibrillation also qualify as long as their resting heart rate is controlled between 60 and 100 bpm. The medical therapy regimen for all patients must be fully titrated, stable for at least 4 weeks, and in compliance with relevant treatment guidelines upon entry.

Patients are randomized in equal proportion to medical therapy or medical therapy with BAT (Fig. 12.5). Efficacy is assessed by evaluating the treatment effect of BAT on NYHA class, QOL, 6MHWd, NTproBNP, and echocardiographic parameters from pre-implant baseline to 6 months. As of this writing, the trial has completed enrollment and patients are being followed in Germany, Italy, France, the United States, and Canada. Results are expected to be available in the first half of 2015. While the results are presently unknown, one might surmise that they are encouraging since it was announced in September 2014 that CE marking for HFrEF was granted on the basis of interim results.

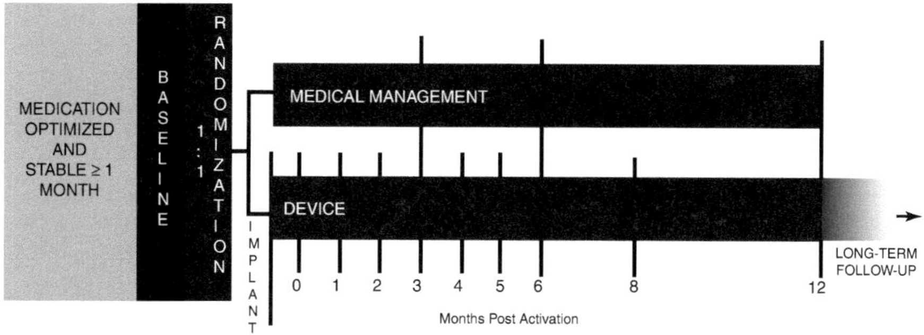

Fig. 12.5 Design of the global randomized BAT in HFrEF trial program, comparing BAT plus guideline-directed medical therapy versus guideline-directed medical therapy alone. Results of the primary efficacy evaluation, assessed following 6 months of therapy, are expected in 2015

12.5.3 BAT in HFpEF with Resistant Hypertension in the Rheos Pivotal Trial

In addition to trials specifically designed to evaluate BAT in HF, experience has also been accumulated serendipitously from the Rheos Pivotal Trial of BAT in resistant hypertension [7, 8]. It has recently been reported [17] that 97 patients in the study cohort were identified as having HF from medical history, elevated BNP, or chart review. As the average baseline EF was>60 %, these would appear to be HFpEF patients. Quality of life using the SF-12 instrument indicated only slight physical impairment at baseline, suggesting that HFpEF was generally not advanced. Nonetheless, in addition to sustained BP reductions of>30 mmHg systolic, a trend toward improved physical quality of life was observed concomitant with a significant reduction in left ventricular mass.

In addition to these intriguing observations, a detailed case report has been published describing the benefits of BAT in a commercially implanted patient with resistant hypertension and HFpEF [12]. Likewise, the invasive human hemodynamic study described earlier was performed in a patient with signs and symptoms of HFpEF [51]. In that study, reductions in pulmonary artery pressure were observed with activation of BAT. Given the prevalence of pulmonary hypertension and right heart dysfunction in HFpEF [41, 45], this may be an important and beneficial effect. The overall experience is sufficient to justify future prospective studies of BAT in HFpEF.

12.6   Conclusions and Future Directions

By virtue of the well-defined mechanism of action validated in proof-of-concept animal and clinical studies, BAT is expected to be generally applicable to the HF syndrome as well as related conditions such as hypertension and arrhythmia prevention. Each major indication will need to be individually evaluated to quantify the impact on outcome and associated healthcare economics. At this point in time, significant evidence exists to support the contention that BAT may improve outcomes in HFrEF as well as HFpEF.

Results from the first randomised controlled trial confirmed the pivotal information generated by the pilot study. BAT produced a significant amelioration in all end points of the study [55]. No efficacy might be expected in patients who remained in NYHA class III despite CRT. At this time, it will be appropriate to conduct an outcome-based trial of adequate size for US regulatory approval. Such a study is presently being designed in consultation with FDA. With regard to HFpEF, it is advisable to exercise caution due to the recent series of failed trials of medical therapy in this condition. A study should be initiated to prospectively validate the observations from the Rheos Pivotal Trial. Beyond application to advanced HF, studies and clinical use of BAT in hypertension should continue as a potential preventative measure for HF. The potential for BAT in preventing ventricular arrhythmias should also be explored, both in patients with HF and others predisposed to electrical instability of the myocardium.

References

1. Abboud FM, Thames MD. Interaction of cardiovascular reflexes in circulatory control. Handbook of Physiology, The Cardiovascular system, peripheral circulation and organ blood flow. Comprehensive Physiology. 2011; Suppl 8; p. 675–753. First published in print 1983. doi:10.1002/cphy.cp020319
2. Ahmed A, Rich MW, Love TE, Lloyd-Jones DM, Aban IB, Colucci WS, Adams KF, Gheorghiade M. Digoxin and reduction in mortality and hospitalization in heart failure: a comprehensive post hoc analysis of the DIG trial. Eur Heart J. 2006;27:178–86.
3. Ahmed A, Pitt B, Rahimtoola SH, Waagstein F, White M, Love TE, Braunwald E. Effects of digoxin at low serum concentrations on mortality and hospitalization in heart failure: a propensity-matched study of the DIG trial. Int J Cardiol. 2008;123:138–46.
4. Alzamora-Castro V, Battilana G, Garrido-Lecca G, Rubio C, Abucattas R, Bouroncle J. Acute left ventricular failure and carotid sinus stimulation. JAMA. 1955;157:226–9.
5. Ambrosy AP, Vaduganathan M, Mentz RJ, Greene SJ, Subačius H, Konstam MA, Maggioni AP, Swedberg K, Gheorghiade M. Clinical profile and prognostic value of low systolic blood pressure in patients hospitalized for heart failure with reduced ejection fraction: insights from the Efficacy of Vasopressin Antagonism in Heart Failure: Outcome Study with Tolvaptan (EVEREST) trial. Am Heart J. 2013;165:216–25.
6. Angell-James JE, Lumley JS. Changes in the mechanical properties of the carotid sinus region and carotid sinus nerve activity in patients undergoing carotid endarterectomy. J Physiol. 1975;244:80P–1.
7. Azevedo ER, Kubo T, Mak S, Al-Hesayen A, Schofield A, Allan R, et al. Nonselective versus selective beta-adrenergic receptor blockade in congestive heart failure: differential effects on sympathetic activity. Circulation. 2001;104:2194–9.
8. Bakris GL, Nadim MK, Haller H, Lovett EG, Schafer JE, Bisognano JD. Baroreflex activation therapy provides durable benefit in patients with resistant hypertension: results of long-term follow-up in the Rheos Pivotal Trial. J Am Soc Hypertens. 2012;6:152–8.
9. Bisognano JD, Bakris G, Nadim MK, Sanchez L, Kroon AA, Schafer J, de Leeuw PW, Sica DA. Baroreflex activation therapy lowers blood pressure in patients with resistant hypertension: results from the double-blind, randomized, placebo-controlled rheos pivotal trial. J Am Coll Cardiol. 2011;58:765–73.

10. Borgdorff P, Gross DR, Burattini R, Duijst P, Westerhof N. Short-term systemic autoregulation. Am J Physiol. 1990;258:H1097–102.
11. Borlaug BA, Kass DA. Ventricular-vascular interaction in heart failure. Heart Fail Clin. 2008;4:23–36.
12. Brandt MC, Madershahian N, Velden R, Hoppe UC. Baroreflex activation as a novel therapeutic strategy for diastolic heart failure. Clin Res Cardiol. 2011;100:249–51.
13. Braunwald E, Epstein SE, Glick G, Wechsler AS, Braunwald NS. Relief of angina pectoris by electrical stimulation of the carotid-sinus nerves. N Engl J Med. 1967;277:1278–83.
14. Burgoyne S, Georgakopoulos D, Belenkie I, Tyberg JV. Systemic vascular effects of acute electrical baroreflex stimulation. Am J Physiol Heart Circ Physiol. 2014;307:H236–41.
15. Chan MM, Lam CS. How do patients with heart failure with preserved ejection fraction die? Eur J Heart Fail. 2013;15:604–13.
16. Cohn JN, Pfeffer MA, Rouleau J, Sharpe N, Swedberg K, Straub M, Wiltse C, Wright TJ, MOXCON Investigators. Adverse mortality effect of central sympathetic inhibition with sustained-release moxonidine in patients with heart failure (MOXCON). Eur J Heart Fail. 2003;5:659–67.
17. de Leeuw P, Bakris G, Haller H, Nadim M, Karunaratne H, Lovett E, Bisognano J. Baroreflex activation therapy improves status of resistant hypertension patients with heart failure. Eur Heart J. 2014;35(Suppl):843.
18. de Leeuw PW, Alnima T, Lovett E, Sica D, Bisognano J, Haller H, Kroon AA. Bilateral or unilateral stimulation for baroreflex activation therapy. Hypertension. 2015;65:187–92.
19. Dunning AJ. Electrostimulation of the carotid sinus nerve in angina pectoris. Amsterdam: Excerpta Medica; 1971. p. 84–8.
20. Ferguson DW, Berg WJ, Sanders JS, Roach PJ, Kempf JS, Kienzle MG. Sympathoinhibitory responses to digitalis glycosides in heart failure patients. Direct evidence from sympathetic neural recordings. Circulation. 1989;80:65–77.
21. Floras JS. The "unsympathetic" nervous system of heart failure. Circulation. 2002;105:1753–5.
22. Floras JS. Sympathetic nervous system activation in human heart failure: clinical implications of an updated model. J Am Coll Cardiol. 2009;54:375–85.
23. Georgakopoulos D, Wagner D, Cates AW, Irwin E, Lovett EG. Effects of electrical stimulation of the carotid sinus baroreflex using the Rheos device on ventricular-vascular coupling and myocardial efficiency assessed by pressure-volume relations in non-vagotomized anesthetized dogs. Conf Proc IEEE Eng Med Biol Soc. 2009;2009:2025–9.
24. Georgakopoulos D, Kroon A, Bach DS, Kaufman CL, Abraham WT, Little WC, Zile MR. Improved left ventricular end-systolic myocardial wall stress following chronic baroreflex activation with the rheos system in resistant hypertension. J Card Fail. 2010;16:S25.
25. Georgakopoulos D, Kroon A, Bach DS, Kaufman CL, Abraham WT, Little WC, Zile MR. Improved ventricular-arterial elastance following chronic treatment using the rheos system implantable device in resistant hypertension. J Card Fail. 2010;16:S27.
26. Georgakopoulos D, Little WC, Abraham WT, Weaver FA, Zile MR. Chronic baroreflex activation: a potential therapeutic approach to heart failure with preserved ejection fraction. J Card Fail. 2011;17:167–78.
27. Gomes ME, Lenders JW, Bellersen L, Verheugt FW, Smits P, Tack CJ. Sympathoinhibitory effect of statins in chronic heart failure. Clin Auton Res. 2010;20:73–8.
28. Grassi G, Seravalle G, Cattaneo BM, Lanfranchi A, Vailati S, Giannattasio C, Del Bo A, Sala C, Bolla GB, Pozzi M. Sympathetic activation and loss of reflex sympathetic control in mild congestive heart failure. Circulation. 1995;92:3206–11.
29. Grassi G, Cattaneo BM, Seravalle G, Lanfranchi A, Pozzi M, Morganti A, Carugo S, Mancia G. Effects of chronic ACE inhibition on sympathetic nerve traffic and baroreflex control of circulation in heart failure. Circulation. 1997;96:1173–9.
30. Grassi G, Vincenti A, Brambilla R, Trevano FQ, Dell'Oro R, Cirò A, Trocino G, Vincenzi A, Mancia G. Sustained sympathoinhibitory effects of cardiac resynchronization therapy in severe heart failure. Hypertension. 2004;44:727–31.

31. Gronda E, Seravalle G, Brambilla G, Costantino G, Casini A, Alsheraei A, Lovett EG, Mancia G, Grassi G. Chronic baroreflex activation effects on sympathetic nerve traffic, baroreflex function, and cardiac haemodynamics in heart failure: a proof-of-concept study. Eur J Heart Fail. 2014;16:977–83.

32. Gronda E, Seravalle G, Quarti-Trevano F et al. Long-term chronic baroreflex activation: persistent efficacy in patients with heart failure and reduced ejection fraction. J Hypertens. 2015;33:1704–1708.

33. Heitz DC, Brody MJ. Inhibition of the aortic depressor reflex by continuous carotid sinus nerve stimulation. Proc Soc Exp Biol Med. 1973;143:854–7.

34. Heusser K, Tank J, Engeli S, Menne J, Eckert S, Haller H, Georgakopoulos D, Pichlmaier AM, Luft FC, Jordan J, Heusser K, Tank J, Engeli S, Menne J, Eckert S, Haller H, Georgakopoulos D, Pichlmaier AM, Luft FC, Jordan J. Baroreflex activation therapy acutely improves central arterial properties in resistant hypertension patients. J Hypertens. 2010;28(e-suppl A):29.

35. Heusser K, Tank J, Engeli S, Diedrich A, Menne J, Eckert S, Peters T, Sweep FC, Haller H, Pichlmaier AM, Luft FC, Jordan J. Carotid baroreceptor stimulation, sympathetic activity, baroreflex function, and blood pressure in hypertensive patients. Hypertension. 2010;55:619–26.

36. Hoppe UC, Brandt MC, Wachter R, Beige J, Rump LC, Kroon AA, Cates AW, Lovett EG, Haller H. Minimally invasive system for baroreflex activation therapy chronically lowers blood pressure with pacemaker-like safety profile: results from the Barostim neo trial. J Am Soc Hypertens. 2012;6:270–6.

37. Iliescu R, Tudorancea I, Irwin ED, Lohmeier TE. Chronic baroreflex activation restores spontaneous baroreflex control and variability of heart rate in obesity-induced hypertension. Am J Physiol Heart Circ Physiol. 2013;305:H1080–8.

38. Kouchaki Z, Georgakopoulos D, Butlin M, Avolio AA. Field stimulation of the carotid baroreceptor complex does not compromise baroreceptor function in spontaneously hypertensive rats. Conf Proc IEEE Eng Med Biol Soc. 2014;2014:2944–7.

39. La Rovere MT, Pinna GD, Maestri R, Robbi E, Caporotondi A, Guazzotti G, Sleight P, Febo O. Prognostic implications of baroreflex sensitivity in heart failure patients in the beta-blocking era. J Am Coll Cardiol. 2009;53:193–9.

40. La Rovere MT, Maestri R, Pinna GD, Sleight P, Febo O. Clinical and haemodynamic correlates of heart rate turbulence as a non-invasive index of baroreflex sensitivity in chronic heart failure. Clin Sci (Lond). 2011;121:279–84.

41. Lam CS, Roger VL, Rodeheffer RJ, Borlaug BA, Enders FT, Redfield MM. Pulmonary hypertension in heart failure with preserved ejection fraction: a community-based study. J Am Coll Cardiol. 2009;53:1119–26.

42. Liao K, Yu L, Yang K, Saren G, Wang S, Huang B, Jiang H. Low-level carotid baroreceptor stimulation suppresses ventricular arrhythmias during acute ischemia. PLoS One. 2014;9(10):e109313.

43. Liao K, Yu L, He B, Huang B, Yang K, Saren G, Wang S, Zhou X, Jiang H. Carotid baroreceptor stimulation prevents arrhythmias induced by acute myocardial infarction through autonomic modulation. J Cardiovasc Pharmacol. 2014;64:431–7.

44. Lu Y, Ma X, Sabharwal R, Snitsarev V, Morgan D, Rahmouni K, Drummond HA, Whiteis CA, Costa V, Price M, Benson C, Welsh MJ, Chapleau MW, Abboud FM. The ion channel ASIC2 is required for baroreceptor and autonomic control of the circulation. Neuron. 2009;64:885–97.

45. Melenovsky V, Hwang SJ, Lin G, Redfield MM, Borlaug BA. Right heart dysfunction in heart failure with preserved ejection fraction. Eur Heart J. 2014;35(48):3452–62. Pii: ehu193. [Epub ahead of print].

46. Mortara A, La Rovere MT, Pinna GD, Prpa A, Maestri R, Febo O, Pozzoli M, Opasich C, Tavazzi L. Arterial baroreflex modulation of heart rate in chronic heart failure: clinical and hemodynamic correlates and prognostic implications. Circulation. 1997;96:3450–8.

47. Rathore SS, Curtis JP, Wang Y, Bristow MR, Krumholz HM. Association of serum digoxin concentration and outcomes in patients with heart failure. JAMA. 2003;289:871–8.

48. Reed SD, Li Y, Dunlap ME, Kraus WE, Samsa GP, Schulman KA, Zile MR, Whellan DJ. In-hospital resource use and medical costs in the last year of life by mode of death (from the HF-ACTION randomized controlled trial). Am J Cardiol. 2012;110:1150–5.
49. Sabbah HN, Gupta RC, Imai M, Irwin ED, Rastogi S, Rossing MA, Kieval RS. Chronic electrical stimulation of the carotid sinus baroreflex improves left ventricular function and promotes reversal of ventricular remodeling in dogs with advanced heart failure. Circ Heart Fail. 2011;4:65–70.
50. Sabbah HN. Baroreflex activation for the treatment of heart failure. Curr Cardiol Rep. 2012;14:326–33.
51. Segers P, Vermeersch SJ, Wachter R, Georgakopoulos D. Effect of carotid baroreceptor activation on ventricular function and central hemodynamics: a case report based on invasive pressure-volume loop analysis. Artery Res. 2011;5:166–7.
52. Thomas GD. Neural control of the circulation. Adv Physiol Educ. 2011;35:28–32.
53. Wustmann K, Kucera JP, Scheffers I, Mohaupt M, Kroon AA, de Leeuw PW, Schmidli J, Allemann Y, Delacrétaz E. Effects of chronic baroreceptor stimulation on the autonomic cardiovascular regulation in patients with drug-resistant arterial hypertension. Hypertension. 2009;54:530–6.
54. Zucker IH, Hackley JF, Cornish KG, Hiser BA, Anderson NR, Kieval R, Irwin ED, Serdar DJ, Peuler JD, Rossing MA. Chronic baroreceptor activation enhances survival in dogs with pacing-induced heart failure. Hypertension. 2007;50:904–10.
55. Zile MR, Abraham WT, Weaver FA et al. Baroreflex activation therapy for the treatment of heart failure with a reduced ejection fraction: safety and efficacy in patients with and without cardiac resynchronization therapy. Eur J Heart Fail. 2015;17:1066–74.

Renal Reflexes and Denervation in Heart Failure

13

Federico Pieruzzi

Heart failure (HF) is associated with the activation of the sympathetic nervous system which presumably results in a progression of the syndrome and thereby in poor outcome.

Autonomic dysfunction is characterised by enhanced sympathetic activity, peripheral adrenoceptor downregulation and reduced efferent parasympathetic heart rate control. The sustained increase in sympathetic outflow in HF, along with the activation of the renin–angiotensin–aldosterone system and the consequent vasoconstriction, precipitates a positive feedback mechanism that leads to worsening of HF with progressive deterioration of left ventricular (LV) function, LV remodelling, end-organ damage and death. The mechanisms responsible of the sympathetic excitation in HF are not fully elucidated yet.

Sympathetic activation involving renal afferent and efferent sympathetic nerves regulates cardiovascular function and in particular cardiac output, heart rate and blood pressure in order to overcome acute stresses such as volume depletion or excessive vasodilatation. However, in chronic cardiovascular disease, sympathetic activation is chronically activated and is involved in the maintenance of the pathological state and in end-organ damage such as in hypertension, sleep apnoea, type 2 diabetes mellitus, end-stage renal disease and heart failure [1].

The heart and kidney interact in terms of haemodynamics and neurohumoral regulatory mechanisms, and this helps to maintain circulatory homeostasis under normal conditions. However, the normal regulatory mechanisms become inappropriate in the setting of congestive heart failure (CHF), and significant renal dysfunction often develops in CHF patients. Activation of renal sympathetic efferent nerves causes renin release, sodium and water retention and reduced renal blood flow, which are hallmarks of the renal involvement in CHF. An increase in plasma levels of angiotensin II that is

F. Pieruzzi
Università degli Studi di Milano-Bicocca, Dipartimento di Medicina e Chirurgia
Via Cadore, 48-78738, Monza (MB), Italy
e-mail: federico.pieruzzi@unimib.it

E. Gronda et al. (eds.), *Heart Failure Management: The Neural Pathways*,
DOI 10.1007/978-3-319-24993-3_13

mediated in part by the renal sympathetic activation has an effect on the central nervous system to further increase global sympathetic tone. Renal sympathetic activity can be assessed clinically by renal norepinephrine spillover, and an increase in renal norepinephrine spillover in CHF predicts reduced survival. In addition to the efferent sympathetic activation, renal sensory nerves activation in CHF may cause a reflex increase in sympathetic tone that contributes to elevated peripheral vascular resistance and vascular remodelling as well as left ventricular remodelling and dysfunction [2]. In animal models of heart failure, surgical renal denervation has been shown to improve both renal and ventricular function. Although surgical renal denervation has long been known to lower blood pressure and improve survival in patients with hypertension, the invasive nature of this approach and its associated complications has limited its clinical impact however, a novel catheter-based device has recently been introduced that specifically interrupts both efferent and afferent renal nerves, and there is significant interest in the use of this device to treat both hypertension and CHF [3].

Renal dysfunction plays a fundamental role in the development and progression of congestive heart failure (CHF). The majority of patients hospitalised for acute decompensated CHF have been shown to have some degree of renal dysfunction. The renal nerves are thought to play an important role in the renal dysfunction that occurs in CHF, since renal sympathetic efferent activation causes renin release, sodium and water retention and reduced renal blood flow (RBF). Renal sympathetic activation has important prognostic value in CHF patients, since increased renal norepinephrine spillover predicts reduced survival. In addition to efferent sympathetic activation, renal afferent sympathetic activation in CHF may cause a reflex increase in sympathetic tone that contributes to the progression of CHF [4] (Fig. 13.1).

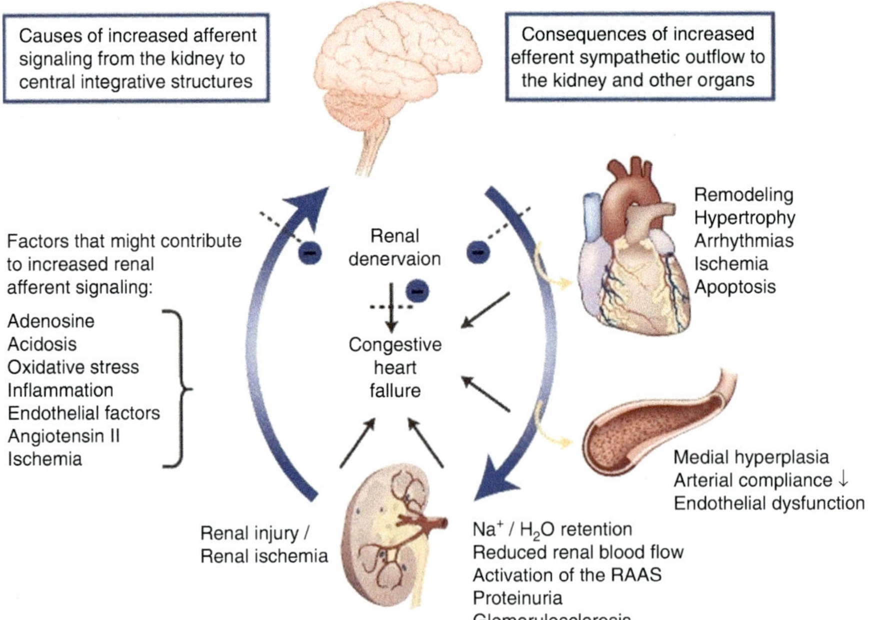

Fig. 13.1 Percutaneous renal denervation procedure. Graphic of catheter tip in distal renal artery. Reproduced with permission from Ardian Inc [19].

13.1   Functional Anatomy of the Renal Nerves

The efferent renal sympathetic nerves modulate renal function through the release of local neurotransmitters. Although immunofluorescent and immunocytochemical methods have identified a large number of substances in renal nerve terminals, only neuropeptide Y and norepinephrine are thought to act as true neurotransmitters. These two substances are released in response to renal nerve activation and bind to specific postjunctional receptors in the kidney. Direct stimulation of the renal sympathetic nerves results in frequency-dependent renal vasoconstriction. Sympathetic activation causes greater constriction of afferent arterioles to the glomerulus than efferent arterioles, causing a drop in glomerular pressure and glomerular filtration rate (GFR). In addition, sympathetic activation reduces blood flow to both the renal cortex and medulla. The renal vasoconstriction induced by sympathetic efferent stimulation results from norepinephrine acting predominantly on α1-adrenergic receptors and neuropeptide Y acting on Y1 receptors [5].

Since changes in renal sympathetic tone may influence RBF and GFR, which in turn influence sodium and water excretion, it is difficult to determine whether there is any direct effect of renal nerve activity on the tubular handling of salt and water. In animal models of sodium overload, blockade of renal α-adrenergic receptors or renal denervation increases urinary sodium excretion in the absence of changes in renal haemodynamic parameters. These findings suggest that there exists a level of efferent renal sympathetic nerve activity that can directly affect renal tubular sodium and water reabsorption independent of changes in GFR, RBF or the intrarenal distribution of blood flow. When the renal sympathetic nerves are directly stimulated at a frequency that is subthreshold for renal vasoconstriction, there is a reversible decrease in urinary sodium excretion without a change in renal perfusion pressure, GFR, RBF or the intrarenal distribution of blood flow (Table 13.1) [6].

This direct antinatriuretic effect of sympathetic activation appears to be mediated by α1-adrenergic receptors.

In addition to neural influences on blood flow and tubular secretion of sodium, the renal sympathetic nerves also stimulate the release of renin from juxtaglomerular cells, which is thought to be meditated by activation of β1-adrenergic receptors with a subsequent increase in cAMP. This mechanism of renin release is independent from but complementary to the release of renin mediated by the vascular baroreceptor mechanism in the afferent arterioles of the juxtaglomerular apparatus and the tubular macula densa mechanism that responds to the sodium load in the distal

Table 13.1 Changes in renal function at different frequencies of renal nerve stimulation

Frequency of RNS, Hz	Renin release	Na+ excretion	GFR	RBF
0.25	NC	NC	NC	NC
0.50	↑	NC	NC	NC
1.00	↑	↓	NC	NC
2.00	↑	↓	↓	↓

With permission from DiBona et al. [6]
Up arrow (↑) increase; down arrow (↓) decrease
GFR glomerular filtration rate, *NC* no change, *RBF* renal blood flow, *RNS* renal nerve stimulation

tubule. Moreover renal sympathetic tone appears to modulate the expression of renin mRNA in the kidney.

The efferent sympathetic activity mediates changes in renal function, but the kidney has also an extensive network of afferent unmyelinated fibres that transmit important sensory information to the central nervous system (CNS). Afferent fibres from the kidney have been shown to travel along with the sympathetic nerves at the level of the kidney and then enter the dorsal roots and project to neurons at both spinal and supraspinal levels. Most of the brainstem regions involved in cardiovascular control including the hypothalamus receive inputs from the renal afferents. Renal afferents are thought to carry information to the CNS from renal chemoreceptors that respond to changes in the composition of the interstitial fluid environment and mechanoreceptors that monitor hydrostatic pressure changes within the kidneys [7]. Mechanoreceptors are located both in the renal cortex and in the renal pelvis, whereas chemoreceptive nerve endings are found primarily in the submucosal layers of the renal pelvis. Direct electrical stimulation of the renal afferent nerves in animals may produce both sympathoinhibitory and sympathoexcitatory reflexes, which reflect the diverse functional nature of various populations of renal receptors [8].

Whether activation of afferent renal nerves contributes to the regulation of arterial pressure and sodium balance has been long overlooked. In normotensive rats, activating renal mechanosensory nerves decreases efferent renal sympathetic nerve activity (ERSNA) and increases urinary sodium excretion, suggesting an inhibitory renorenal reflex. There is an interaction between efferent and afferent renal nerves, whereby increases in ERSNA increase afferent renal nerve activity (ARNA), leading to decreases in ERSNA by activation of the renorenal reflexes to maintain low ERSNA to minimise sodium retention. Increased renal ANG II reduces the responsiveness of the renal sensory nerves in physiological and pathophysiological conditions, including hypertension, congestive heart failure and ischemia-induced acute renal failure. Impairment of inhibitory renorenal reflexes in these pathological states would contribute to the hypertension and sodium retention. When the inhibitory renorenal reflexes are suppressed, excitatory reflexes may prevail. Renal denervation is associated with a fall in muscle sympathetic nerve activity, suggesting that there may be increased renal afferent activity prior to ablation that causes a reflex increase in global sympathetic tone [9].

Although removal of both renal sympathetic and afferent renal sensory nerves most likely contributes to the overall renal and haemodynamic effects initially, additional mechanisms may be involved in long-term effects since sympathetic and sensory nerves may reinnervate renal tissue in a similar time-dependent fashion following renal denervation [10].

Much less is known about the normal function of the renal afferent nerves than the efferent nerves, but there is evidence that renal afferents play a role in the reflex increase in sympathetic tone that occurs in hypertension. Presumably, the renal afferents also mediate a reflex increase in sympathetic tone in CHF, but this has not yet been confirmed in humans or experimental animals.

The increase in sympathetic activity may start as a compensatory response to ventricular dysfunction and reduced cardiac output, but may become part of a pathological positive feedback cycle with the progression of CHF. Although there is a global increase in sympathetic tone in CHF that is due to CNS integration of all afferent input, sympathetic outflow does not increase equally to all organs. Some vascular beds such as the renal vasculature receive greater sympathetic activation than others in the presence of CHF. A disproportionate increase in renal sympathetic activity results in increased renal vascular resistance compared with other systemic vascular beds, and this results in increased plasma renin activity as well as sodium and water retention. The disproportionate increase in renal sympathetic activity may be an important mechanism that reduces GFR and prevents a compensatory natriuresis during the progression of CHF [11].

13.2 Interventions that Reduce Renal Sympathetic Activation in CHF

Although bilateral renal denervation has little effect on kidney function in normal animals, several studies in animal models of heart failure have established the beneficial effects of renal denervation. In a rat model of heart failure induced by left anterior descending artery ligation, increased sodium retention was abolished by surgical renal denervation. Surgical renal denervation in dogs with an arteriovenous fistula and compensated high-output heart failure improved the postprandial natriuresis in response to a sodium load (125 mEq). The therapeutic value of renal denervation was demonstrated in two other rat models of heart failure induced by coronary ligation. Surgical renal denervation was performed prior to coronary ligation and resulted in reduced ventricular filling pressures and improved ventricular function after ligation compared to nondenervated control animals. Renal denervation was also shown to restore the diuresis and natriuresis in response to exogenously administered atrial natriuretic peptide in rats with heart failure induced by coronary ligation. In a rabbit model of pacing-induced heart failure, there was a decrease in RBF, an increase in renal vascular resistance, an increase in the expression of angiotensin II type 1 receptors in renal cortical vessels and a decrease in the expression of angiotensin II type 2 receptors. All of these changes were prevented by renal denervation prior to the induction of heart failure. Taken together, the results of these animal studies suggest that renal denervation may be particularly useful in the treatment of CHF [12].

Although there is little information on the effects of renal denervation in CHF patients, there is indirect evidence for the beneficial effects of interventions that reduce renal sympathetic activation. The observation of a natriuresis in response to acute intrarenal α-adrenergic blockade in CHF patients supports a therapeutic role for reducing the effects of increased renal sympathetic nerve activity on sodium and water retention. Renin release from the kidneys is influenced by β1-adrenergic receptors, and the administration of β-blockers without intrinsic sympathomimetic activity has been shown to reduce plasma renin activity in CHF patients. Furthermore, the beneficial effects of angiotensin-converting enzyme inhibitors and angiotensin II receptor blockers in CHF patients may be mediated in part by reducing or attenuating the negative effects of renal sympathetic activation [13].

Even the efficacy of loop diuretics may be influenced by renal sympathetic activity. A recent study showed that total urine volume and sodium excretion were considerably greater when CHF patients received the same dose of furosemide after lying down for 90 min, as opposed to being active (sitting or walking on a tread-mill). Plasma norepinephrine and renin were higher with the upright posture, and these results suggest that the reduced response to furosemide was due to an increase in renal sympathetic tone. These findings suggest that renal denervation may enhance the efficacy of exogenous diuretics administered to CHF patients [14].

13.3 Afferent Renal Nerve Activation in CHF

The afferent nerves in the kidney may also play a role in CHF. The precise population of afferent nerves that are activated and the mechanisms responsible for their activation are unknown. However, it is likely that increased renal afferent nerve signals travel to the CNS and induce a reflex increase in renal sympathetic tone (renorenal reflex), thereby causing renal vasoconstriction, renin secretion and sodium and water retention. Moreover, increased renal afferent nerve signals that travel to the CNS may also cause a reflex increase in sympathetic tone to other organs that have a dense sympathetic innervation, such as the heart and the peripheral vasculature. The CNS in this case serves as the central component of the reflex arc. It is possible that a pathological positive feedback cycle at the level of the kidney may exist, whereby an increase in renal efferent sympathetic tone leads to an increase in renal afferent nerve activity, which further increases efferent sympathetic outflow from the CNS [15].

Although several substances (nitric oxide, calcitonin gene-related peptide, substance P, H+, adenosine) have been postulated to stimulate chemosensitive renal afferents under various conditions, adenosine is of particular interest, since it is readily released by renal proximal tubular cells directly into the tubular fluid during increased metabolic activity. Furthermore, intrarenal adenosine has been shown to be elevated in patients with CHF, and it may activate renal afferents resulting in a reflex increase in sympathetic tone.

Although studies of renal afferent activity in animals or patients with CHF are limited, there is evidence of renal afferent activation in other types of kidney dysfunction. In humans with end-stage renal disease, nephrectomy in patients with or without kidney transplantation resulted in a reduction of muscle sympathetic nerve activity and total body norepinephrine spillover, confirming the role of renal afferents in mediating a reflex increase in sympathetic tone [16].

13.3.1 Renal Denervation Technique

Renal sympathetic denervation in the management of hypertension has previously been explored in man via surgical nephrectomy and even radical surgical sympathectomy. Surgical renal denervation has been shown to be an effective means of reducing sympathetic outflow to the kidneys, augmenting natriuresis and diuresis, and reducing renin release, without adversely affecting other functions of the kidney such as GFR and RBF. However, these early surgical approaches (e.g.

splanchnicectomy) were complicated by severe orthostatic hypotension, impotence and incontinence [17, 18].

A minimally invasive, catheter-based approach to directly target sympathetic nerves adjacent to the renal artery has therefore been developed in an attempt to overcome the above surgery-related problems (Fig.13.2).

The renal denervation procedure itself involves femoral or radial artery catheterization, with the tip of the catheter being placed in the distal renal artery. The principle is based on the delivery of high-frequency energy applied to the endothelial lining. This procedure is repeated 4–5 times in the individual renal artery and then the same energy is applied to the contralateral renal artery, which interrupts sympathetic nerves located in the adventitia of the renal arteries, whilst the vessel is cooled by the high intraluminal blood flow [21, 22].

Renal imaging should be undertaken to exclude atherosclerotic renal artery disease prior to catheterization and a contrast renal angiogram performed at the time of catheterization (but pre-procedure) to ensure again that no major renovascular disease was present as well as to exclude dual renal arteries and other anatomical abnormalities.

Peri-procedural problems at the time of radiofrequency (RF) energy application include loin pain. This is usually treated with prophylactic use of intravenous analgesia. Potential longer-term complications such as vessel thrombosis have been

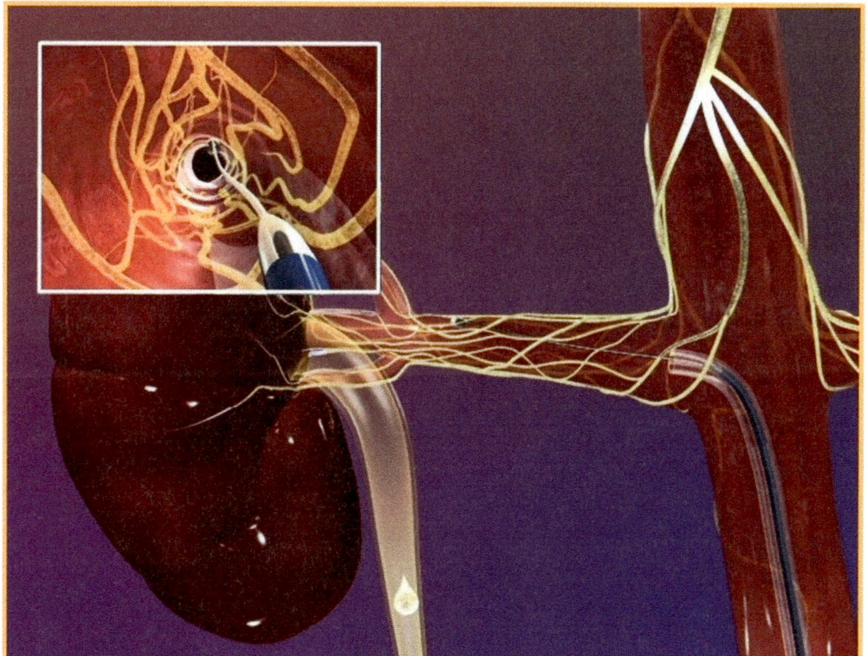

Fig. 13.2 Reflex axe of the effects of sympathetic tone activation in chronic heart failure on the kidneys, heart and peripheral vasculature (Modified with permission from Sobotka et al. [20])

mitigated with the prophylactic use of aspirin and clopidogrel. Evaluation of development of catheter-related complications to the treated vessel was performed using various angiographic techniques, including computed tomography and magnetic resonance angiography. Very few peri-procedural complications have been reported in the wide experience in resistant hypertensive patients so far such as vessel thrombosis, kidney embolisation or renal artery dissection upon placement of the catheter for RF energy delivery. Sporadic clinical evidences of renal artery stenosis in the follow-up period have been reported.

A key issue with this RF energy denervation approach is whether anatomical and/or functional regrowth of renal sympathetic nerves occurs. Studies in rats subjected to renal surgical denervation have shown that functional reinnervation of the renal vasculature begins to occur between 14 and 24 days after denervation, with complete return of neural function by 8 weeks. It is likely that some efferent sympathetic reinnervation occurs in patients after catheter-based renal denervation, although the time course of this response is unknown. Furthermore, it is difficult to clinically evaluate the amount of reinnervation, since there are no simple diagnostic tests that can evaluate the functional innervation of the kidneys. In contrast to efferent nerves, the afferent nerves may have less capacity to regenerate. Thus, the removal of renal afferent activity with renal denervation and the subsequent effects on central sympathetic outflow may be sustained [19].

It is unknown whether it is disruption of the afferent or the efferent traffic that is the more important element of the treatment, but the effect is a substantial reduction in blood pressure. The first procedure has been performed in patients with resistant hypertension. In patients with uncontrolled hypertension, despite 4.7 ± 1.5 antihypertensive drugs, with average baseline blood pressure levels of 177/110 mmHg, there was a reduction of blood pressure by up to 27/17 mmHg at 12 months. These reductions were sustained over 2 years [23, 24].

The reduction of renal afferent signalling is additionally expected to reduce efferent sympathetic drive, including that to the kidney itself. Furthermore, a reduction in central sympathetic drive via central integration of altered signalling from the denervated kidney is expected to beneficially influence sympathetic outflow to other organs (reduction of left ventricular hypertrophy, reduction of ventricular rates in patients with atrial fibrillation, abrogation of lethal arrhythmias and slowing of progression of deterioration of renal function in chronic kidney disease) [25]. A reduction in renal renin release may also be of particular relevance to diseases characterised by a marked RAAS activation such as chronic heart failure.

13.4   Evaluation of Renal Denervation in CHF Patients

In heart failure sympathetic activation, in particular, renal norepinephrine release is closely associated with morbidity and mortality [26]. Initial studies have shown that renal denervation is able to reduce not only blood pressure but also heart rate and is associated with a reduction in myocardial hypertrophy, improved glucose tolerance and ameliorated microalbuminuria. There is also experimental and clinical evidence that renal denervation might play a therapeutic role in arrhythmias often occurring in chronic heart failure [27].

Renal denervation should reverse the effects of increased α-adrenergic tone on renal blood flow, tubular excretion of sodium and systemic vasoconstriction. In addition, renal denervation should eliminate the release of other transmitters such as neuropeptide Y that might also contribute to sympathetically mediated renal vasoconstriction.

13.5   Heart Failure

Renal denervation in experimental models after myocardial infarction showed an improvement of sodium excretion, increased cardiac output, improved renal blood flow and a downregulation of angiotensin AT1 receptors [28, 29].

Renal denervation in patients with resistant hypertension and hypertrophy, in part fulfilling the European Society of Cardiology (ESC) criteria for heart failure with preserved EF (HFPEF), showed a reduction of LV mass and an improvement of diastolic function as evaluated by tissue Doppler measurements.

Interestingly, the antiremodelling effect has recently been shown to be at least in part independent of blood pressure, which could be of particular importance, because the majority of heart failure patients present with normal or low blood pressure.

Given the fact that renal spillover of norepinephrine is activated and is predictive of mortality in heart failure and renal denervation in humans reduces renal and total body norepinephrine spillover, it is conceivable that renal denervation might have a positive impact on heart failure symptoms and outcomes.

Although in principle renal denervation could be beneficial for improving the neurohormonal dysregulation of chronic heart failure, there are concerns in practice because heart failure patients typically have normal or low blood pressure and might therefore become symptomatically worse following renal denervation should blood pressure be lowered further. The first-in-man study of seven patients with chronic systolic heart failure, undergoing bilateral renal denervation, was performed with an intensive protocol of observation and assessment comprising a 5-day hospital stay post-procedure and 6 months of regular outpatient follow-up [30]. There were no procedural complications or symptomatic adverse effects. The 5-day inpatient monitoring revealed non-acute deleterious haemodynamic disturbances. In the longer term, there was a trend towards blood pressure reduction over the 6-month follow-up period which was small and did not achieve statistical significance. In all subjects, markers of renal function remained stable with no clinical or symptomatic deterioration. Whilst there may be a theoretical concern that patients with heart failure may be relying upon contributions from their renal nerves to sustain blood pressure and organ perfusion, data from this study suggest that bilateral renal denervation can be carried out safely in patients with chronic systolic heart failure.

Diastolic heart failure, which shares some characteristics of hypertension and some of systolic heart failure, is another condition for which renal denervation might offer potential benefits. However, future studies are needed to evaluate whether renal artery denervation can achieve symptomatic improvements and increase objective functional measures.

Therefore, some pilot studies for renal denervation and heart failure are planned or ongoing, the majority being performed in patients with heart failure with reduced EF (HFREF) (Table 13.2) [20].

Since CHF patients should already be on optimal doses of β-adrenergic blockers, and angiotensin-converting enzyme inhibitors or angiotensin II receptor blockers when they undergo renal denervation, it is possible that these drugs may attenuate

Table 13.2 List of the ongoing trials or those at the planning stage in heart failure

Title	Primary outcome	Secondary outcome	Sponsor	Number
Heart failure with preserved ejection fraction				
Denervation of the renal sympathetic nerves in heart failure with normal LV ejection fraction (DIASTOLE)	Change from baseline E/E' at 12 months (time frame: 12 months after treatment)	Number of participants with adverse events, in-depth analysis of diastolic function (e.g. MR, pressure–volume curves)	UMC Utrecht	NCT01583681
Renal denervation in heart failure with preserved ejection fraction (RDT-PEP)	Primary outcome measure: change in symptoms, change in exercise function, change in heart failure biomarkers, change in LV filling pressure, change in LV remodelling, change in left atrial size	Change in autonomic function, change in renal function, change in vascular function, change in neurohormones, change in renal blood flow, change in blood pressure, change in endothelial function	Royal Bromptom & Harefield NHS Foundation Trust	NCT01840059
heart failure with impaired ejection fraction				
Renal denervation in patients with chronic heart failure and renal impairment clinical trial (SymplicityHF)	Safety of renal denervation in heart failure patients as measured by adverse events	Ventricular function as measured by echocardiography, renal function as measured by GFR	Medtronic Vascular	NCT01392196
Renal denervation in patients with heart failure and severe left ventricular dysfunction	Change in serum NT-proBNP at 6 months and 1 year from baseline in both groups	Reduction in the number of hospitalizations and/ or death due to cardiovascular causes	University Hospital Olomouc	NCT01870310

Table 13.2 (continued)

Study of renal denervation in patients with heart failure (PRESERVE)	Urine sodium excretion	Urine volume, urine volume following furosemide therapy after sodium loading, 24 h urine sodium excretion, GFR, serum cystatin C, BUN level, creatinine clearance, urine albumin, renal resistive index, LV function symptoms, neuroendocrine markers, heart rate parameters	Adrian Hernandez	NCT01954160
Renal artery denervation in chronic heart failure (REACH-Pilot)	Number of participants with adverse events	NYHA classification to assess NYHA classification of dyspnoea, 6-min walk test, cardiopulmonary testing, NT-proBNP, urinary excretion of renal hormones	Imperial College London	NCT01584700
Renal artery denervation in chronic heart failure study (REACH)	Improvement of symptomatology	Improvement in peak VO$_2$ cardiopulmonary exercise testing, improvement in self-paced exercise distance, change in chemoreflex sensitivity, change in NYHA functional classification	Imperial College London	NCT01639378
Renal sympathetic modification in patients with heart failure	Composite cardiovascular events, comprising myocardial infarction, heart failure, sudden death, cardiogenic death		Jiangsu Provincial People's Hospital Chongqing Medical University	NCT01402726

(continued)

Table 13.2 (continued)

Renal sympathetic denervation for patients with chronic heart failure (RSD4CHF)	All-cause mortality, cardiovascular events	Blood pressure, life quality and symptoms, rehospitalisation rate, the recurrence rate of electric storm with ICD, cardiac function and structure	The First Hospital of Nanjing Medical University	NCT01799906
Renal denervation in patients with chronic heart failure (RE-ADAPT-HF)	Safety	Ventricular function, renal function, symptoms (KCCQ)	University of the Saarland, Clinic of Internal Medicine III	Pending

Reproduced with permission from Michael Böhm et al. [31]
BUN blood urea nitrogen, *GFR* glomerular filtration rate, *ICD* implantable cardioverter defibrillator, *MR* magnetic resonance

some of the beneficial effects of renal denervation. However, the doses of these agents used are usually less than the doses needed to eliminate all stimulation of β-receptors and angiotensin II receptors; thus, these patients may still benefit from renal denervation.

The prevalence of co-morbidities in heart failure has gained increased importance in the growing and elderly population. A large proportion of hospitalizations are due to noncardiac co-morbid conditions rather than for cardiovascular reasons in advanced heart failure and they are correlated to mortality and morbidity. Since co-morbidities are dependent on or further stimulate sympathetic activity, it is reasonable to speculate that they could also provide an important target for renal denervation to improve outcomes in the heart failure population.

Sympathetic activation of the renin–angiotensin II–aldosterone system has been shown to be part of the cardiorenal syndrome affecting outcome and occurs in ~50 % of heart failure patients. Renal denervation reduced intrarenal resistive indices and improved microalbuminuria [32].

About 50 % of patients with symptomatic heart failure suffer from insulin resistance and type 2 diabetes. Since insulin resistance is dependent on sympathetic activity, it appears likely that this co-morbidity could also be a target in the treatment of heart failure with renal denervation.

Sleep apnoea is associated with heart failure. Recent studies have shown that renal denervation was able to improve the apnoea–hypopnoea indices in patients with sleep apnoea and resistant hypertension.

Interesting data suggest that any intervention which can modulate the cardiac autonomic nervous system, and reverse the negative remodelling-associated sympathetic overactivity, may result in a reduced risk of recurrent atrial arrhythmias.

The relevance of these presently speculative observations needs to be substantiated in clinical studies in heart failure patients.

Heart rate reduction has become a major therapeutic target in cardiovascular diseases. Indeed resting heart rate is a modifiable risk factor in HF and is related to outcomes. It might also be a clinical sign to predict sympathetic activation and also different norepinephrine handlings of the failing heart. Renal denervation results in a reduction of heart rate of 3–4 b.p.m. However, renal denervation reduces the heart rate in the highest tertile of baseline heart rates, i.e. >71 b.p.m., by 9 b.p.m., in patients with hypertension. This mechanism might also be effective in heart failure because selective heart rate reduction provides a better arterioventricular coupling and unloading of the failing heart and is associated with an improved collateral growth and an improved vascular stiffness in a model of diastolic heart failure. Since the majority of the patients might be on treatment with beta-blockers as recommended by the guidelines, not all patients will be above the critical heart rate threshold. Thus, heart rate reduction might apply only for a part of the heart failure population [33].

13.6 Perspectives

Chronic systolic heart failure is characterised by overactivity of sympathetic pathways, which contributes to a detrimental triad of arterial vasoconstriction, increased chronotropic and inotropic stimulus and enhanced salt and water reabsorption [34].

Renal sympathetic denervation has the potential to positively influence the course and outcome in chronic heart failure. The first proof-of-concept trials in HFREF and HFPEF have been initiated to verify improvement of exercise tolerance and safety and also to provide data on the biological plausibility with marker studies. Furthermore, several subanalyses from these trials will address the question of whether co-morbidities such as renal dysfunction, arrhythmias or metabolic disease can be favourably influenced.

It is fundamental to continue with further appropriately designed renal denervation trials to identify markers for the confirmation that the renal sympathetic denervation clearly occurred and was effective exists.

The renal denervation procedure may be technically easy; however, it is becoming more obvious that the importance of the complex underlying anatomy and physiology as well as the biophysics of radiofrequency lesion formation has been widely underestimated. Investigators and device manufactures should be stimulated to perform rigorous preclinical and clinical studies to resolve essential unanswered questions.

If long-term follow-up shows that renal denervation might determine measurable benefits in terms of harder end points of morbidity and mortality, this new approach could have the potential to become a strong candidate for representing a new device-based standard of care in heart failure.

References

1. Kaplan NM. Resistant hypertension. J Hypertens. 2005;23:1441–4.
2. Patel HC, Rosen SD, Lindsay A, Hayward C, Lyon AR, di Mario C. Targeting the autonomic nervous system: measuring autonomic function and novel devices for heart failure management. Int J Cardiol. 2013;170(2):107–17. doi:10.1016/j.ijcard.2013.10.058. Epub 2013 Oct 25.
3. Shen MJ, Zipes DP. Interventional and device-based autonomic modulation in heart failure. Heart Fail Clin. 2015;11(2):337–48. doi:10.1016/j.hfc.2014.12.010. Epub 2015 Feb 17.
4. Floras JS. Sympathetic nervous system activation in human heart failure: clinical implications of an updated model. J Am Coll Cardiol. 2009;54:375–85.
5. Eppel GA, Luff SE, Denton KM, Evans RG. Type 1 neuropeptide Y receptors and alpha1-adrenoceptors in the neural control of regional renal perfusion. Am J Physiol. 2006;290:R331–40.
6. DiBona GF, Kopp UC. Neural control of renal function. Physiol Rev. 1997;77:75–197.
7. Genovesi S, Pieruzzi F, Camisasca P, Golin R, Zanchetti A, Stella A. Renal afferents responsive to chemical and mechanical pelvic stimuli in the rabbit. Clin Sci (Lond). 1997;92(5):505–10.
8. Stella A, Zanchetti A. Functional role of renal afferents. Physiol Rev. 1991;71(3):659–82.
9. Kopp UC. Role of renal sensory nerves in physiological and pathophysiological conditions. Am J Physiol Regul Integr Comp Physiol. 2015;308(2):R79–95. doi:10.1152/ajpregu.00351.2014. Epub 2014 Nov 19.
10. Kline RL, Mercer PF. Functional reinnervation and development of supersensitivity to NE after renal denervation in rats. Am J Physiol. 1980;238:R353–8.
11. Ramchandra R, Hood SG, Denton DA, Woods RL, McKinley MJ, McAllen RM, May CN. Basis for the preferential activation of cardiac sympathetic nerve activity in heart failure. Proc Natl Acad Sci U S A. 2009;106:924–8.
12. Villarreal D, Freeman RH, Johnson RA, Simmons JC. Effects of renal denervation on postprandial sodium excretion in experimental heart failure. Am J Physiol. 1994;266:R1599–604.
13. Schrier RW. Pathogenesis of sodium and water retention in high-output and low-output cardiac failure, nephrotic syndrome, cirrhosis, and pregnancy (1). N Engl J Med. 1988;319:1065–72.
14. Galiwango PJ, McReynolds A, Ivano J, Chan CT, Floras JS. Activity with ambulation attenuates diuretic responsiveness in chronic heart failure. J Card Fail. 2011;17:797–803.
15. Francis GS, Benedict C, Johnstone DE, et al. Comparison of neuroendocrine activation in patients with left ventricular dysfunction with and without congestive heart failure. A substudy of the Studies of Left Ventricular Dysfunction (SOLVD). Circulation. 1990;82:1724–9.
16. Hausberg M, Kosch M, Harmelink P, Barenbrock M, Hohage H, Kisters K, Dietl KH, Rahn KH. Sympathetic nerve activity in end-stage renal disease. Circulation. 2002;106:1974–9.
17. Smithwick RH, Thompson JE. Splanchnicectomy for essential hypertension: results in 1,266 cases. JAMA. 1953;152:1501–4.
18. Morrissey DM, Brookes VS, Cooke WT. Sympathectomy in the treatment of hypertension; review of 122 cases. Lancet. 1953;1:403–8.
19. Krum H, Schlaich M, Sobotka P, Scheffers I, Kroon AA, de Leeuw PW. Novel procedure and device-based strategies in the management of systemic hypertension. Eur Heart J. 2011;32(5):537–44. doi:10.1093/eurheartj/ehq457. Epub 2011 Jan 18.
20. Sobotka PA, Krum H, Böhm M, Francis DP, Schlaich MP. The role of renal denervation in the treatment of heart failure. Curr Cardiol Rep. 2012;14(3):285–92. doi:10.1007/s11886-012-0258-x.
21. Schlaich MP, Sobotka PA, Krum H, Lambert EA, Esler MD. Renal sympathetic nerve ablation for the treatment of uncontrolled hypertension. N Engl J Med. 2009;361:932–4.
22. Krum H, Schlaich M, Whitbourn R, Sobotka PA, Sadowski J, Bartus K, Kapelak B, Walton A, Sievert H, Thambar S, Abraham WT, Esler M. Catheter-based renal sympathetic denervation for resistant hypertension: a multicentre safety and proof-of-principle cohort study. Lancet. 2009;373:1275–81.

23. Esler MD, Krum H, Sobotka PA, Schlaich MP, Schmieder RE, Böhm M. Renal sympathetic denervation in patients with treatment-resistant hypertension (The Symplicity HTN-2 Trial): a randomized controlled trial. Lancet. 2010;376:1903–9.
24. Symplicity HTN-1 Investigators. Catheter-based renal sympathetic denervation for resistant hypertension: durability of blood pressure reduction out to 24 months. Hypertension. 2011;57:911–7.
25. Schirmer SH, Sayed M, Reil JC, Ukena C, Linz D, Kindermann M, Laufs U, Mahfoud F, Böhm M. Improvements of left-ventricular hypertrophy and diastolic function following renal denervation—effects beyond blood pressure and heart rate reduction. J Am Coll Cardiol. 2014. doi:10.1016/j.jacc.2013.10.073.
26. Hasking GJ, Esler MD, Jennings GL, Burton D, Johns JA, Korner PI. Norepinephrine spillover to plasma in patients with congestive heart failure: evidence of increased overall and cardiorenal sympathetic nervous activity. Circulation. 1986;73:615–21.
27. Ahmed H, Miller MA, Dukkipati SR, Cammack S, Koruth JS, Gangireddy S, Ellsworth BA, D'Avila A, Domanski M, Gelijns AC, Moskowitz A, Reddy VY. Adjunctive renal sympathetic denervation to modify hypertension as upstream therapy in the treatment of atrial fibrillation (H-FIB) study: clinical background and study design. J Cardiovasc Electrophysiol. 2013;24(5):503–9. doi:10.1111/jce.12095. Epub 2013 Feb 19.
28. Nozawa T, Igawa A, Fujii N, Kato B, Yoshida N, Asanoi H, Inoue H. Effects of long-term renal sympathetic denervation on heart failure after myocardial infarction in rats. Heart Vessels. 2002;16:51–6.
29. Souza DR, Mill JG, Cabral AM. Chronic experimental myocardial infarction produces antinatriuresis by a renal nerve-dependent mechanism. Braz J Med Biol Res. 2004;37:285–93.
30. Davies JE, Manisty CH, Petraco R, Barron AJ, Unsworth B, Mayet J, Hamady M, Hughes AD, Sever PS, Sobotka PA, Francis DP. First-in-man safety evaluation of renal denervation for chronic systolic heart failure: primary outcome from REACH-Pilot study. Int J Cardiol. 2013;162:189–92.
31. Böhm M, Ewen S, Kindermann I, Linz D, Ukena C, Mahfoud F. Renal denervation and heart failure. Eur J Heart Fail. 2014;16:608–13. doi:10.1002/ejhf.83.
32. Napoli C, Casamassimi A, Crudele V, Infante T, Abbondanza C. Kidney and heart interactions during cardiorenal syndrome: a molecular and clinical pathogenic framework. Future Cardiol. 2011;7:485–97.
33. Ukena C, Mahfoud F, Spies A, Kindermann I, Linz D, Cremers B, Laufs U, Neuberger HR, Böhm M. Effects of renal sympathetic denervation on heart rate and atrioventricular conduction in patients with resistant hypertension. Int J Cardiol. 2013;167:2846–51.
34. Fong MW, Shavelle D, Weaver FA, Nadim MK. Renal denervation in heart failure. Curr Hypertens Rep. 2015;17(3):17. doi:10.1007/s11906-014-0528-7.

Back to the Future

14

Emilio Vanoli and Edoardo Gronda

To Donatella (1958–2010)

If you have made it here by skipping the entire book, to read just the end of it, well, our suggestion is to give it a try from the beginning and you may find good reasons to justify yourself for the time spent on these pages. If you have gotten here after reading through it, we hope you enjoyed this book.

How many times did we hear: back to the future? Many times, probably, and the fortune of that great movie will never fade away. Here, once more, the same common recall of a great hit? Well, try to think about reading great science of the 1950s through the 1970s telling us how much damage would an uncontrolled sympathetic activation do to a wounded heart. Back to the future now, we wonder how much benefit can be given to the heart controlling such outrage.

Back to the future because after so many years of misunderstanding that hampered the development of dedicated research to integrated physiology, we are now using a more comprehensive approach, yet far from being satisfactory, to the autonomic nervous system. This book speaks of symphony orchestra, harmony, and serenades, but when harmony is broken and it is replaced by restless hyperactivity, swelling, and pain, then failure is about to come.

The key word is indeed ANS activation, which is not the consequence but, mostly, the cause of left ventricle dysfunction evolving towards heart failure. This is because an unrestrained acceleration is the killer of any engine, even the most sophisticated ones, like the human heart and the cardiovascular system. The burden

E. Vanoli
Department of Molecular Medicine, University of Pavia, Pavia, Italy

IRCCS MultiMedica, Sestso S Giovanni, Italy

E. Gronda (⊠)
Cardiology and Heart Failure Research Unit, IRCCS MultiMedica - Sesto San Giovanni, Milan, Italy
e-mail: edoardo.gronda@multimedica.it

© Springer International Publishing Switzerland 2016
E. Gronda et al. (eds.), *Heart Failure Management: The Neural Pathways*,
DOI 10.1007/978-3-319-24993-3_14

of the failing and dying heart triggers a genetic remodeling, which prompts cardiac cells to express new proteins with diuretic and vasodilating actions or to remodel contractile proteins. However, if we lose the capability to control the drive, then the horse race can only have a fatal end.

There are now new molecules able to modulate the effects of endogenous diuretics/vasodilators, namely, brain natriuretic peptides, and new devices are now able to modulate the neural traffic to the two major players of the game: the heart and the kidneys. This while the central nervous system is standing by, expecting to see its needs of oxygen fulfilled.

This is a book we all (editors and authors) are proud of, and we sincerely hope that it will bring a small but strong contribution to a novel thinking of heart failure and the autonomic nervous system.